As founder and president of Life Fitness, makers of the Lifecycle® aerobic trainer and two dozen other computerized fitness machines, I've seen remarkable changes in scores of individuals who have lost weight by adding something to their diets—regular exercise.

That's why I think *The Exercise Exchange Program* by Dr. James Rippe should be required reading by all people who are—or want to be—serious about their health and well-being. Finally, here's a practical guide to losing weight that proves why fad diets don't work: Starve away pounds and you're not only losing fat, but important calorie-burning lean muscle as well. But, exercise while dieting and you'll preserve almost all of that lean muscle and actually burn more calories even after you stop dieting.

Far from being a fad diet, Dr. Rippe's program offers you a sensible, simple way to ensure that you exercise and eat right. The program makes losing weight and keeping it off a lifestyle choice you can live with, rather than the lost cause offered by those starvation diets.

*The Exercise Exchange Program* involves no deprivation or quick-fix promises. It simply provides the realistic combination of good nutrition and a sensible amount of exercise to help you stay in shape. It's not only for those who want to lose weight. Its principles can help anyone feel better, be more energized and just enjoy life to the fullest.

*The Exercise Exchange Program* should not be merely read; it should be lived. Use it as your lifetime guide to responsible eating and exercise. Feel comfortable that it's based on scientific research conducted at Dr. Rippe's world-renowned Exercise Physiology and Nutrition Laboratory at the University of Massachusetts Medical School in Worcester.

I'm proud to say that we at Life Fitness have relied upon Dr. Rippe's research for years to help us design our fitness equipment, now used successfully by millions of people in health clubs and homes across the United States and around the world.

I feel strongly about the book's message of combining a balanced diet with sensible exercise to lose weight and, more importantly, to keep it off. I'm convinced that Dr. Rippe has outlined a life plan in this book that is easy to follow and destined to help you succeed.

Like Dr. Rippe, I am committed to making regular exercise a lifestyle for everyone in America. I'm excited about *The Exercise Exchange Program* and its potential for having such a positive effect on the lives of those who read it. Feeling better, looking better, living longer—these are attainable goals that this book brings closer to reality for everyone.

*The Exercise Exchange Program* gives you a safe, practical plan for simple, yet potentially life-altering changes. Whether you want to lose weight and keep it off, or simply feel better every day, reading *The Exercise Exchange Program* is your first important step.

Augie Nieto, Founder and President, Life Fitness

OTHER BOOKS BY JAMES M. RIPPE, M.D.:

The Rockport Walking Program (with
    exercise physiologist Ann Ward,
    Ph.D., and Karla Dougherty)
Dr. James M. Rippe's Complete Book of
    Fitness Walking (with exercise
    physiologist Ann Ward, Ph.D.)
Dr. James M. Rippe's Fit for Success
Fitness Walking for Women
The Sports Performance Factors (with
    William Southmayd, M.D.)

# THE EXERCISE EXCHANGE PROGRAM

JAMES M. RIPPE, M.D.
with
PATRICIA AMEND

*Recipes by*
*Judy Fredal Pang, M.P.H., R.D.*

SIMON & SCHUSTER
New York London Toronto Sydney Tokyo Singapore

**Simon & Schuster**
Simon & Schuster Building
Rockefeller Center
1230 Avenue of the Americas
New York, New York 10020

Designed by Stanley S. Drate / Folio Graphics Co. Inc.
Manufactured in the United States of America

1   3   5   7   9   10   8   6   4   2

Library of Congress Cataloging-in-Publication Data

Rippe, James M.
    The exercise exchange program/by James M. Rippe with Patricia
Amend.
      p.    cm.
    Includes index.
    ISBN 0-671-76117-X
    1. Reducing diets.  2. Exercise.  3. Reducing.  I. Amend,
Patricia.  II. Title.
RM222.2.R55   1992
613.7—dc20                        91-26196   CIP

The charts in Appendix D and E and the chart in Appendix F are reprinted courtesy of Life
Fitness, Inc.

The graphs in Appendix C are reprinted courtesy of The Rockport Walking Institute. ©
1986.

Lifecycle, Lifestep, and Lifecircuit are registered trademarks of Life Fitness, Inc. The
Lifestep FIT Test and The Lifestep Electronic FIT Test are service marks of Life Fitness, Inc.
The Rockport Fitness Walking Test is a trademark of The Rockport Company. © 1986.

# Acknowledgments

A project of the size and complexity of *The Exercise Exchange Program* requires the enthusiasm, dedication, and energy of many talented people. While it would be impossible to list everyone who has helped along the way, a number of people stand out whose special contributions made possible this book and the underlying research project at the Exercise Physiology and Nutrition Laboratory at the University of Massachusetts Medical School.

First and foremost, I have been privileged to be associated with Dr. Ann Ward over the past six years. Dr. Ward serves as the codirector of the laboratory and is largely responsible for the research design and general execution of this project, as well as most other research projects in our laboratory.

Dr. Bonita Marks supervised the daily progress of *The Exercise Exchange Program* research study as the major project of her postdoctoral fellowship in our laboratory and served as the consulting physiologist for all aspects of exercise testing and prescription in this book.

Judy Fredal Pang, M.P.H., R.D., served as chief nutritionist for the book, in addition to developing the 101 new low-fat recipes for it.

Many members of our laboratory staff devoted untold hours to the diverse tasks that make scientific research possible. Laurie Fortlage, R.D., served as nutrition coordinator for the research project and as a nutrition consultant for the book. David Brown, Ph.D., director of sport psychology in our laboratory, supervised psychological testing. Diane Morris, Ph.D., R.D., offered important advice on research design for the nutrition portion. Elaine Puleo, Ph.D., and Sadri Ahmadi,

5

M.S., developed the statistical framework for the research project and analyses for the resultant research papers. Linda Teuwen, R.D., Paula Cuneo, R.D., Linda Botelho, M.S., R.D., and Merry Yarmartino, M.S., R.D., provided dietary counseling and help with recruitment. John Castellani, M.S., David Kelleher, B.S., Lauri Webber, M.S., and Lynn Ahlquist, Ph.D., all contributed to subject recruitment and testing. James Bradley, M.D., Harvey Goldfine, M.D., Mahmoud Nimer, M.D., and John Baga, M.D., supervised exercise tests.

To these individuals and other laboratory staff who were helpful, enthusiastic, patient, and courteous to our research subjects, I am very grateful.

A number of people helped to test the recipes in the book, including Melinda Morris, R.D., Linda Armstrong, R.D., Stephanie Larmour Sanders, M.S., R.D., and Marcella Theeman, M.S., R.D.

My office staff, who by now are "old hands" at both research and book projects and the multiple demands they place on my time and attention, deserve a special word of thanks. First, Beth Porcaro, managing editor, never fails to amaze me with her organizational skills, her calmness "under fire," and her unfailing good humor. Sherri Herland, my administrative assistant, coordinates the multiple details of writing, travel, patient care, and research with efficiency approaching wizardry. Maureen Bonardi and Susan Casey manage the schedules of a bustling twenty-five-member research laboratory with great skill and patience.

Research requires both vision and enormous financial resources. Throughout the last five years, I have been privileged to work closely with Augie Nieto, president of Life Fitness, Inc.; he is one of the true visionaries and leaders of the fitness industry. Augie has shared in and helped develop a vision of fitness and health for the 1990s and has committed substantial resources from Life Fitness to help get the job done. Without the support of Life Fitness, *The Exercise Exchange Program* would still be on the drawing board. In addition, Craig Hannah, executive vice-president for marketing and sales, lent his ample enthusiasm and insight to this project. Bob Hood, executive vice president of Life Fitness, has been a strong, consistent supporter. Jeff Hills, Michael Hoffman, Bryan Andrus, and Bill Fleming, Ph.D., and many others on the Life Fitness team have offered their wisdom along the way.

Many of the concepts in this book represent "cutting edge" thinking in the fitness industry. I have been privileged to learn from and be inspired by top fitness leaders such as John McCarthy, executive director of IRSA, and Rick Devereux, Amy Allison, and Cathy McNeil, as well as many others in this leading organization of health clubs.

My editors and publisher at Simon and Schuster continue to support, inspire, cajole, and prod me in equal measure to produce the best and most readable book. Paul Aron, editor for all of my Prentice Hall Press/Simon and Schuster books, offers great creativity, attention to detail, and remains a pleasure to work with. Marilyn Abraham, John Paul Jones, and Liz Perle have been wonderfully supportive of all of my book projects for Simon and Schuster.

Last but certainly not least, I am deeply grateful to the sixty-five individuals who participated in the research project that provided the new insights described in this book. I am particularly grateful to the individuals who consented to extensive interviews based on their belief in the benefits of the program and their desire to share them with others: Helene Freed, Ann Marie Nelson, Molly Woodbury, Paula Schofield, and Helen Morin.

To all of these individuals and the many others who helped along the way, I am deeply grateful. I hope that what has emerged is a book that will inspire others to take charge of their lives with proper nutritional and exercise choices and thereby lead happier, healthier, and more successful lives.

James M. Rippe, M.D.

# Contents

# Preface

When I chose to study medicine fifteen years ago, I did so for one main reason: to help people learn to take better care of their own health. You see, many of us were never taught to manage our lifestyles—and perhaps our own health—effectively because most of our well-intentioned parents, teachers, and even our doctors didn't know how to do so themselves.

And so the weight comes on as we get older, and we find ourselves locked in a constant battle to change mindless eating and sporadic exercise habits—if we exercise at all. It's been a losing battle.

The reason? Until now, no one had ever developed a *workable* system to make sense of the chaos. One that was easy to learn and would blend into each day.

*The Exercise Exchange Program* is just that. It's a life plan that organizes both food and exercise into units called exchanges.

All you do is eat the proper number of food exchanges and perform the proper number of exercise exchanges each day, and forget about it. You will lose weight—if that is your goal—and you'll feel relaxed, refreshed, satisfied, organized, and in control every day. There's no deprivation here. In fact, the program calls for you to eat at least twelve hundred calories a day, precisely the minimum nutrition the body requires to maintain good health.

If you have ten to fifty pounds to lose, or if you would just like to balance your lifestyle, I urge you to try this program. It's safe, easy, reliable, and backed by seven years of research at my Exercise Physiology and Nutrition Laboratory at the University of Massachusetts Medical School. It is both gratifying and energizing. And it is truly the first step toward a better life.

Best wishes in your efforts!

JAMES M. RIPPE, M.D.

# 1

# THE PRINCIPLES

Broken promises. How many times have you vowed to change your eating and exercise habits to feel better, and failed to keep that oath?

If your answer is "too often," I'll bet you feel a bit out of control.

You try to watch what you eat, and yet you find yourself gaining more weight each year.

You try to get enough sleep and manage the stress in your life, and yet you find yourself constantly tired and overly stressed.

It doesn't matter if you have as few as ten pounds to lose. It doesn't matter if you're only "a little tired." If you're concerned about food, if you can't control your diet enough to lose the weight you want to lose permanently, if you ever find yourself off on a binge, if you've tried to exercise without success, then you need to take action.

If followed carefully, *The Exercise Exchange Program* will, with its Thirty-Day Eating and Exercise Starter Plan, show you how easy it is to prepare delicious, low-fat meals (snacks included), and incorporate moderate activity (both exercise and recreation) into your day. And if you stay with it for twenty weeks, as we suggest, you will enjoy a substantial, lasting weight loss—all without the deprivation, fatigue, high cost, and inconvenience that accompany so many other programs. And you'll feel nourished, rested, and relaxed at the same time.

The program was developed through seven years of research with thousands of people—and *The Exercise Exchange Program* study in particular—at the Exercise Physiology and Nutrition Laboratory at the University of Massachusetts Medical School. It's for you if you have ten to fifty pounds to lose. It's also for you if you're happy with your weight but still yearn to enjoy a healthier, more balanced lifestyle.

How does it work?

As its name implies, *The Exercise Exchange Program* is a plan based on a system of exchanges for both diet *and* exercise.

The nutrition side of the program calls for a moderate eating plan of 1,200, 1,500, or 1,800 calories that is based on a system of "exchanges," or units that help you keep track of what you're eating. The food exchange system is a proven method of weight control used and endorsed by both the American Dietetic and American Diabetes associations.

Foods are grouped together into six exchange categories: starch/bread, meat, vegetables, fruit, milk, and fat. Within each category, each exchange contains about the same amount of protein, fat, carbohydrates, and calories as the others, so any one of these foods can be traded with any other in that category.

The 1,200-calorie plan, for example, calls for four starch/bread, four meat, three vegetable, three fruit, two milk, and three fat exchanges.

The 1,500-calorie plan lists five starch/bread, five meat, three vegetable, four fruit, two milk, and three fat exchanges.

The 1,800-calorie plan allows for six starch/bread, six meat, four vegetable, four fruit, two milk, and four fat exchanges.

*And for the first time anywhere, we've set up a similar exchange system for exercise and other calorie-burning activities, including everything from leaf-raking to Ping-Pong to car repair.*

Exchange activities have been grouped into five categories: *outdoor work*, which includes repairing the car, chopping wood, gardening, and mowing the lawn; *indoor work* such as baking, carpentry, painting, various housecleaning activities, and clothes-washing; *leisure activities* such as archery, badminton, bowling, canoeing, cycling, sailing, and table tennis; *recreational* sports such as football, handball, karate, soccer, squash, and tennis; and *cardiovascular fitness activities* such as aerobic dance, running, cycling, swimming and stair-climbing.

In addition, there are separate exchange lists for the Lifecycle stationary cycle and Lifestep stair-climbing machines, since both are now found in many homes, health clubs, and recreational facilities.

We also include options for strength training—either in a health club, for those who have access to one, or at home. Our research shows that the optimal exercise exchange program includes both aerobic conditioning and strength training.

As you'll discover, the food and exercise exchange systems allow you tremendous flexibility and variety in your food and exercise choices. They allow you, in effect, to design your own diet and exercise program, one that suits your tastes and schedule. Exchanges take the drudgery out of eating well and staying active.

If, for example, you want to try a variety of fruits while they're in season, you could have two tangerines, or two plums, or a whole cup of raspberries as one of your fruit exchanges. Or if you find you've got a yen for a bowl of pasta with spicy tomato sauce for dinner, and you're on the 1,500-calorie meal plan, you can "save up" two or three of your starch exchanges and "spend" them on that meal.

Let's say you're tired of walking forty-five minutes five times a week. Do something fun or different—substitute the appropriate amount of tennis, housepainting, or wood-chopping if you want. My hope is that you'll learn to be flexible about getting and staying in shape. Play—if you do it long enough—can be physically healthy. And it's a great attitude-booster and stress-reducer as well.

In the chapters that follow, we'll help you assess your current diet, plan better meals, gauge your fitness level, and choose the exercise that's best for you. We'll teach you how to provide yourself with moral support and show you how to measure your progress.

You'll quickly discover that proper diet and weight control depend more on good management than "willpower." And you'll realize that what you really needed all along to get these habits under control was a workable program.

Instead of dozing off in front of the TV set, you'll Lifecycle as you watch TV, take an invigorating walk after dinner, or mow the lawn. As a result, you'll sleep better and feel prepared for the next day. You'll also be glad you did the lawn.

Rather than skipping breakfast or lunch or both, you'll enjoy low-fat meals that leave you neither starved nor stuffed but satisfied.

Instead of eating erratically when you're overly hungry, and choosing the first fatty food you can get your hands on, you'll learn to carry healthy snacks from the list of food exchanges. At night you'll feel pleased that you ate moderately, not angry with yourself for overdoing it.

Instead of eating because you're bored, tired, or need a break from work, you'll take a walk, call a friend, or read a magazine article to get that break.

Finally, instead of finding that food and your lack of exercise are things you can't get off your mind, you'll put those issues to rest for good. And you'll feel like a strong person for having accomplished that.

Briefly, the program calls for:

■ Keeping track of what you're eating for a short time to reveal hidden sources of fat.

■ Eating three balanced, low-fat meals a day, plus snacks, with the flexibility to enjoy the foods you like in moderation—including occasional treats.

■ Adding a moderate amount of exercise and activity to your routine to help you relax, preserve muscle, burn more calories, elevate your mood, and provide more energy.

■ Making a commitment to follow the program for at least twenty weeks, but at the same time giving yourself adequate time—at least thirty days—to adjust to it.

■ Accepting a *gradual* weight loss of one-half to one pound of *fat* per week, which is in keeping with the latest dietary guidelines set forth by the U.S. Department of Agriculture and the U.S. Department of Health and Human Services. If you were to lose more quickly, there's a very good chance that you'd be losing muscle along with fat. As long as you follow both the eating and exercise plans, the weight you lose will be nearly all fat.

By implementing these simple lifestyle changes, you'll be setting the stage for long-term healthy living and weight control. In fact, this is the program I follow and the one I recommend to all of my patients, whether they're overweight or not.

Does it work? Paula Schofield—one of the sixty-five subjects who participated in *The Exercise Exchange Program* study, on which this book is based—is living, slimmed-down proof that it does.

A bubbly, busy, intense, energetic mother of three grown children, Paula was feeling desperate in the fall of 1989 when she called us at the University of Massachusetts after seeing our newspaper ad calling for study volunteers.

In twenty-one years of marriage and childrearing, Paula had gained seventy pounds—a tremendous amount for her five-one frame. She had tried most of the major diet plans and met with failure each time. At age forty-five, Paula sensed that her time to do something about her weight was running out.

"I didn't feel good as an overweight person," Paula remembers. "I felt I was sending a negative message to my three children about health. How could I tell them to eat healthy and be healthy if I wasn't doing so?"

But once Paula entered our program, her life began to move in a new direction.

While in the five-month study, Paula learned to moderate both the portion size and fat content of her meals to meet the requirements of the 1,200-calorie eating plan prescribed for her. She also rode a Lifecycle stationary cycle three times a week and strength trained three times a week, in keeping with the latest exercise guidelines set forth by the American College of Sports Medicine.

As Paula began to eat better and exercise regularly, the pounds started to come off. Slowly her body took on a new shape and tone. Her spirits soared as she began to feel more *in control*. She lost a total of nineteen pounds during the five months of the study, and eleven pounds more on her own after the study ended, for a total of thirty pounds. And she plans to lose more.

But weight loss—in terms of pounds—is just one part of Paula's success with *The Exercise Exchange Program*. Virtually all of Paula's pound loss during the study was fat. And she *added* nearly two pounds in muscle. That's important because muscle is the most metabolically active tissue in the body. So from now on, Paula will burn more calories with everything she does. Without exercise, some of Paula's weight loss would surely have been muscle.

Paula lost a lot of "emotional weight" as well. A worrywart all of her life, she has finally begun to relax. Problems seem to bother her less. She sleeps more restfully, and she greets the day with more energy. She now enjoys taking extended bicycling and cross-country ski trips with her husband.

In addition, Paula—and many others like her in the study—gained self-esteem, confidence, and the knowledge that the "problem" of food has been solved for life. Says Paula: "I tend to walk fast, and it's nice that my legs don't bounce. I feel firm. It's a good feeling. . . . I don't shy away from the mirror anymore. I look at it!"

Why did our program work for Paula when so many others failed? For several reasons:

■ *The Exercise Exchange Program* is a simple concept to grasp. All she had to do was consume the correct number of food exchanges and perform the correct amount of exercise, which made it possible for her to change habits acquired over a lifetime. (Our thirty-day plan calculates your exchanges for you to get you started.) She lost about a pound a week.

■ It calls for a sensible, nutritionally balanced, low-fat diet rather than starvation. So Paula felt satisfied rather than deprived on her 1,200-calorie plan.

■ It calls for exercise to reduce stress and improve mood, to burn calories, and to preserve or add lean muscle mass—the tissue in the body that metabolizes the most calories and gives the body its shape and tone. So not only did Paula see her weight slowly drop, she saw her body change as well.

## Why an Eating Plan with 1,200, 1,500 or 1,800 Calories?

The experience of millions has proved that deprivation dieting doesn't work.

While it's true that just about anybody can lose weight on 600 calories a day, such a limited diet simply isn't safe. Your body can't get the nutrients it needs on less than 1,200 calories per day. We need to eat to live. Too many of us have been conditioned to think we don't.

I'm sure you know someone who has lost fifty pounds but is afraid to look at food. It's sad to see that. You know they can't go on that way for long. It's as if they live in a diet prison. And they want out. Badly.

The problem is, they never really learned to manage food, and once they're faced with making choices, they end up bingeing. They find themselves in prison once more, this time with a heavier sentence. And they've lost precious lean muscle besides.

That's no way to make a lifestyle change. So, sooner or later, the body will rebel.

When you deprive your body of adequate fuel by skipping meals or severely restricting your calorie intake, it begins to think it's starving. So it slows the metabolism and stores fat. The less you eat, the slower your metabolism becomes, and the more efficient your body becomes at conserving fat—ironically, the exact opposite of what you intended!

Is it any wonder that dieting alone results in permanent weight loss for less than 5 percent of the population?

## Why Reduce Dietary Fat?

The Exercise Exchange Program emphasizes cutting back on the amount of fat you consume. Reducing fat is important, not just for weight control but for generally better health as well.

For one thing, fat is the most concentrated source of calories. Fat contains about nine calories per gram, more than double that of protein and carbohydrates. So eating high-fat foods is the quickest way to "spend" the calories you've allocated yourself for the day.

In addition, a diet high in fat, especially saturated fat, has been linked to high blood-cholesterol levels—a well-known risk factor for heart disease. Too much body fat has also been associated with high blood pressure, diabetes, certain gastrointestinal problems, and certain forms of cancer.

That is not to say that fat doesn't have a place in a healthy diet. It does. As nature's most concentrated source of energy, fat is essential for proper growth and development. It aids in the absorption and digestion of vitamins A, D, E, and K. It cushions our bones and vital organs. It insulates us against the cold.

Saturated fats are the villains to watch out for. They tend to raise the level of LDL cholesterol or "bad" cholesterol in the blood, a known risk factor for heart disease. These fats are usually solid at room temperature and come primarily from animal sources. You know them: butter, lard, solid shortening, and the fats found in meat, poultry, and dairy products. In addition, some plant oils—including coconut and palm oil—are also high in saturated fat.

You should also try to limit your consumption of polyunsaturated fats. Recent studies have shown that these fats tend to lower HDL, the "good" cholesterol in the blood. Polyunsaturated fats include safflower, sunflower, soybean, cottonseed, and sesame oils.

Monounsaturated fats, on the other hand, tend to help lower LDL cholesterol. Monounsaturated fats are liquid at room temperature and are obtained primarily from plants and vegetables. They include canola oil and olive oil, and the fat present in avocados and nuts.

Overall, the American Heart Association recommends keeping the amount of fat in your diet at 30 percent or less, with equal parts saturated and polyunsaturated, and slightly more emphasis on the monounsaturated fat. These same guidelines have been incorporated into *The Exercise Exchange Program*.

## Why Both Diet *and* Exercise Exchanges?

If you're dieting without getting regular exercise, much of what you're losing is muscle—10 to 30 percent of your weight loss each time you diet. In a thirty-pound-weight loss, that could mean four and a half pounds of lost muscle. The loss of muscle and addition of fat lead to so-called middle-aged spread.

Even if you aren't dieting, you do, like most adults, lose five pounds of lean tissue—muscle—each decade simply by being less active. That's important because lean muscle is the body's "engine." As the most metabolically active tissue, it burns more calories than any other tissue in the body.

The more you diet without exercise, the less active you become in your lifestyle, the more you shrink this engine. So, at this lower weight, you'll burn even fewer calories. You become, in effect, a fat person in a temporarily thin body, doomed to regain the weight you lost—and more—as 95 percent of us who try to diet without changing our basic lifestyle do.

And if you don't exercise, you're completely missing out on one of the best ways of handling stress. Without a reliable means of dealing with it, stress often builds to a point where small problems seem insurmountable. It can rob you of a good night's rest. When it does, you're left with vague feelings of fatigue and general malaise that make just getting through the day—not to mention staying on any weight-control program—a major effort.

Can low-fat eating and moderate, regular exercise stem the tide of middle-age spread? *The Exercise Exchange Program* research study, completed in the Fall of 1990 at my laboratory at the University of

Massachusetts with the support of Life Fitness, Inc., a major manufacturer of exercise equipment, proved that it can.

It compared weight loss and changes in body fat and lean muscle content of sixty-five subjects, some of whom dieted alone, some of whom dieted and strength-trained, and some of whom dieted in combination with aerobic exercise and strength training.

Just as we thought:

■ Those who dieted alone lost weight, an average of nine pounds. But 11 percent of their weight loss was lean muscle. Because of that loss of muscle, sometime in the future they'll be more likely to regain the weight they lost.

■ The subjects who dieted and performed aerobic exercise on the Lifecycle stationary cycle lost an average of ten pounds, 99 percent of which was fat. Aerobic exercise helped them preserve the lean muscle tissue they had. They also strengthened their cardiovascular systems in the process, and they experienced a variety of psychological benefits as well.

■ The people who dieted and used the Lifecircuit strength training system lost an average of nine pounds, 109 percent of which was fat. How can you lose more than 100 percent fat? By gaining lean muscle through exercise as you selectively lose fat.

■ Those who dieted and engaged in aerobic exercise and strength training lost an average of thirteen pounds. This powerful combination resulted in the greatest total weight loss among the study subjects. In addition, 104 percent of their loss was fat, meaning they added 4 percent in lean muscle.

But fat loss and muscle gain are only part of the story. Like Paula, the people who exercised also made tremendous psychological and emotional gains. Many have told me that they now feel calmer, happier, and better than they ever have before. As one woman who had lost twenty pounds of fat said, "This plan isn't really about losing anything. It's about gaining something—control over your life."

## How Much and What Kind of Exercise Do You Need?

So you don't want to run a marathon. How much exercise do you need to stay healthy and fit?

Your goal for this program will be to perform some kind of activity—walking, cycling, stair-stepping, strength-training, and one or more of the exercise exchanges each day, to the tune of 200 calories.

Regular aerobic exercise is necessary for cardiovascular health. Aerobic exercise is also the best way to burn calories and improve your mood. There is even some evidence that it helps lower blood pressure indirectly through weight loss, that it raises the level of HDL or "good cholesterol," and that it helps to preserve lean muscle and bone mass.

However, if you're looking to preserve as much muscle as you can or even add some, then I suggest doing strength training along with your aerobic exercise.

Let me give you more background on both.

Walking, cycling, swimming, and other such activities improve your aerobic capacity—your VO2max, a measure of the maximum amount of oxygen you can consume per minute. The reason: As you begin to exercise, your muscles call for more energy. Your brain complies by stimulating the heart to deliver oxygenated blood to the exercising muscles via the red blood cells. This oxygen combines with glucose, glycogen, or free fatty acids, which are then broken down to produce more energy.

When you exercise at 60 to 80 percent of capacity, you're slightly "overloading," or safely stressing your system, which increases your heart's ability to pump oxygenated blood through your body. And your muscles become increasingly efficient at extracting oxygen from your blood. So walking up a steep hill, mowing the lawn, or lugging laundry up the stairs no longer wears you out. That's why exercise will give you more energy for everything you do.

What I encourage is duration, consistency, and enjoyment, not intensity. Walking, stationary cycling, or stair-stepping at a comfortable brisk pace for forty-five minutes is a lot better than jogging for fifteen, especially if you're new to exercise. If you like what you're doing, you're bound to stay with it longer. And you'll want to do it more frequently, so you'll burn more calories overall.

And don't forget to use the exercise exchange program to add variety to your exercise day. Chapter 5 has a long list, so you can vary your exercise regimen to suit your individual tastes and lifestyle.

We also encourage strength training because it can, among other things, help keep you thinner, stronger, and more flexible.

How?

If it's not being used, any muscle in your body will begin to atrophy or get smaller. I'm sure you've seen an arm or leg that's been bound in a cast. It's smaller and weaker through lack of use.

To a lesser extent, that's exactly what happens, although gradually, to the major muscle groups in your body as you get older. Your muscles slowly shrink, due to inactivity and a variety of health and biological factors, to the tune of one-half pound per year for people thirty years and older.

While that may not sound like a lot, that level of muscle loss can actually lead to a noticeable weight gain, the dreaded "middle-age spread."

As I said earlier, muscle is the most metabolically active tissue in your body. And a half-pound loss can lead to a slowdown in your resting metabolism of as much as 0.5 percent per year. So even though you may be eating the same amount of food, you're burning what you eat more slowly; hence, fat accumulates.

Weak muscles can also lead to a variety of other problems: more frequent sprains and strains, low back pain, and an overall feeling that routine, daily tasks require too much energy.

When it comes to strength training, I suggest gradually building up to a moderate fifteen- or twenty-minute workout, three times a week at home, using two- or five-pound weights if you're a woman, or ten pound weights if you're a man. Or join a health club or recreational facility and do high-repetition, low-weight circuit training for fifteen to twenty minutes on the equipment provided three times a week. This amount of training will build strength, tone, and endurance. It will not build bulk.

So, even though at age forty-three, my exercise program centers on what I enjoy most—walking, cycling, stair-stepping, running, tennis, and windsurfing when I can fit it in—I make sure that I do strength-training exercises at least two or three times a week to prevent the kind of muscle loss that we've been talking about. It makes me feel and look better and decreases my risk of injury in daily life, as well as in the sports I enjoy.

While I can do my training on a Lifecircuit strength-training system at my own laboratory, some of you, I realize, may not have such equipment available to you because you don't belong to a health club. If you would like to find a reputable one, I suggest contacting IRSA, The Association of Quality Clubs, toll-free at 1-800-228-4772. This Boston-based nonprofit trade association will send you a free guide to choosing a club that best suits your needs.

What's the best way for you to start exercising?

Find something you like to do. And start off gently. Many people choose walking because it's the easiest and most natural exercise—all you need is a decent pair of shoes. Walk alone, walk with your spouse, walk your dog. Forget the notion that exercise needs to be punishing to be good for you. In fact, that's completely the wrong approach. Don't focus on forcing yourself to exercise. Think of ways you can *blend* it into your day.

In just a few weeks you won't want to go without exercise because you'll have learned the difference between feeling just "so-so" and feeling the best you can. You'll wonder why you didn't start years ago.

Says Ann Marie Nelson, another of our study participants: "Just try it and give it a chance. Just do it. You've got nothing to lose. In my case, the only thing I had to lose was weight, and in the process of doing this, I gained a lot more self-confidence, energy . . . and the list goes on and on."

## The Framework

Briefly, here's what you'll do:

■ Read Chapter 2 to find out how to reduce the fat in your diet, to find a starting point for the exercise of your choice, by taking either *The Rockport Fitness Walking Test*, the *Lifecycle FIT Test*, or the *Lifestep Electronic FIT Test*, and the sit-up and push-up tests to assess your strength. In addition, you will measure the circumference of your waist, hips, and thighs, which will help you assess changes in your body fat later on.

■ Complete the Thirty-Day Eating and Exercise Starter Plan in Chapter 3 to acquaint you with the program. You'll find convenient daily menus, plus daily exercise goals for walking, for the Lifecycle, for the Lifestep, and for strength training on Lifecircuit or other types of equipment in a club setting, or at home, and for the exercise exchanges.

■ Once you finish with the thirty-day plan, you can design your own menus using the 101 delicious recipes in the last section.

For exercise, you'll continue in Chapter 4 with week five of the twenty-week walking, Lifecycle, Lifestep, Lifecircuit strength training, generic strength training, or home strength training programs.

*Your overall goal is to keep eating properly and to perform some kind of activity—walking, cycling, stair-stepping, strength-training, and one or more of the exercise exchanges each day, to the tune of 200 calories.* Exercise exchanges are listed in Chapter 5, food exchanges in Chapter 6.

■ At week ten, you'll retake *The Rockport Fitness Walking Test*, the *Lifecycle FIT Test*, or the *Lifestep Electronic FIT Test* to assess the gains you've made in aerobic capacity, as well as the sit-up and push-up tests to see if you're stronger. In addition, you'll remeasure your circumferences to note changes in body fat.

■ When you've completed week twenty, you'll test yourself again to gauge your progress—*and celebrate your accomplishments.* Then read Chapter 7 for tips on keeping up the good work.

# 2

# THE STEPS

Planning. It's essential to lifestyle change. But you really can't plan if you don't know what areas of your life need attention. That's why, in this chapter, I've outlined five simple steps that will:

- increase your knowledge about your diet and your level of fitness and
- give you a starting point to help you set goals.

You'll find, as many of our *Exercise Exchange Program* research subjects have, that it's much easier to reorganize your life if you break it down into bite-size pieces.

Let's get started by looking at your diet.

## STEP ONE: Assessing Your Diet

First, a brief "fat quiz":

1. _____True. _____False. When eating out, the diet plate is the best choice on the menu.

2. _____True. _____False. Salad bars are a healthy choice.

3. _____True. _____False. Food labeled "low cholesterol" or "no cholesterol" are low in fat and calories as well.

**4.** _____True. _____False. A typical fast-food fish sand-wich is likely to be lower in fat than a typical fast-food quarter-pound hamburger.

**5.** _____True. _____False. A vegetarian diet is a low-fat diet.

Is the answer to all of these true? Not necessarily. Here's why:

1. Though some are getting better, many diet plates are outmoded; many still consist of hamburger, cottage cheese, and egg—too much saturated fat and cholesterol.

2. Salad bars are not a healthy choice if you load on the extras and high-fat dishes. Salad dressings have an average of seventy-five calories and eight grams of fat per tablespoon, and can easily add 300 calories—or more—and thirty-two grams of fat to your plate. Without your realizing it, that "smart" salad bar meal with all of the fixings may carry 1,200 to 1,500 calories per serving.

3. Fat and cholesterol content don't automatically go together. Shrimp, for example, is low in fat but relatively high in cholesterol. Margarine, which is made from vegetable oil, is cholesterol-free but high in both fat and calories.

4. Hamburgers and fish sandwiches can be close. However, the fish sandwich is often higher, with approximately twenty-five grams of fat due to the oil used in frying, the cheese, and the tartar sauce. A quarter-pound hamburger without cheese contains about twenty-two grams of fat. In addition, fried chicken cutlet sandwiches, chicken nuggets, and grilled chicken sandwiches are also fatty unless you remove the skin.

5. A vegetarian diet that includes lots of cheese or fried foods may actually have a higher fat content than diets that include meat. One ounce of Cheddar cheese, for example, has 9.4 grams of fat. For a person on a 1,200-calorie diet, that is 25 percent of one day's fat allotment.

If any of these questions caught you by surprise, I strongly suggest that you take advantage of the food diary, the Food Frequency Chart and the sample, completed food diary in Appendix A. The simple exercises in this section will help you become more aware of what you're eating every day, and awareness alone will help you cut down on fat.

Fill out the food diary for a few days, including the time, place, item, and quantity of food as accurately as possible.

Continue with the Food Frequency Chart, which lists common categories of foods and how often you need to eat these foods each week for a balanced, low-fat diet. Compare this chart to your diary to see just how balanced your diet is.

Also, compare your diary to the completed, sample food diary, which highlights "visible" and "invisible" sources of fat and gives step-by-step instructions for calculating the percentage of fat in your diet. The American Heart Association recommends that your diet consist of no more than 30 percent fat. Don't be surprised if your total exceeds that figure. Americans consume an average of 37 percent fat.

To cut down on the fat you're consuming, you can follow the meal plans in Chapter 3 and use the food exchange system in Chapter 6 and the fat and cholesterol comparison charts in Appendix A. All of these will aid you in making better food choices.

## STEP TWO: Choosing Your Meal Plan

For those wishing to lose weight, The Exercise Exchange Program calls for a weight loss of one-half to one pound per week, using a 1,200-, 1,500-, or 1,800-calorie meal plan in conjunction with exercise. This is in keeping with the most recent dietary guidelines set forth by the U.S. government. Every scientific study ever done over the last twenty years on highly restrictive weight-loss diets has shown that virtually everyone who uses them eventually gains all of the weight they lost back—usually sooner rather than later.

To calculate the appropriate calorie level you need to achieve this weight loss, simply take your present body weight and multiply it by ten. The answer is the number of calories for your diet plan.

For example, if you now weigh 150 pounds, yours would be the 1,500-calorie meal plan ($150 \times 10 = 1500$ calories).

At that calorie level, your body will have adequate nutrition while you lose weight, mostly fat. If you consume less than the appropriate amount of calories, your body may begin storing fat because it thinks it's starving.

What if you're between plans? No problem.

To allow for flexibility, the program includes a certain number of "open calories" you can use at your own discretion, provided they're not all fat.

The 1,200-calorie plan has 1,120 calories in the main plan and 80 open calories; the 1,500-calorie plan has 1,300 calories in the main plan and 200 open calories; and the 1,800-calorie plan has 1,500 calories in the main plan and 300 open calories.

To get to the appropriate calorie level, simply add or subtract open calories to give the appropriate calorie level for safe and appropriate weight loss:

1,300 calories: Follow the 1,200-calorie plan and add an additional 100 open calories to the standard plan ($1,200 + 100 = 1,300$).

1,400 calories: Follow the 1,500-calorie plan but subtract 100 calories from the 200 open calories allowed under the standard plan ($1,500 - 100 = 1,400$).

1,600 calories: Follow the 1,800-calorie plan but *subtract* 200 calories from the 300 open calories allowed under the standard plan (1,800 − 200 = 1,600).

1,700 calories: Follow the 1,800-calorie plan but *subtract* 100 open calories from the 300 allowed under the standard plan (1,800 − 100 = 1,700).

1,900 calories: Follow the 1,800-calorie plan but *add* one starch exchange to the standard menu (1, 800 + 80 = 1,880).

Over 1,900 calories: Follow the 1,800-calorie plan but *add* one meat, one starch, and one fruit exchange to the standard menu (1,800 + 215 = 2,015).

(Note: As we said earlier, this program is designed for people who wish to lose ten to fifty pounds. If you believe you need to lose more than that, we suggest you consult a physician or a registered dietitian for advice.)

## STEP THREE: Choosing Your Exercise

I can't emphasize the importance of exercise enough. If you lose fifteen, twenty, or thirty pounds with this program, the toning effects of exercise will make you *look and feel* as if you've lost much, much more. But what kind of exercise is best for you?

The one you like the best, not the one you think you *should* do.

If you took part in a sport when you were in high school or college, try it again. If you were good at it then, chances are you'll be good at it now. But if you haven't a clue as to what to do, consider the following:

■ Your schedule: If your schedule is erratic, walking may be the most practical activity because you can do it nearly anywhere at virtually any time. Keep your walking shoes in the car, and whenever you know you have idle time between meetings or sales appointments, put on those shoes and walk. It will improve your mood and help you collect your thoughts for the next meeting. But at the same time, don't be haphazard about it. Plan for it by jotting it down in your daily planner, just as you would any other appointment.

■ The environment you prefer: If you like a quiet, peaceful routine, try walking or indoor cycling on a Lifecycle. If, instead, you enjoy the challenge of "mastering" the wind and weather, try outdoor cycling or jogging.

■ Your interest in competition: If you're competitive, you might try running or cycling. But if you prefer cooperative, noncompetitive events, try an aerobics class or cross-country skiing with friends.

■ Your stress level: If you're generally calm, a brisk walk at lunch or after work may help you gather your thoughts. On the other hand, "beating up a bike" at home or at a health club may help you relax if you've had a stressful day.

■ Desire to be alone or with others: If you enjoy time alone, walking, jogging, outdoor cycling, or indoor stationary cycling at home may be for you. If you need others, consider joining a health club or recreational facility. In a few weeks you'll start to identify familiar faces and develop a feeling of "belonging" that can help motivate you. Another option is to find an "exercise buddy" to work out with.

If none of these options seems possible, you may want to consider purchasing a couple of pieces of exercise equipment—perhaps a rowing machine for your upper body and a Lifecycle for your legs—and doing your exercise at home. For variety you can invite your exercise buddy to your home to work out with you.

Still another option is to combine your at-home workouts with workouts at a health club. In that way you get the convenience and solitude of home when you need it and companionship, a change of scene, or a large array of equipment at your club when you want that. It's truly the best of both worlds.

And don't forget about the exercise exchanges, which, as we have said, are designed to add variety to this program and help you to blend exercise and activity into your life.

The exercise portion of the Thirty-Day Starter Plan requires that you burn at least 200 calories a day. To start, approximately 100 of those calories will be burned through aerobic exercise, and 100 will be burned through doing other activities on the exercise exchange list in Chapter 5.

As you think about the aerobic exercise you'd like to do, it might also be a good idea to scan the list in Chapter 5 and consider which of the exchanges will fit best in your life.

## STEP FOUR: Measurements

Next I'd like you to measure the circumference of your waist, your abdomen, your buttocks, and the middle of one thigh, and record these figures in Appendix G. Do the same in ten and twenty weeks to check your progress. Any loss in inches reflects the fat you'll have lost, the muscle you'll have saved, and the toning of your muscles that's taken place.

Ideally, body fat should be 15 to 18 percent for men and 20 to 25 percent for women. Ordinarily, measuring body fat is a fairly exact science that takes some pretty sophisticated equipment. However, a simple tape measure will give you a general idea of how you're doing. All measurements should be taken to the nearest eighth of an inch. Here some tips for accurate measuring:

THE WAIST. To find your natural waistline, look in the mirror and find the narrowest spot just below your rib cage. Place the tape measure around your waist so it's slightly taut.

THE ABDOMEN. Place the tape measure directly over your belly button and draw the tape around the abdomen, making sure it's even all around.

THE BUTTOCKS. Look in the mirror once again to find the widest section of your buttocks. Place the tape around you at that spot, again making sure the tape is even and hasn't slipped up or down in the back or sides.

THE MIDDLE OF THE THIGH. This one is the hardest to locate. To find that spot, place the tape measure at the crease at the top of the thigh, directly in line with the hip bone. Then extend the tape down to the kneecap. Mark the part of the thigh that's at the halfway point of the tape. That is the section of the thigh you should measure.

## STEP FIVE: Simple Exercise Tests

Now it's time to take a simple exercise test to determine your starting level in the exercise you've chosen.

The test results will determine the color of your program for the the Thirty-Day Eating and Exercise Starter Plan in the next chapter. Don't forget to record your test results in Appendix G.

■ If you've chosen to walk, turn to Appendix C to take the *Rockport Fitness Walking Test*, which requires a brisk one-mile walk.

■ If you want to do stationary cycling, turn to Appendix D for the *Lifecycle FIT Test*, which requires a five-minute cycle ride on a Lifecycle stationary cycle.

■ If you want to stair-step, the *Lifestep Electronic FIT Test* appears in Appendix E. It requires approximately three minutes of stepping on a Lifestep machine.

If you don't have a Lifecycle or a Lifestep and still want to take either test, contact a local health club or recreational facility.

The *Rockport Fitness Walking Test*, the *Lifecycle FIT Test*, and the *Lifestep Electronic FIT Test* were developed by researchers in my laboratory at the University of Massachusetts Medical School and have been demonstrated to yield highly accurate estimates of aerobic capacity.

A note to those on medication: If you are on a class of drugs called beta blockers, which slow the heart rate response to exercise, the *Rockport Fitness Walking Test*, the Lifecycle FIT Test, and the *Lifestep Electronic FIT Test* may overestimate your fitness level and make it impossible for you to achieve the training rates recommended for your age. If you are on such medication, talk to your physician about an appropriate exercise program.

For those who want to strength-train, we offer three options:

A *Lifecircuit program* that offers information on how to use Lifecircuit strength training equipment.

A *generic program* that can be used with any other type of strength-training equipment.

A *home program* of eleven strengthening exercises you can do in about twelve minutes.

To test yourself for any of these three programs, simply perform the sit-up and push-up tests in Appendix F, record your results in Appendix G, then use those results to determine the color of your strength-training program for the Thirty-Day Eating and Exercise Starter Plan in Chapter 3.

## Exercising Safely

Whatever you choose, you need to do it safely.

I support the view of the American Heart Association and the American College of Sports Medicine that if you've been inactive and are over age forty-five, you should see or talk with your physician prior to starting a program. A little guidance from your doctor is also in order if you're over thirty-five and have a major risk factor for heart disease, such as cigarette smoking, high blood pressure, or elevated blood cholesterol.

Be sure to exercise in your target heart-rate zone. To get many of the fitness benefits from exercise, you need to exercise without strain, but at the same time within your target heart-rate zone. To determine your maximum heart rate, subtract your age from 220 heartbeats per minute (see Table 1). Then multiply it by 60 percent and 80 percent to get your range.

For example, a man or a woman thirty-five years old would have a range of 111 to 148 (220 − 35 = 185; 185 × .60 = 111; 185 × .80 = 148).

While these numbers are helpful guidelines that should keep you in the safe range, you should at all times monitor the way you feel. A good rule of thumb: If you can't carry on a conversation, or feel any dizziness or shortness of breath at all while you're exercising, or if you're very tired two hours after your workout, you're pushing too hard.

To monitor your progress as you start, I suggest taking your pulse every five minutes for ten seconds (multiply that number by 6 to get your pulse for one minute). And take it *immediately* after you stop. If you're below your target heart rate, *gradually* increase your pace; if you're above your target, *gradually* decrease the intensity of your workout.

## TABLE 1: DETERMINING TARGET HEART RATE ZONE

| Age (years) | Average Maximum Heart Rate (beats/minute) | Target Training Zone (beats/minute) 60% | 80% | 70% Maximum Heart Rate (beats/minute) |
|---|---|---|---|---|
| 20 | 200 | 120 | 160 | 140 |
| 25 | 195 | 117 | 156 | 137 |
| 30 | 190 | 114 | 152 | 133 |
| 35 | 185 | 111 | 148 | 130 |
| 40 | 180 | 108 | 144 | 126 |
| 45 | 175 | 105 | 140 | 123 |
| 50 | 170 | 102 | 136 | 119 |
| 55 | 165 | 99 | 132 | 116 |
| 60 | 160 | 96 | 128 | 112 |
| 65 | 155 | 93 | 124 | 109 |
| 70 | 150 | 90 | 120 | 105 |

*You'll note that, after a few weeks, the same amount of exercise will no longer raise your heart rate into your training zone.* That's a good sign. It means your cardiovascular system and your muscles have become stronger and more efficient. You'll need to increase your intensity slightly to keep your heart rate in the desirable training range. The Thirty-Day Starter Plan will help you increase your exertion level safely.

Do warm-ups, cool-downs, and stretching regularly. Just as a cold car is sluggish when it starts, so your muscles will be sluggish—and more prone to injury—if you don't warm them up gradually before exercising vigorously. Exercising with warmed-up muscles feels better. And it's essential for cardiac safety.

You don't have to do much to warm up—just walk, cycle, or stair-step at a slower pace than usual for five minutes or so, then speed it up. Do the same thing to cool down. For both warming up and cooling down, add a few stretching exercises.

Warm-ups and cool-downs have another value: They give you a chance to prepare yourself mentally for your workout, and enjoy the good feelings afterward. If you rush into and out of your program without paying attention to how you feel, you'll miss out on some of the most important benefits, besides setting yourself up for injury.

Stretching your muscles is also important to reduce soreness *and increase flexibility.* While some people argue that stretching is the same thing as warm-ups and cool-downs, it isn't. You need at least five minutes of stretching after exercise as well.

Use the simple, eight-step stretching program in Appendix B along with your workout. You can also use portions of it during the day to relieve stress.

## Planning Exercise into Your Day

The key to fitting exercise into your schedule is—once again—to know yourself.

When will you be most likely to exercise consistently without interruption? Answering this question may take some experimenting. Many of the top executives I interviewed for my book *Fit for Success* found that they needed to exercise first thing in the morning because it was the only time they had control of their time. Many working parents have the same problem.

My situation is a little different. I've never been able to exercise consistently at dawn when I get up, or at night when I finish work. I'm often just too tired. So I try to exercise in the middle of the day. Because it's so important as a stress reducer and as a way of organizing my thoughts, it's often the most creative time I have. So I *make an appointment with myself to exercise.*

Occasionally I do get caught up with responsibilities and don't keep my exercise appointment. I always feel the worse for it when that happens. But I try to remember that the next day is a new day. If you fall off the wagon, be kind to yourself. Say to yourself, "There's no reason to stop altogether."

To stay on track, I encourage people to keep a simple exercise log. Jot down the exercise you do in a little notebook and carry it with you. Or, if you like, you can use the sample walking exercise, Lifecycle, Lifestep, or the strength training log, all of which appear in the appendixes. Then, if you miss one day, you can look at the rest of the week—or the rest of the month—and say to yourself, "Maybe I've lost one day. But overall I'm doing fine."

That's it. You've tested your aerobic capacity, your strength, and your willingness to change. You're ready for your thirty-day plan. Best of luck to you!

# 3

# THE STARTER PLAN

Balance. That should be your overall goal with *The Exercise Exchange Program*. That means not obsessing about the extra cookie you've eaten, about what the scale says, or about missing one workout.

Obsessive behavior is the wrong approach. If you're obsessed about what you eat and do for exercise, you'll soon start to feel anxious, burned out, deprived, and tired of the whole process. You'll give up because you're miserable.

Instead, the Thirty-Day Eating and Exercise Starter Plan is just what it says—a plan to get you started toward achieving an overall *balance* in the food you eat and the exercise you do, a balance that favors weight loss and an improved outlook. The nutrient content of the meal plans is about 54 percent carbohydrate, 23 percent protein, and 23 percent fat. This is well within the general nutritional guidelines recommended by the nation's major health organizations and is far below the guideline for fat, which is 30 percent. The exercise plan strives for a mix of both exercise and activities through the exchange system.

Once you've finished the first month, you can continue with week five of the twenty-week walking, Lifecycle, Lifestep, Lifecircuit, ge-

33

neric strength training, or home strength training programs in the next chapter.

The plan will show you how to use the food exchanges to see that you have the right mix of protein, carbohydrates, and fat in your meals; and the exercise exchanges to make sure you have enough aerobic exercise and enjoyable, calorie-burning activities in your exercise "diet" to achieve long-term weight loss. You don't have to hit the target every time, just most of the time. If you don't achieve a perfect mix one day, concentrate on achieving it the next.

## Tips for Using the Meal Plans

■ Each meal plan offers a certain number of "open calories" that you can "spend" on a food item of your choice. For suggestions, choose items from the food exchange lists in Chapter 6 (pages 172–189) and the fat and cholesterol comparison charts in Appendix A. Enjoy the flexibility. Just make sure you don't consistently choose more fat.

■ All meats used in the meal plan are lean meats, which means they contain three grams of fat or less per cooked ounce. If you use meats that are higher in fat, you must count an additional fat exchange. See the meat section of the food exchange list in Chapter 6 (page 174) for information on the fat content of various meats.

■ When turkey and chicken are listed on the lunch menu, use hot or cold, freshly cooked, skinless chicken or turkey. Or use luncheon meat with no more than three grams of fat per ounce. It will be described on the package as "extra lean" or as 95 to 98 percent fat-free.

■ Most of the cheeses listed in the meal plans are low-fat cheeses, or cheeses with two to three grams of fat per ounce. If you use regular cheese instead, you must count it as one lean meat exchange (because of the protein content) and one fat exchange. See page 179 of the food exchange list for the fat content of various cheeses.

■ If you can't get the fruits listed in the meal plans, simply substitute from these lists:

For vitamin A: cantaloupe, apricots, mango, papaya, and persimmon. For vitamin C: orange, orange juice, grapefruit, grapefruit juice, papaya, strawberries, cantaloupe, tangerines, kiwi, guava, and lichees. For iron: prunes, prune juice, figs, watermelon, raisins, dates, apricots, dried apricots, dried peaches, blackberries, boysenberries, raspberries, strawberries, and mulberries.

In addition, apples, bananas, cherries, grapes, nectarines, peaches, pears, pineapples, plums, and pomegranates are also rich in vitamins and minerals.

■ When choosing cookies or crackers, make sure you're choosing the low-fat varieties. Low-fat cookies include graham bears, fig bars, vanilla wafers, animal crackers, and gingersnaps.

Low-fat crackers include Wasa Extra Crisp, Wasa Crispbread Savory Sesame, Finn Crisp, Ak-Mak Sesame Crackers, Kavli Norwegian Crispbread, Manischewitz Whole Wheat Matzos, Premium Saltines, Premium Unsalted Tops, Stoned Corn Crackers, Stoned Rye Crackers, Stoned Wheat Thins, Triscuit Wafers, and Ry-Krisp.

■ When it comes to beverages, skim or nonfat milk should be used whenever milk is called for. The "noncaloric beverages" mentioned in the meal plans refer to coffee, hot tea, or ice tea with no milk, cream, or sugar; and water, seltzer water, or diet beverages.

■ Low-fat frozen yogurt is frequently suggested as a dessert or snack in the meal plans. If you like, you can substitute nonfat or low-fat ice milk or similar desserts from the milk section of the additional exchange list on page 188 of Chapter 6.

■ Dishes in your meal plan that require recipes are indicated by upper-case letters (e.g., Sautéed Chicken, page 306). You'll find them in the section "The Recipes" in this book.

■ Tempted to buy the "healthy" frozen dinners and other prepared foods because you don't have time to cook? Check the package for calorie and fat information, then use the following equation to determine if the product exceeds the 30 percent guideline:

Let's say the dinner has 400 calories. Multiply the total calories by 0.30, the maximum amount of fat you should be consuming, and divide the answer by 9, the number of calories in a gram of fat:

$$400 \times .30 = 120; 120 \text{ divided by } 9 = 13.3 \text{ grams of fat}$$

To be safe, any 400-calorie dinner you buy should have no more than 13 grams of fat.

■ The foods for days 4, 12, 20 and 28 were specifically chosen so that they can be eaten either at home or at a restaurant. For example, Day 4's lunch can be eaten at a fast food restaurant, and dinner at a steak house or similar establishment. Just remember, days used for eating out are interchangeable, as long as the whole day is swapped, not just one meal.

Should you decide to eat out, keep these tips in mind:

1. Simple foods are usually lower in fat (or the fat is more obvious) than mixed dishes such as casseroles, stews, and quiches.

2. Restaurant portions will be larger than the portions in your eating plan, so make sure you have the wait staff bag the extra food at the beginning of the meal (so you won't be tempted to eat all of it) or consider leaving some food behind.

3. Get in the habit of ordering your foods prepared without fat and ask for dressings, sauces, and butter on the side.

4. Choose broth soups instead of cream soups; tomato-based pasta dishes instead of cream-based ones.

5. For smaller portions, order pastas from the appetizer menu and

fill in with dinner salad. If all of the salads have high-fat ingredients, a sandwich may be a better choice.

6. Beware of specialty breads such as muffins, croissants, cornbread, and "grilled bread." Some can add as many as 500 calories to your meal.

7. To make the best choice, don't go to a restaurant starved. Eat some fruit, a piece of bread, or drink a glass of milk to tame your appetite beforehand.

## Tips for Using the Exercise Plan

■ This plan calls for burning a minimum of 200 calories a day to start. Approximately 100 of these calories will be burned through the walking, the Lifecycle, or the Lifestep program; 100 will be burned through doing exercise exchanges. Consult Chapter 5 for a list of suggested activities.

■ The Lifecycle and Lifestep have three settings or "profiles": hill, random, or manual. The programs in this book are designed for use with the hill profile.

■ Some workouts for the Lifecycle and Lifestep are broken up into two or three time slots (6 + 6 + 6, 12 + 6, or 12 + 12). That gives you a chance to rest for two minutes or less during your workout if you need to, and still complete the total time allotted. If you stop for longer than that, your heart rate will drop below your training range, and you won't get the same cardiovascular benefits you would from an uninterrupted workout.

■ While the Lifecircuit program calls for multiple sets of repetitions, research has shown that only one set is necessary for a good workout. The additional sets are for those who may be accustomed to doing more than one.

■ The generic program can be done on any type of strength-training equipment available (other than Lifecircuit, of course) at a health club or recreational facility. The home program can be done using the strength-training exercises in Appendix F.

■ If you run into problems sticking with your eating or exercise plan, read—and reread—Chapter 7. It discusses the major mental roadblocks to lifestyle change, as well as how to get past them.

In the meantime, good luck . . . and enjoy!

# DAY 1

**ALL PROGRAMS** eight to ten minutes of warm-ups and cool-downs, including stretching exercises in Appendix B. See Chapter 2 and Appendices C, D, E, or F for self-testing and exercise program information.

## WALKING

BLUE: 1.1 miles in 22 minutes (3.0 mph) for 86 calories.
GREEN: 1.3 miles in 25 minutes (3.0 mph) for 97 calories.
YELLOW: 1.4 miles in 27 minutes (3.0 mph) for 106 calories.
ORANGE: 1.5 miles in 26 minutes (3.5 mph) for 122 calories.
RED: 1.6 miles in 24 minutes (4.0 mph) for 140 calories.

## LIFECYCLE

PURPLE: level 1 for 12 minutes (4 + 4 + 4) for 83 calories.
BLUE: level 2 for 12 minutes for 86 calories.
GREEN: level 4 for 12 minutes for 97 calories.
YELLOW: level 6 for 12 minutes for 106 calories.
ORANGE: level 8 for 12 minutes for 122 calories.
RED: level 10 for 12 minutes for 140 calories.

## LIFESTEP

PURPLE: level 1 for 18 minutes (6 + 6 + 6) for 73 calories.
BLUE: level 1 for 18 minutes (12 + 6) for 73 calories.
GREEN: level 2 for 18 minutes (12 + 6) for 101 calories.
YELLOW: level 3 for 18 minutes (12 + 6) for 112 calories.
ORANGE: level 4 for 18 minutes for 122 calories.
RED: level 6 for 18 minutes for 142 calories.

**LIFECIRCUIT.** All colors take the day off.

**GENERIC/HOME STRENGTH TRAINING.** All colors take the day off.

**EXERCISE EXCHANGE.** One exchange for all color groups, which will burn 100 calories. See Chapter 5 for suggestions.

# DAY 1

## 1,200-Calorie Meal Plan

| | |
|---|---|
| 4 meat | 3 fruit |
| 4 bread | 3 fat |
| 3 vegetable | 2 milk |

80 open calories

BREAKFAST
1 orange
1 slice whole-wheat toast
1 teaspoon margarine
1 cup milk
coffee or tea (optional)

LUNCH
¼ cup water-pack tuna mixed with
1 tablespoon reduced-calorie mayonnaise* on
2 cups garden salad
1 (1-ounce) whole-wheat roll
1¼ cup watermelon
1 cup milk

   *Nonfat yogurt can be mixed in for a moister dressing.

DINNER
3 ounces Sautéed Chicken, page 306*
1 serving Oven-Crisped Potatoes, page 283
½ cup cooked broccoli
½ cup summer squash
1 fresh peach or ½ cup water-pack canned peaches
noncaloric beverage

   *Make extra for day 3 dinner.

SNACK
3 cups plain popcorn with 1 teaspoon margarine
noncaloric beverage

*Open Calorie Suggestions:*

Increase toast at breakfast to 2 slices, or add a medium apple for a
snack, or add ½ cup lowfat frozen yogurt for dessert at dinner.

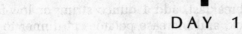

# DAY 1

## 1,500 Calorie Meal Plan

| | |
|---|---|
| 5 meat | 4 fruit |
| 5 bread | 3 fat |
| 3 vegetable | 2 milk |

200 open calories

---

BREAKFAST
1 orange
2 slices whole-wheat toast
1 teaspoon margarine
1 cup milk
coffee or tea (optional)

LUNCH
½ cup water-pack tuna mixed with
1 tablespoon reduced-calorie mayonnaise* on
2 cups garden salad
1 (1-ounce) whole-wheat roll
1¼ cup watermelon
1 cup milk

*Nonfat yogurt can be mixed in for a moister dressing.

SNACK
1 small pear
noncaloric beverage

DINNER
3 ounces Sautéed Chicken, page 306*
1 serving Oven-Crisped Potatoes, page 283
½ cup cooked broccoli
½ cup summer squash
1 fresh peach or ½ cup water-pack canned peaches
noncaloric beverage

*Make extra for day 3 dinner.

SNACK
3 cups plain popcorn with
1 teaspoon margarine
noncaloric beverage

*Open calorie suggestions:*

Add ½ tablespoon jelly at breakfast, add 1 ounce string or low-fat cheese to the afternoon snack, and increase potatoes at dinner to 2 servings.

## D A Y   1

# 1,800-Calorie Meal Plan

| | |
|---|---|
| 6 meat | 4 fruit |
| 6 bread | 4 fat |
| 4 vegetable | 2 milk |

300 open calories

### BREAKFAST
1 orange
2 slices whole-wheat toast
½ tablespoon (1 pat) margarine
1 cup milk
coffee or tea (optional)

### LUNCH
½ cup water-pack tuna mixed with 1 tablespoon reduced-calorie
    mayonnaise* on 2 cups garden salad
1 (1-ounce) whole-wheat roll
1¼ cup watermelon
1 cup milk

  *Nonfat yogurt can be mixed in for a moister dressing.

### SNACK
1 small pear
noncaloric beverage

### DINNER
1 tomato, sliced
4 ounces Sautéed Chicken, page 306*
2 servings Oven-Crisped Potatoes, page 283
½ cup cooked broccoli
½ cup summer squash
1 fresh peach or ½ cup water-pack canned peaches
noncaloric beverage

  *Make extra for day 3 dinner.

SNACK
3 cups plain popcorn with 1 teaspoon margarine
noncaloric beverage

*Open calorie suggestions:*

Add 1 tablespoon jelly at breakfast, omit roll at lunch and add 2 slices rye bread for a tuna sandwich, add 1 ounce string or low-fat cheese to the afternoon snack, increase popcorn to 5 cups, and increase margarine to 2 teaspoons at the evening snack.

# DAY 2

**ALL PROGRAMS** eight to ten minutes of warm-ups and cool-downs, including stretching exercises in Appendix B.

**WALKING.** Take the day off.

**LIFECYCLE.** Take the day off.

**LIFESTEP.** Take the day off.

**LIFECIRCUIT**

BLUE: 1 set of 12 repetitions.
GREEN: 1 set of 12 repetitions.
YELLOW: 1 set of 12 repetitions.
ORANGE: 2 sets of 12 repetitions.
RED: 2 sets of 12 repetitions.

**GENERIC/HOME STRENGTH TRAINING**

BLUE: 1 set of 8 to 10 repetitions.
GREEN: 1 set of 10 repetitions.
YELLOW: 1 set of 12 repetitions.
ORANGE: 3 sets of 10 repetitions.
RED: 3 sets of 12 repetitions.

**EXERCISE EXCHANGE.** Two exchanges for all color groups today (see Chapter 5).

# DAY 2

## 1,200-Calorie Meal Plan

| | |
|---|---|
| 4 meat | 3 fruit |
| 4 bread | 3 fat |
| 3 vegetable | 2 milk |

80 open calories

BREAKFAST
½ grapefruit
¾ cup iron-fortified cold flake cereal
1 cup milk
coffee or tea (optional)

LUNCH
1 tablespoon peanut butter
1 (1-ounce) bagel
1 cup carrot/celery sticks
1 small apple
noncaloric beverage

DINNER
2 cups salad with spinach, tomato, green pepper, and
    2 tablespoons reduced-calorie dressing
1 serving Trout Almondine, page 246
½ cup brown rice
⅓ cup mixed vegetables
1 teaspoon margarine
1 cup milk

SNACK
1 cup cantaloupe cubes
noncaloric beverage

*Open calorie suggestions:*

Increase peanut butter at lunch to 2 tablespoons, or increase bagel at lunch to 2 ounces, or add ¾ ounce low-fat crackers as a snack (see page 176 for suggestions).

# DAY 2

## 1,500-Calorie Meal Plan

| | |
|---|---|
| 5 meat | 4 fruit |
| 5 bread | 3 fat |
| 3 vegetable | 2 milk |

200 open calories

BREAKFAST
½ grapefruit
¾ cup iron-fortified, cold flake cereal
1 cup milk
coffee or tea (optional)

LUNCH
2 tablespoons peanut butter
1 (2-ounce) bagel
1 cup carrot/celery sticks
1 small apple
noncaloric beverage

SNACK
1 nectarine
noncaloric beverage

DINNER
2 cups salad with spinach, tomato, green pepper, and
    2 tablespoons low-cal dressing (free food, see page 186)
1 serving Trout Almondine, page 246
½ cup brown rice
⅓ cup mixed vegetables
1 teaspoon margarine
1 cup milk

SNACK
1 cup cantaloupe cubes
noncaloric beverage

*Open calorie suggestions:*

Increase cereal at breakfast to 1½ cups and add ¾ cup nonfat frozen
yogurt as a dessert or snack.

# DAY 2

## 1,800-Calorie Meal Plan

| | |
|---|---|
| 6 meat | 4 fruit |
| 6 bread | 4 fat |
| 4 vegetable | 2 milk |

300 open calories

BREAKFAST
½ grapefruit
1½ cups iron-fortified, cold flake cereal
1 cup milk
coffee or tea (optional)

LUNCH
2 tablespoons peanut butter
1 (2-ounce) bagel
1 cup carrot/celery sticks
1 small apple
noncaloric beverage

SNACK
1 nectarine
noncaloric beverage

DINNER
2 cups salad with spinach, tomato, green pepper, and
    1 ounce low-fat cheese, shredded
    2 tablespoons reduced-calorie dressing
1 serving Trout Almondine, page 246
½ cup brown rice
⅔ cup mixed vegetables
1 teaspoon margarine
1 cup milk

SNACK
1 cup cantaloupe cubes
noncaloric beverage

*Open calorie suggestions:*

Add 1 cup nonfat frozen yogurt as a dessert or snack and increase rice
to 1 cup at dinner.

## DAY 3

ALL PROGRAMS eight to ten minutes of warm-ups and cool-downs, including stretching exercises in Appendix B.

### WALKING

BLUE: 1.1 miles in 22 minutes (3.0 mph) for 86 calories.
GREEN: 1.3 miles in 25 minutes (3.0 mph) for 97 calories.
YELLOW: 1.4 miles in 27 minutes (3.0 mph) for 106 calories.
ORANGE: 1.5 miles in 26 minutes (3.5 mph) for 122 calories.
RED: 1.6 miles in 24 minutes (4.0 mph) for 140 calories.

### LIFECYCLE

PURPLE: level 1 for 12 minutes (4 + 4 + 4) for 83 calories.
BLUE: level 2 for 12 minutes for 86 calories.
GREEN: level 4 for 12 minutes for 97 calories.
YELLOW: level 6 for 12 minutes for 106 calories.
ORANGE: level 8 for 12 minutes for 122 calories.
RED: level 10 for 12 minutes for 140 calories.

### LIFESTEP

PURPLE: level 1 for 18 minutes (6 + 6 + 6) for 73 calories.
BLUE: level 1 for 18 minutes (12 + 6) for 73 calories.
GREEN: level 2 for 18 minutes (12 + 6) for 101 calories.
YELLOW: level 3 for 18 minutes (12 + 6) for 112 calories.
ORANGE: level 4 for 18 minutes for 122 calories.
RED: level 6 for 18 minutes for 142 calories.

LIFECIRCUIT. A day off for all color groups.

GENERIC/HOME STRENGTH TRAINING. A day off for all color groups.

EXERCISE EXCHANGE. One exchange for all color groups today (see Chapter 5).

# DAY 3

## 1,200-Calorie Meal Plan

| | |
|---|---|
| 4 meat | 3 fruit |
| 4 bread | 3 fat |
| 3 vegetable | 2 milk |

80 open calories

BREAKFAST
1 (1-ounce) bagel
½ tablespoon cream cheese
½ banana, sliced
1 cup milk
coffee or tea (optional)

LUNCH
½ 6-inch pita bread filled with
    1 ounce shredded low-fat Cheddar or jack cheese
    shredded lettuce, tomato, and onion slices
    grated carrot or jicama
    1 tablespoon seeds or chopped nuts
    2 tablespoons reduced-calorie salad dressing
1 small pear
noncaloric beverage

DINNER
1 serving Chicken with Chinese Peas, page 242
⅓ cup rice
1 cup milk

SNACK
1 cup honeydew melon cubes
noncaloric beverage

*Open calorie suggestions:*

Increase bread at lunch to 1 6-inch pita, or increase cheese at lunch to 2 ounces and add raw vegetables for a snack, or increase rice at dinner to ⅔ cup.

# DAY 3

## 1,500-Calorie Meal Plan

| 5 meat | 4 fruit |
|--------|---------|
| 5 bread | 3 fat |
| 3 vegetable | 2 milk |

200 open calories

BREAKFAST
1 (1-ounce) bagel
½ tablespoon cream cheese
½ banana, sliced
1 cup milk
coffee or tea (optional)

LUNCH
1 6-inch pita bread filled with
    2 ounces shredded low-fat Cheddar or jack cheese
    shredded lettuce, tomato, and onion slices
    grated carrot or jicama
    1 tablespoon seeds or chopped nuts
    2 tablespoons reduced-calorie salad dressing
1 small pear
noncaloric beverage

SNACK
4 fresh apricots or 7 dried apricot halves
noncaloric beverage

DINNER
1 serving Chicken with Chinese Peas, page 242
⅓ cup rice
1 cup milk

SNACK
1 cup honeydew melon cubes
noncaloric beverage

*Open calorie suggestions:*

Increase bagel at breakfast to 2 ounces and cream cheese to 1 tablespoon, and increase rice to ⅔ cup and add 1 small sliced tomato to
dinner.

## D A Y   3

## 1,800-Calorie Meal Plan

| | |
|---|---|
| 6 meat | 4 fruit |
| 6 bread | 4 fat |
| 4 vegetable | 2 milk |

300 open calories

BREAKFAST
1 egg, cooked any style
1 (2-ounce) bagel
1 tablespoon cream cheese
½ banana, sliced
1 cup milk
coffee or tea (optional)

LUNCH
1 6-inch pita bread filled with
     2 ounces shredded low-fat Cheddar or jack cheese
     shredded lettuce, tomato, and onion slices
     grated carrot or jicama
     1 tablespoon seeds or chopped nuts
     2 tablespoons reduced-calorie salad dressing
1 small pear
noncaloric beverage

SNACK
4 fresh apricots or 7 dried apricot halves
noncaloric beverage

DINNER
1 small tomato, sliced
1 serving Chicken with Chinese Peas, page 242
⅓ cup rice
1 cup milk

SNACK
1 cup honeydew melon cubes
noncaloric beverage

*Open calorie suggestions:*

Increase rice to 1 cup at dinner and add ½ sandwich with 1 ounce
sliced turkey, mustard, and lettuce leaves to evening snack.

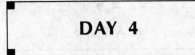

# DAY 4

**ALL PROGRAMS** eight to ten minutes of warm-ups and cool-downs, including stretching exercises in Appendix B.

## WALKING

BLUE: Day off.
GREEN: Day off.
YELLOW: Day off.
ORANGE: 1.5 miles in 26 minutes (3.5 mph) for 122 calories.
RED: 1.6 miles in 24 minutes (4.0 mph) for 140 calories.

## LIFECYCLE

PURPLE: Day off.
BLUE: Day off.
GREEN: Day off.
YELLOW: Day off.
ORANGE: level 8 for 12 minutes for 122 calories.
RED: level 10 for 12 minutes for 140 calories.

## LIFESTEP

PURPLE: Day off.
BLUE: Day off.
GREEN: Day off.
YELLOW: Day off.
ORANGE: level 4 for 18 minutes for 122 calories.
RED: level 6 for 18 minutes for 142 calories.

**LIFECIRCUIT.** Day off for everyone.

**GENERIC/HOME STRENGTH TRAINING.** Day off for everyone.

**EXERCISE EXCHANGE.** Two exchanges for Purple, Blue, Green, and Yellow; one exchange for Orange and Red.

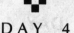

# DAY 4

## 1,200-Calorie Meal Plan

| | |
|---|---|
| 4 meat | 3 fruit |
| 4 bread | 3 fat |
| 3 vegetable | 2 milk |

80 open calories

BREAKFAST
½ cup grapefruit juice
½ cup shredded wheat or similar cereal
1 cup milk
coffee or tea (optional)

LUNCH
2 cups mixed vegetable salad (such as fast-food salad bar) with
    2 ounces lean ham
    2 tablespoons reduced-calorie dressing, or vinegar and 1
        teaspoon oil
4 low-fat whole-grain crackers (¾ ounce)
2 tablespoons raisins or dates
noncaloric beverage

DINNER
2 cups mixed green salad with 2 tablespoons reduced-calorie salad
    dressing, or vinegar and 1 teaspoon oil
2 ounces lean steak (such as round, sirloin, tenderloin, or London
    broil)
1 medium (6-ounce) baked potato
½ cup steamed vegetable
1 teaspoon margarine
noncaloric beverage

SNACK
½ cup low-fat frozen yogurt with
1 cup sliced strawberries

*Open calorie suggestions:*

Increase steak at dinner to 3½ ounces, or add 1 slice dry toast at
breakfast or a roll at dinner, or add 1 small glass wine at dinner.

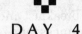

# DAY 4

## 1,500-Calorie Meal Plan

| | |
|---|---|
| 5 meat | 4 fruit |
| 5 bread | 3 fat |
| 3 vegetable | 2 milk |

200 open calories

BREAKFAST
½ cup grapefruit juice
½ cup shredded wheat or similar cereal
1 slice whole-wheat toast
1 cup milk
coffee or tea (optional)

LUNCH
2 cups mixed vegetable salad (such as fast-food salad bar) with
    2 ounces lean ham
    2 tablespoons reduced-calorie salad dressing, or vinegar and 1
        teaspoon oil
    2 tablespoons raisins or dates
4 low-fat, whole-grain crackers (¾ ounce)
noncaloric beverage

SNACK
1 small apple
noncaloric beverage

DINNER
2 cups mixed green salad with 2 tablespoons reduced-calorie salad
    dressing or vinegar and 1 teaspoon oil
3 ounces lean steak (such as round, sirloin, tenderloin, or London
    broil)
1 medium (6-ounce) baked potato
½ cup steamed vegetable
1 teaspoon margarine
noncaloric beverage

SNACK
½ cup low-fat frozen yogurt with 1 cup sliced strawberries

*Open calorie suggestions:*

Add 1 teaspoon margarine at breakfast and ¼ cup croutons to salad at lunch; increase steak to 4 ounces and add 1 small glass wine at dinner.

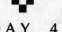

## D A Y   4

### 1,800-Calorie Meal Plan

| | |
|---|---|
| 6 meat | 4 fruit |
| 6 bread | 4 fat |
| 4 vegetable | 2 milk |

300 open calories

BREAKFAST
½ cup grapefruit juice
½ cup shredded wheat or similar cereal
1 slice whole-wheat toast
1 teaspoon margarine
1 cup milk
coffee or tea (optional)

LUNCH
1 cup raw carrot sticks
2 cups mixed vegetable salad (such as fast-food salad bar) with
    2 ounces lean ham
    ½ cup pasta salad
    2 tablespoons raisins or dates
4 low-fat whole-grain crackers (¾ ounce)
noncaloric beverage

SNACK
1 small apple
noncaloric beverage

DINNER
2 cups mixed green salad with 2 tablespoons reduced-calorie salad
    dressing, or vinegar and 1 teaspoon oil
4 ounces lean steak (such as round, sirloin, tenderloin, or London
    broil)
1 medium (6-ounce) baked potato
½ cup steamed vegetable

1 teaspoon margarine
noncaloric beverage

SNACK
½ cup low-fat frozen yogurt with
1 cup sliced strawberries

*Open calorie suggestions:*

Add 1 (1-ounce) roll, 1 teaspoon margarine, and 1 small glass wine to dinner, and increase frozen yogurt to 1 cup for evening snack.

# DAY 5

**ALL PROGRAMS** eight to ten minutes of warm-ups and cool-downs, including stretching exercises in Appendix B.

## WALKING

BLUE: 1.1 miles in 22 minutes (3.0 mph) for 86 calories.
GREEN: 1.3 miles in 25 minutes (3.0 mph) for 97 calories.
YELLOW: 1.4 miles in 27 minutes (3.0 mph) for 106 calories.
ORANGE: 1.5 miles in 26 minutes (3.5 mph) for 122 calories.
.RED: 1.6 miles in 24 minutes (4.0 mph) for 140 calories.

## LIFECYCLE

PURPLE: level 1 for 12 minutes (4 + 4 + 4) for 83 calories.
BLUE: level 2 for 12 minutes for 86 calories.
GREEN: level 4 for 12 minutes for 97 calories.
YELLOW: level 6 for 12 minutes for 106 calories.
ORANGE: level 8 for 12 minutes for 122 calories.
RED: level 10 for 12 minutes for 140 calories.

## LIFESTEP

PURPLE: level 1 for 18 minutes (6 + 6 + 6) for 73 calories.
BLUE: level 1 for 18 minutes (12 + 6) for 73 calories.
GREEN: level 2 for 18 minutes (12 + 6) for 101 calories.
YELLOW: level 3 for 18 minutes (12 + 6) for 112 calories.
ORANGE: level 4 for 18 minutes for 122 calories.
RED: level 6 for 18 minutes for 142 calories.

**LIFECIRCUIT**

BLUE: 1 set of 12 repetitions.
GREEN: 1 set of 12 repetitions.
YELLOW: 1 set of 12 repetitions.
ORANGE: 2 sets of 12 repetitions.
RED: 2 sets of 12 repetitions.

**GENERIC/HOME STRENGTH TRAINING**

BLUE: 1 set of 8 to 10 repetitions.
GREEN: 1 set of 10 repetitions.
YELLOW: 1 set of 12 repetitions.
ORANGE: 3 sets of 10 repetitions.
RED: 3 sets of 12 repetitions.

**EXERCISE EXCHANGE.** One exchange for all colors.

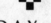

# DAY 5

## 1,200-Calorie Meal Plan

| | |
|---|---|
| 4 meat | 3 fruit |
| 4 bread | 3 fat |
| 3 vegetable | 2 milk |
| 80 open calories | |

BREAKFAST
¾ cup cold oat bran cereal
2 tablespoons raisins
1 cup milk
coffee or tea (optional)

LUNCH
green salad with 2 tablespoons reduced-calorie salad dressing
grilled open-face hamburger with
    2 ounces extra-lean ground beef
    ½ hamburger bun
    fresh tomato and onion slices
    ⅛ medium avocado, sliced
melon wedges
noncaloric beverage

<u>DINNER</u>
1 serving Oriental Noddles, page 251*
1 orange, sliced
1 cup milk

*Make enough for day 6 lunch.

<u>SNACK</u>
1½ cups plain popcorn
1 teaspoon margarine
noncaloric beverage

*Open calorie suggestions:*

Increase cereal at breakfast to 1 cup and popcorn to 3 cups for the
evening snack, or add ½ hamburger bun at lunch, or add ¾ ounce
low-fat (less than 30 percent fat) cookies for an afternoon snack. See
page 188 for suggestions.

## D A Y   5

### 1,500-Calorie Meal Plan

| 5 meat | 4 fruit |
|---|---|
| 5 bread | 3 fat |
| 3 vegetable | 2 milk |

200 open calories

<u>BREAKFAST</u>
¾ cup cold oat bran cereal
2 tablespoons raisins
1 cup milk
coffee or tea (optional)

<u>LUNCH</u>
green salad with 2 tablespoons reduced-calorie salad dressing
grilled hamburger with
    3 ounces extra-lean ground beef
    1 hamburger bun
    fresh tomato and onion slices
    ⅛ medium avocado, sliced
melon wedges
noncaloric beverage

SNACK
1 large kiwi or 1 small pear
noncaloric beverage

DINNER
1 serving Oriental Noodles, page 251*
1 orange, sliced
1 cup milk

*Make enough for day 6 lunch.

SNACK
1½ cups plain popcorn
1 teaspoon margarine
noncaloric beverage

*Open calorie suggestions:*

Increase cereal at breakfast to 1½ cups, add 1 cup Miso Soup, page 223, or vegetable soup to dinner, and increase popcorn to 3 cups for the evening snack.

---

# DAY 5

## 1,800-Calorie Meal Plan

| | |
|---|---|
| 6 meat | 4 fruit |
| 6 bread | 4 fat |
| 4 vegetable | 2 milk |

300 open calories

---

BREAKFAST
1½ cups cold oat bran cereal
2 tablespoons raisins
1 cup milk
coffee or tea (optional)

LUNCH
green salad with 2 tablespoons reduced-calorie salad dressing
grilled hamburger with
    3 ounces extra-lean ground beef
    1 ounce Cheddar or Swiss cheese
    1 hamburger bun

fresh tomato and onion slices
⅛ medium avocado, sliced
melon wedges
noncaloric beverage

SNACK
1 large kiwi or 1 small pear
noncaloric beverage

DINNER
1 cup fresh sliced cucumber and cherry tomatoes
1 serving Oriental Noodles, page 251*
1 orange, sliced
1 cup milk

*Make enough for day 6 lunch.

SNACK
1½ cups plain popcorn
1 teaspoon margarine
noncaloric beverage

*Open calorie suggestions:*

Add ¾ ounce pretzels for afternoon snack, increase Oriental Noodles
at dinner to 1½ servings, and increase popcorn at evening snack to 4
cups.

```
┌─────────────────────────┐
│                         │
│        DAY  6           │
│                         │
└─────────────────────────┘
```

ALL PROGRAMS eight to ten minutes of warm-ups and cool-downs,
including stretching exercises in Appendix B.

WALKING. Day off.

LIFECYCLE. Day off.

LIFESTEP. Day off.

LIFECIRCUIT. Day off for everyone.

**GENERIC/HOME STRENGTH TRAINING.** How about a nice, hot bath to relax tonight?

**EXERCISE EXCHANGE.** Two exchanges for all colors. See Chapter 5 to pick something you really like doing.

# DAY 6

## 1,200-Calorie Meal Plan

| | |
|---|---|
| 4 meat | 3 fruit |
| 4 bread | 3 fat |
| 3 vegetable | 2 milk |

80 open calories

BREAKFAST
1 cup honeydew melon cubes
1 (1-ounce) bagel
1 teaspoon margarine
1 cup milk
coffee or tea (optional)

LUNCH
½ serving Oriental Noodles (leftovers from day 5)
1 small granola bar
1 nectarine
noncaloric beverage

DINNER
1 serving Simmered Halibut, page 244
½ cup white rice
½ cup cooked carrots
1 teaspoon margarine
1 cup milk
coffee or tea (optional)

SNACK
1 small apple
noncaloric beverage

*Open calorie suggestions:*

Increase bagel for breakfast to 2 ounces, or add 20 grapes for a snack, or add 1 cup milk at lunch, or add additional ⅓ cup rice at dinner.

# DAY 6

## 1,500-Calorie Meal Plan

| | |
|---|---|
| 5 meat | 4 fruit |
| 5 bread | 3 fat |
| 3 vegetable | 2 milk |

200 open calories

BREAKFAST
1 cup honeydew melon cubes
1 (1-ounce) bagel
1 teaspoon margarine
1 cup milk
coffee or tea (optional)

LUNCH
1 serving Oriental Noodles (leftovers from day 5)
1 small granola bar
1 nectarine
noncaloric beverage

SNACK
1 small apple
noncaloric beverage

DINNER
1 serving Simmered Halibut, page 244
½ cup white rice
½ cup cooked carrots
1 teaspoon margarine
1 cup milk

SNACK
1¼ cup strawberries
noncaloric beverage

*Open calorie suggestions:*

Increase bagel to 2 ounces and margarine to 2 teaspoons at breakfast
and add ½ cup nonfat frozen yogurt to evening snack.

## D A Y   6

### 1,800-Calorie Meal Plan

| | |
|---|---|
| 6 meat | 4 fruit |
| 6 bread | 4 fat |
| 4 vegetable | 2 milk |

300 open calories

BREAKFAST
1 cup honeydew melon cubes
1 (2-ounce) bagel
2 teaspoons margarine
1 cup milk
coffee or tea (optional)

LUNCH
1 serving Oriental Noodles (leftovers from day 5)
1 small granola bar
1 nectarine
noncaloric beverage

SNACK
1 ounce low-fat cheese
1 small apple
noncaloric beverage

DINNER
½ steamed artichoke with fresh lemon wedges
1 serving Simmered Halibut, page 244
½ cup white rice
½ cup cooked carrots
1 teaspoon margarine
1 cup milk

SNACK
1¼ cup strawberries
noncaloric beverage

*Open calorie suggestions:*

Add 1 (1-ounce) roll and 1 teaspoon margarine to dinner, and 1 (1-ounce) muffin and ½ cup milk to evening snack.

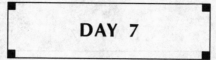

# DAY 7

ALL PROGRAMS eight to ten minutes of warm-ups and cool-downs, including stretching exercises in Appendix B.

## WALKING

BLUE: Day off.
GREEN: 1.3 miles in 25 minutes (3.0 mph) for 97 calories.
YELLOW: 1.4 miles in 27 minutes (3.0 mph) for 106 calories.
ORANGE: 1.5 miles in 26 minutes (3.5 mph) for 122 calories.
RED: 1.6 miles in 24 minutes (4.0 mph) for 140 calories.

## LIFECYCLE

PURPLE: Day off.
BLUE: Day off.
GREEN: level 4 for 12 minutes for 97 calories.
YELLOW: level 6 for 12 minutes for 106 calories.
ORANGE: level 8 for 12 minutes for 122 calories.
RED: level 10 for 12 minutes for 140 calories.

## LIFESTEP

PURPLE: Day off.
BLUE: Day off.
GREEN: level 2 for 18 minutes (12 + 6) for 101 calories.
YELLOW: level 3 for 18 minutes (12 + 6) for 112 calories.
ORANGE: level 4 for 18 minutes for 122 calories.
RED: level 6 for 18 minutes for 142 calories.

LIFECIRCUIT. Day off.

GENERIC/HOME STRENGTH TRAINING. Day off.

EXERCISE EXCHANGE. Two exchanges for Purple and Blue. Other colors, one exchange.

# DAY 7

## 1,200-Calorie Meal Plan

| | |
|---|---|
| 4 meat | 3 fruit |
| 4 bread | 3 fat |
| 3 vegetable | 2 milk |

80 open calories

BREAKFAST
½ cup orange juice
1 egg, cooked any style
1 slice whole-wheat toast
1 teaspoon margarine (use on toast or to cook egg)
coffee or tea (optional)

LUNCH
1 cup nonfat plain yogurt
½ banana, sliced
1 (1-ounce) bran muffin
noncaloric beverage

DINNER
1 serving Beef Tomato, page 259
2 6-inch flour tortillas, warmed
1 cup milk

SNACK
4 fresh or ½ cup water-pack canned apricots
noncaloric beverage

*Open calorie suggestions:*

Increase toast at breakfast to 2 slices, or increase orange juice to ¾ cup at breakfast and banana to 1 whole at lunch, or add ½ cup low-fat frozen yogurt for snack.

# DAY 7

## 1,500-Calorie Meal Plan

| | |
|---|---|
| 5 meat | 4 fruit |
| 5 bread | 3 fat |
| 3 vegetable | 2 milk |

200 open calories

---

BREAKFAST
½ cup orange juice
1 egg, cooked any style
1 slice whole-wheat toast
1 teaspoon margarine (use on toast or to cook egg)
coffee or tea (optional)

LUNCH
½ sandwich with
    1 ounce chicken
    1 slice whole-wheat bread
    lettuce and mustard
1 cup nonfat plain yogurt with 1 sliced banana
noncaloric beverage

SNACK
1 (1-ounce) bran muffin
noncaloric beverage

DINNER
1 serving Beef Tomato, page 259
2 6-inch flour tortillas, warmed
1 cup milk

SNACK
4 fresh or ½ cup water-pack canned apricots
noncaloric beverage

*Open calorie suggestions:*

Increase toast at breakfast to 2 slices and add ½ tablespoon jelly, and add 6 vanilla wafers for a dessert or snack anytime.

# DAY 7

## 1,800-Calorie Meal Plan

| | |
|---|---|
| 6 meat | 4 fruit |
| 6 bread | 4 fat |
| 4 vegetable | 2 milk |

300 open calories

BREAKFAST
½ cup orange juice
1 egg, cooked any style
1 slice whole-wheat toast
1 teaspoon margarine (use on toast or to cook egg)
coffee or tea (optional)

LUNCH
1 sandwich with
    2 ounces chicken
    2 slices whole-wheat bread
    lettuce and mustard
1 cup nonfat plain yogurt with 1 sliced banana
noncaloric beverage

SNACK
1 (1-ounce) bran muffin
1 teaspoon margarine
noncaloric beverage

DINNER
1 cup green salad with seasoned vinegar or low-cal dressing (free
    food, see page 186)
1 serving Beef Tomato, page 259
2 6-inch flour tortillas, warmed
1 cup milk

SNACK
4 fresh or ½ cup water-pack canned apricots
noncaloric beverage

*Open calorie suggestions:*

Increase toast at breakfast to 2 slices and add 1 teaspoon margarine,
increase afternoon snack to 1½ ounce muffin, and add 6 vanilla
wafers for a dessert or snack.

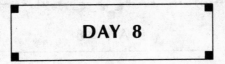

# DAY 8

**ALL PROGRAMS** eight to ten minutes of warm-ups and cool-downs, including stretching exercises in Appendix B.

## WALKING

BLUE: 1.1 miles in 22 minutes (3.0 mph) for 86 calories.
GREEN: 1.3 miles in 25 minutes (3.0 mph) for 97 calories.
YELLOW: 1.7 miles in 33 minutes (3.0 mph) for 132 calories.
ORANGE: 1.9 miles in 33 minutes (3.5 mph) for 152 calories.
RED: 2.0 miles in 30 minutes (4.0 mph) for 175 calories.

## LIFECYCLE

PURPLE: level 1 for 12 minutes (6 + 6) for 83 calories.
BLUE: level 2 for 12 minutes for 86 calories.
GREEN: level 4 for 12 minutes for 97 calories.
YELLOW: level 6 for 15 minutes (12 + 3) for 132 calories.
ORANGE: level 8 for 15 minutes (12 + 3) for 152 calories.
RED: level 10 for 15 minutes (12 + 3) for 175 calories.

## LIFESTEP

PURPLE: level 1 for 18 minutes (12 + 6) for 73 calories.
BLUE: level 1 for 18 minutes for 73 calories.
GREEN: level 2 for 18 minutes for 101 calories.
YELLOW: level 4 for 18 minutes for 122 calories.
ORANGE: level 4 for 24 minutes for 163 calories.
RED: level 6 for 24 minutes for 189 calories.

**LIFECIRCUIT.** Day off.

**GENERIC/HOME STRENGTH TRAINING.** Day off.

**EXERCISE EXCHANGE.** One exchange for all color groups.

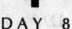

# DAY 8

## 1,200-Calorie Meal Plan

| | |
|---|---|
| 4 meat | 3 fruit |
| 4 bread | 3 fat |
| 3 vegetable | 2 milk |

80 open calories

BREAKFAST
½ cup shredded wheat
2 tablespoons raisins
1 cup milk
coffee or tea (optional)

LUNCH
1 6-inch pita bread filled with
    2 ounces low-fat shredded Cheddar or jack cheese
    tomato and onion slices
    grated carrot or jicama
    shredded lettuce
    1 tablespoon reduced-calorie mayonnaise
1 peach
noncaloric beverage

DINNER
2 ounces turkey cutlet
½ cup pasta with 1 teaspoon olive oil
1 serving Asparagus with Mild Peanut Sauce, page 268
1 orange, sliced
noncaloric beverage

SNACK
½ cup sugar-free pudding made with nonfat milk
noncaloric beverage

*Open calorie suggestions:*

Increase shredded wheat at breakfast to 1 cup, or increase turkey at
dinner to 3½ ounces, or increase pasta at dinner to 1 cup, or add 1
medium apple for a snack.

# DAY 8

## 1,500-Calorie Meal Plan

| | |
|---|---|
| 5 meat | 4 fruit |
| 5 bread | 3 fat |
| 3 vegetable | 2 milk |

200 open calories

BREAKFAST
1 cup shredded wheat
2 tablespoons raisins
1 cup milk
coffee or tea (optional)

LUNCH
1 6-inch pita bread filled with
    2 ounces low-fat shredded Cheddar or jack cheese
    tomato and onion slices
    grated carrot or jicama
    shredded lettuce
    1 tablespoon reduced-calorie mayonnaise
1 peach
noncaloric beverage

SNACK
½ cup applesauce
noncaloric beverage

DINNER
3 ounces turkey cutlet
½ cup pasta with 1 teaspoon olive oil
1 serving Asparagus with Mild Peanut Sauce, page 268
1 orange, sliced
noncaloric beverage

SNACK
½ cup sugar-free pudding made with nonfat milk
noncaloric beverage

*Open calorie suggestions:*

Increase pasta at dinner to 1 cup, have pudding for dessert at dinner instead of in evening snack, and add 3 cups plain popcorn and 1 teaspoon margarine for evening snack.

## DAY 8

### 1,800-Calorie Meal Plan

| | |
|---|---|
| 6 meat | 4 fruit |
| 6 bread | 4 fat |
| 4 vegetable | 2 milk |

300 open calories

BREAKFAST
½ cup vegetable juice
1 cup shredded wheat
2 tablespoons raisins
1 cup milk
coffee or tea (optional)

LUNCH
1 6-inch pita bread filled with
    2 ounces low-fat shredded Cheddar or jack cheese
    tomato and onion slices
    grated carrot or jicama
    shredded lettuce
    1 tablespoon reduced-calorie mayonnaise
1 peach
noncaloric beverage

SNACK
½ cup applesauce
noncaloric beverage

DINNER
4 ounces turkey cutlet
½ cup pasta with 1 teaspoon olive oil
1 serving Asparagus with Mild Peanut Sauce, page 268
1 orange, sliced
½ cup sugar-free pudding made with nonfat milk
noncaloric beverage

SNACK
3 cups plain popcorn
1 teaspoon margarine
noncaloric beverage

*Open calorie suggestions:*

Increase shredded wheat at breakfast to 1½ cups, add 1 cup milk at lunch, increase pasta at dinner to 1 cup, and increase popcorn in evening snack to 5 cups.

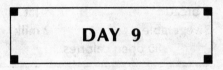

# DAY 9

**ALL PROGRAMS** eight to ten minutes of warm-ups and cool-downs, including stretching exercises in Appendix B.

**WALKING.** Day off for all colors.

**LIFECYCLE.** Day off for all colors.

**LIFESTEP.** Day off for all colors.

## LIFECIRCUIT

BLUE: 1 set of 12 repetitions.
GREEN: 1 set of 12 repetitions.
YELLOW: 1 set of 12 repetitions.
ORANGE: 2 sets of 12 repetitions.
RED: 2 to 3 sets of 12 repetitions.

## GENERIC/HOME STRENGTH TRAINING

BLUE: 1 set of 8 to 10 repetitions.
GREEN: 1 set of 10 repetitions.
YELLOW: 1 set of 12 repetitions.
ORANGE: 3 sets of 10 repetitions.
RED: 3 sets of 12 repetitions.

**EXERCISE EXCHANGE.** Two aerobic exchanges today. Why not try one outdoor and one indoor activity?

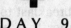

## DAY 9

### 1,200-Calorie Meal Plan

| | |
|---|---|
| 4 meat | 3 fruit |
| 4 bread | 3 fat |
| 3 vegetable | 2 milk |

80 open calories

BREAKFAST
½ cup orange juice
1 ounce Canadian bacon
1 slice whole-grain toast
1 teaspoon margarine
coffee or tea (optional)

LUNCH
1 small serving Tuna Salad, page 224
1 ounce whole-wheat crackers
    or roll with 1 teaspoon margarine
1 small pear
1 cup milk

DINNER
¼ cup low-fat cottage cheese with ⅓ cup water-pack canned
    pineapple or lettuce leaves
1 serving T.J.'s Vegetarian Chili, page 218
noncaloric beverage

SNACK
½ cup low-fat frozen yogurt
1 tablespoon chopped nuts
noncaloric beverage

*Open calorie suggestions:*

Increase toast at breakfast to 2 slices, or add a 1-ounce roll at dinner,
or increase cottage cheese and pineapple to ½ cup each at dinner, or
add 3 plums for snack.

# DAY 9

## 1,500-Calorie Meal Plan

| | |
|---|---|
| 5 meat | 4 fruit |
| 5 bread | 3 fat |
| 3 vegetable | 2 milk |

200 open calories

BREAKFAST
½ cup orange juice
1 ounce Canadian bacon
1 slice whole-grain toast
1 teaspoon margarine
coffee or tea (optional)

LUNCH
1 open-face sandwich with
    1 small serving Tuna Salad, page 224
    1 slice whole-grain bread
    lettuce leaves
1 small pear
1 cup milk

SNACK
2 plums
noncaloric beverage

DINNER
½ cup low-fat cottage cheese with ⅓ cup water-pack canned
    pineapple on lettuce leaves
1 serving T.J.'s Vegetarian Chili, page 218
1 ounce whole-wheat crackers, or
    1 (1-ounce) roll with 1 teaspoon margarine
noncaloric beverage

SNACK
½ cup low-fat frozen yogurt with 1 tablespoon chopped nuts
noncaloric beverage

*Open calorie suggestions:*

Add 1 slice toast and ½ tablespoon jelly at breakfast, and 1 cup milk
at breakfast or dinner.

## D A Y   9

### 1,800-Calorie Meal Plan

| | |
|---|---|
| 6 meat | 4 fruit |
| 6 bread | 4 fat |
| 4 vegetable | 2 milk |

300 open calories

BREAKFAST
½ cup orange juice
1 ounce Canadian bacon
2 slices whole-grain toast
2 teaspoons margarine
coffee or tea (optional)

LUNCH
1 open-face sandwich with
     1 large serving Tuna Salad, page 224
     1 slice whole-grain bread
     lettuce leaves
1 small pear
1 cup milk

SNACK
2 plums
noncaloric beverage

DINNER
½ cup low-fat cottage cheese with ⅓ cup water-pack canned
     pineapple on lettuce leaves
1 serving T.J.'s Vegetarian Chili, page 218
1 ounce whole-wheat crackers, or 1 (1-ounce) roll with 1 teaspoon
     margarine
noncaloric beverage

SNACK
½ cup low-fat frozen yogurt with
     1 tablespoon chopped nuts
noncaloric beverage

*Open calorie suggestions:*

Increase T.J.'s Vegetarian Chili at dinner to 1½ servings, add 1 cup
milk at dinner, and increase frozen yogurt for evening snack to 1 cup.

# DAY 10

**ALL PROGRAMS** eight to ten minutes of warm-ups and cool-downs, including stretching exercises in Appendix B.

## WALKING

BLUE: 1.1 miles in 22 minutes (3.0 mph) for 86 calories.
GREEN: 1.3 miles in 25 minutes (3.0 mph) for 97 calories.
YELLOW: 1.7 miles in 33 minutes (3.0 mph) for 132 calories.
ORANGE: 1.9 miles in 33 minutes (3.5 mph) for 152 calories.
RED: 2.0 miles in 30 minutes (4.0 mph) for 175 calories.

## LIFECYCLE

PURPLE: level 1 for 12 minutes (6 + 6) for 83 calories.
BLUE: level 2 for 12 minutes for 86 calories.
GREEN: level 4 for 12 minutes for 97 calories.
YELLOW: level 6 for 15 minutes (12 + 3) for 132 calories.
ORANGE: level 8 for 15 minutes (12 + 3) for 152 calories.
RED: level 10 for 15 minutes (12 + 3) for 175 calories.

## LIFESTEP

PURPLE: level 1 for 18 minutes (12 + 6) for 73 calories.
BLUE: level 1 for 18 minutes for 73 calories.
GREEN: level 2 for 18 minutes for 101 calories.
YELLOW: level 4 for 18 minutes for 122 calories.
ORANGE: level 4 for 24 minutes for 163 calories.
RED: level 6 for 24 minutes for 189 calories.

**LIFECIRCUIT.** All colors take the day off.

**GENERIC/HOME STRENGTH TRAINING.** All colors take the day off.

**LIFETIME EXERCISE EXCHANGE.** All colors choose one exchange today.

## D A Y   10

## 1,200-Calorie Meal Plan

| | |
|---|---|
| 4 meat | 3 fruit |
| 4 bread | 3 fat |
| 3 vegetable | 2 milk |

80 open calories

<u>BREAKFAST</u>
1 cup cantaloupe cubes
1 (1-ounce) bran muffin
1 cup milk
coffee or tea (optional)

<u>LUNCH</u>
½ sandwich with
     1½ ounces lean roast reef
     1 slice whole-wheat bread
     tomato and onion slices
     lettuce leaves and mustard
1 cup julienned jicama
1 small apple
noncaloric beverage

<u>DINNER</u>
2 cups garden salad with 2 tablespoons reduced-calorie dressing
1 serving Quick Crab Cakes, page 248
1 4-inch corn on the cob
1 sourdough roll
1 teaspoon margarine
1 cup milk

<u>SNACK</u>
1 orange or 1 large kiwi
noncaloric beverage

*Open calorie suggestions:*

Increase bread at lunch to 2 slices, or add ¾ ounce low-fat (less than 30 percent) cookies for snack.

## D A Y   10

# 1,500-Calorie Meal Plan

| | |
|---|---|
| 5 meat | 4 fruit |
| 5 bread | 3 fat |
| 3 vegetable | 2 milk |

200 open calories

**BREAKFAST**
1 cup cantaloupe cubes
1 (1-ounce) bran muffin
1 cup milk
coffee or tea (optional)

**LUNCH**
1 sandwich with
    2½ ounces lean roast beef
    2 slices whole-wheat bread
    tomato and onion slices
    lettuce leaves and mustard
1 cup julienned jicama
1 small apple
noncaloric beverage

**SNACK**
½ cup apple juice or cider

**DINNER**
2 cups garden salad with 2 tablespoons reduced-calorie dressing
1 serving Quick Crab Cakes, page 248
1 4-inch corn on the cob
1 sourdough roll
1 teaspoon margarine
1 cup milk

**SNACK**
1 orange or 1 large kiwi
noncaloric beverage

*Open calorie suggestions:*

Add 2 Peanut Butter Cookies, page 296, to afternoon snack, increase corn at dinner to 6-inch cob, and add 1 teaspoon margarine to meal of choice.

## D A Y  10

## 1,800-Calorie Meal Plan

| | |
|---|---|
| 6 meat | 4 fruit |
| 6 bread | 4 fat |
| 4 vegetable | 2 milk |

300 open calories

BREAKFAST
1 cup cantaloupe cubes
1 (2-ounce) bran muffin
1 cup milk
coffee or tea (optional)

LUNCH
1 sandwich with
    2½ ounces lean roast beef
    2 slices whole-wheat bread
    tomato and onion slices
    lettuce leaves and mustard
1 cup julienned jicama
1 small apple
noncaloric beverage

SNACK
½ cup apple juice or cider

DINNER
2 cups garden salad with 2 tablespoons reduced-calorie dressing
1½ servings Quick Crab Cakes (3 cakes), page 248
1 4-inch corn on the cob
1 sourdough roll
1 teaspoon margarine
1 cup milk

SNACK
1 orange or 1 large kiwi
noncaloric beverage

*Open calorie suggestions:*

Add 1 tablespoon reduced-calorie mayonnaise to lunch, add 2 Peanut
Butter Cookies, page 296, to afternoon snack, and increase corn to 8-

inch cob and add 1 tablespoon tartar sauce or ½ tablespoon margarine to dinner.

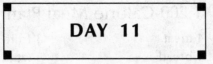

# DAY 11

**ALL PROGRAMS** eight to ten minutes of warm-ups and cool-downs, including stretching exercises in Appendix B.

## WALKING

BLUE: Day off.
GREEN: Day off.
YELLOW: 1.7 miles in 33 minutes (3.0 mph) for 132 calories.
ORANGE: 1.9 miles in 33 minutes (3.0 mph) for 152 calories.
RED: 2.0 miles in 30 minutes (4.0 mph) for 175 calories.

## LIFECYCLE

PURPLE: Day off.
BLUE: Day off.
GREEN: Day off.
YELLOW: level 6 for 15 minutes (12 + 3) for 132 calories.
ORANGE: level 8 for 15 minutes (12 + 3) for 152 calories.
RED: level 10 for 15 minutes (12 + 3) for 175 calories.

## LIFESTEP

PURPLE: Day off.
BLUE: Day off.
GREEN: Day off.
YELLOW: Day off.
ORANGE: level 4 for 24 minutes for 163 calories.
RED: level 6 for 24 minutes for 189 calories.

**LIFECIRCUIT.** Take another day off.

**GENERIC/HOME STRENGTH TRAINING.** A day off here, too.

**EXERCISE EXCHANGE.** Purple, Blue, and Green choose two exchanges. Yellow, Orange, and Red choose one exchange.

# DAY 11

## 1,200-Calorie Meal Plan

| | |
|---|---|
| 4 meat | 3 fruit |
| 4 bread | 3 fat |
| 3 vegetable | 2 milk |

80 open calories

---

BREAKFAST
¾ cup bran flakes
½ banana, sliced
1 cup milk
coffee or tea (optional)

LUNCH
2 cups garden salad with
    1 ounce shredded chicken breast
    2 tablespoons low-calorie dressing (free food, see page 186)
4 Ry-Krisp crackers
1 small pear
½ cup low-fat frozen yogurt
noncaloric beverage

DINNER
1 tomato sliced, with 1 tablespoon reduced-calorie salad dressing
1 small serving Veal Piccata on Fresh Pasta, page 264
½ cup summer squash
noncaloric beverage

SNACK
1 cup honeydew melon
noncaloric beverage

*Open calorie suggestions:*

Increase bran flakes at breakfast to 1½ cups, or increase chicken at lunch to 1½ ounces and add 1 ounce low-fat cheese, or increase Ry-Krisp crackers to 8 at lunch, or add 1 cup milk at dinner.

## D A Y   11

### 1,500-Calorie Meal Plan

| | |
|---|---|
| 5 meat | 4 fruit |
| 5 bread | 3 fat |
| 3 vegetable | 2 milk |

200 open calories

BREAKFAST
1½ cups bran flakes
½ banana, sliced
1 cup milk
coffee or tea (optional)

LUNCH
2 cups garden salad with
    2 ounces shredded chicken breast
    2 tablespoons low-calorie dressing (free food, see page 186)
4 Ry-Krisp crackers
1 large pear
noncaloric beverage

SNACK
½ cup low-fat frozen yogurt
noncaloric beverage

DINNER
1 tomato sliced, with 1 tablespoon reduced-calorie salad dressing
1 small serving Veal Piccata on Fresh Pasta page 264
½ cup summer squash
noncaloric beverage

SNACK
1 cup honeydew melon
noncaloric beverage

*Open calorie suggestions:*

Add 1 ounce low-fat cheese to salad at lunch, increase frozen yogurt
to 6 ounces for afternoon snack, and add 1 cup milk to dinner.

## DAY  11

### 1,800-Calorie Meal Plan

| | |
|---|---|
| 6 meat | 4 fruit |
| 6 bread | 4 fat |
| 4 vegetable | 2 milk |

300 open calories

BREAKFAST
½ cup vegetable juice
1½ cups bran flakes
½ banana, sliced
1 cup milk
coffee or tea (optional)

LUNCH
2 cups garden salad with
    2½ ounces shredded chicken breast
    2 tablespoons low-calorie dressing (free food, see page 186)
4 Ry-Krisp crackers
1 large pear
noncaloric beverage

SNACK
½ cup low-fat frozen yogurt
noncaloric beverage

DINNER
1 tomato sliced, with 1 tablespoon reduced-calorie salad dressing
1 large serving Veal Piccata on Fresh Pasta, page 264
½ cup summer squash
noncaloric beverage

SNACK
1 cup honeydew melon
noncaloric beverage

*Open calorie suggestions:*

Increase frozen yogurt to 1 cup at afternoon snack, add 1 cup milk or
1 glass wine to dinner, and add 1 ounce pretzels or low-fat crackers to
evening snack.

# DAY 12

ALL PROGRAMS eight to ten minutes of warm-ups and cool-downs, including stretching exercises in Appendix B.

## WALKING

BLUE: 1.1 miles in 22 minutes (3.0 mph) for 86 calories.
GREEN: 1.3 miles in 25 minutes (3.0 mph) for 97 calories.
YELLOW: 1.7 miles in 33 minutes (3.0 mph) for 132 calories.
ORANGE: 1.9 miles in 33 minutes (3.5 mph) for 152 calories.
RED: 2.0 miles in 30 minutes (4.0 mph) for 175 calories.

## LIFECYCLE

PURPLE: level 1 for 12 minutes (6 + 6) for 83 calories.
BLUE: level 2 for 12 minutes for 86 calories.
GREEN: level 4 for 12 minutes for 97 calories.
YELLOW: level 6 for 15 minutes (12 + 3) for 132 calories.
ORANGE: level 8 for 15 minutes (12 + 3) for 152 calories.
RED: level 10 for 15 minutes (12 + 3) for 175 calories.

## LIFESTEP

PURPLE: level 1 for 18 minutes (12 + 6) for 73 calories.
BLUE: level 1 for 18 minutes for 73 calories.
GREEN: level 2 for 18 minutes for 101 calories.
YELLOW: level 4 for 18 minutes for 122 calories.
ORANGE: level 4 for 24 minutes for 163 calories.
RED: level 6 for 24 minutes for 189 calories.

## LIFECIRCUIT

BLUE: 1 set of 12 repetitions.
GREEN: 1 set of 12 repetitions.
YELLOW: 1 set of 12 repetitions.
ORANGE: 2 sets of 12 repetitions.
RED: 2 to 3 sets of 12 repetitions.

## GENERIC/HOME STRENGTH TRAINING

BLUE: 1 set of 8 to 10 repetitions.

GREEN: 1 set of 10 repetitions.
YELLOW: 1 set of 12 repetitions.
ORANGE: 3 sets of 10 repetitions.
RED: 3 sets of 12 repetitions.

**EXERCISE EXCHANGE.** All colors choose one exchange today. How about something social, such as bowling?

# DAY 12

## 1,200-Calorie Meal Plan

| | |
|---|---|
| 4 meat | 3 fruit |
| 4 bread | 3 fat |
| 3 vegetable | 2 milk |

80 open calories

### BREAKFAST
½ grapefruit
½ English muffin
1 teaspoon margarine
1 cup milk
coffee or tea (optional)

### LUNCH
1 tostada with
    4 tablespoons shredded Cheddar cheese
    ⅓ cup refried beans
    1 6-inch tortilla (not fried)
    tomato slices and shredded lettuce
    salsa
fresh fruit slices
noncaloric beverage

### DINNER
½ steamed artichoke with lemon wedges
3 ounces salmon (prepared without added fat)
⅓ cup rice
½ cup steamed broccoli
1 cup fresh raspberries
noncaloric beverage

SNACK
½ cup nonfat frozen yogurt
noncaloric beverage

*Open calorie suggestions:*

Increase English muffin to 1 whole muffin at breakfast, or add 1½ ounces chicken to tostada at lunch, or add 1 small glass wine at dinner, or increase rice to ⅔ cup or add 1 (1-ounce) roll at dinner.

## DAY 12

### 1,500-Calorie Meal Plan

| | |
|---|---|
| 5 meat | 4 fruit |
| 5 bread | 3 fat |
| 3 vegetable | 2 milk |

200 open calories

BREAKFAST
½ grapefruit
1 English muffin
1 teaspoon margarine
1 cup milk
coffee or tea (optional)

LUNCH
1 tostada with
    1 ounce chicken
    4 tablespoons shredded Cheddar cheese
    ⅓ cup refried beans
    1 6-inch tortilla (not fried)
    tomato slices and shredded lettuce
    salsa
fresh fruit slices
noncaloric beverage

SNACK
1 small pear
noncaloric beverage

DINNER
½ steamed artichoke with lemon wedges

3 ounces salmon (prepared without added fat)
⅓ cup rice
½ cup steamed broccoli
1 cup fresh raspberries
noncaloric beverage

SNACK
½ cup nonfat frozen yogurt
noncaloric beverage

*Open calorie suggestions:*

Add ½ tablespoon jelly at breakfast, and 1 ounce salmon, 1 (1-ounce) roll, and 1 teaspoon margarine at dinner.

---

## D A Y   12

## 1,800-Calorie Meal Plan

| | |
|---|---|
| 6 meat | 4 fruit |
| 6 bread | 4 fat |
| 4 vegetable | 2 milk |

300 open calories

---

BREAKFAST
½ grapefruit
1 English muffin with 1 teaspoon margarine
1 cup milk
coffee or tea (optional)

LUNCH
1 tostada with
    1 ounce chicken
    4 tablespoons shredded Cheddar cheese
    ⅓ cup refried beans
    1 6-inch tortilla (not fried)
    tomato slices and shredded lettuce
    salsa
fresh fruit slices
noncaloric beverage

SNACK
1 cup carrot sticks

1 small pear
noncaloric beverage

DINNER
½ steamed artichoke with lemon wedges
4 ounces salmon (prepared without added fat)
⅓ cup rice
1 (1-ounce) whole-wheat bread
½ cup steamed broccoli with 1 teaspoon margarine
1 cup fresh raspberries
noncaloric beverage

SNACK
½ cup nonfat frozen yogurt
noncaloric beverage

*Open calorie suggestions:*

Add 1 tablespoon jelly at breakfast, 1 ounce tortilla chips at lunch,
and increase rice to ⅔ cup and margarine to ½ tablespoon at dinner.

## DAY 13

ALL PROGRAMS eight to ten minutes of warm-ups and cool-downs, including stretching exercises in Appendix B.

WALKING. Take a day off.

LIFECYCLE. Take a day off.

LIFESTEP. Take a day off.

LIFECIRCUIT. Take a day off.

GENERIC/HOME STRENGTH TRAINING. Take a day off.

EXERCISE EXCHANGE. All colors choose two exchanges today.

# DAY 13

## 1,200-Calorie Meal Plan

| | |
|---|---|
| 4 meat | 3 fruit |
| 4 bread | 3 fat |
| 3 vegetable | 2 milk |

80 open calories

---

BREAKFAST
½ cup oatmeal or oat bran with cinnamon
2 tablespoons raisins or 1½ dried figs, chopped
1 cup milk
coffee or tea (optional)

LUNCH
1 tablespoon peanut butter
¾ ounce matzo or crispbread crackers
1 cup sliced celery
2 plums
noncaloric beverage

DINNER
3 ounces baked or Sautéed Chicken, page 306*
1 serving Vegetable Medley with Honeyed Potatoes, page 281
1 whole-wheat roll with 1 teaspoon margarine
1 cup sliced papaya
noncaloric beverage


*Prepare extra for day 15's luncheon salad.

SNACK
½ cup nonfat fruited yogurt with 2 tablespoons granola
noncaloric beverage

*Open calorie suggestions:*

Increase oatmeal to 1 cup at breakfast, or increase peanut butter to 1½ tablespoons and crackers to 1¼ ounces at lunch, or add 1 large peach for a snack, or add 1 cup milk at lunch or dinner.

# DAY 13

## 1,500-Calorie Meal Plan

| 5 meat | 4 fruit |
|--------|---------|
| 5 bread | 3 fat |
| 3 vegetable | 2 milk |

200 open calories

BREAKFAST
½ cup oatmeal or oat bran with cinnamon
2 tablespoons raisins or 1½ dried figs, chopped
1 cup milk
coffee or tea (optional)

LUNCH
1 sandwich with
     2 tablespoons peanut butter
     2 slices whole-grain bread
1 cup sliced celery
2 plums
noncaloric beverage

SNACK
1 peach
noncaloric beverage

DINNER
3 ounces baked or Sautéed Chicken, page 306*
1 serving Vegetable Medley with Honeyed Potatoes, page 281
1 whole-wheat roll
1 cup sliced papaya
noncaloric beverage

*Prepare extra for day 15's luncheon salad.

SNACK
½ cup nonfat fruited yogurt with 2 tablespoons granola
noncaloric beverage

*Open calorie suggestions:*

Increase oatmeal to 1 cup at breakfast, add 1 cup milk to lunch or dinner, and add 1 teaspoon margarine to dinner.

## D A Y  13

## 1,800-Calorie Meal Plan

| | |
|---|---|
| 6 meat | 4 fruit |
| 6 bread | 4 fat |
| 4 vegetable | 2 milk |

300 open calories

BREAKFAST
¾ cup oatmeal or oat bran with cinnamon
2 tablespoons raisins or 1½ dried figs, chopped
1 cup milk
coffee or tea (optional)

LUNCH
1 sandwich with
    2 tablespoons peanut butter
    2 slices whole-grain bread
1 cup sliced celery
2 plums
noncaloric beverage

SNACK
1 peach
noncaloric beverage

DINNER
4 ounces baked or Sautéed Chicken, page 306*
1½ servings Vegetable Medley with Honeyed Potatoes, page 281
1 whole-wheat roll
1 teaspoon margarine
1 cup sliced papaya
noncaloric beverage

  *Prepare extra for day 15's luncheon salad.

SNACK
½ cup nonfat fruited yogurt with 2 tablespoons granola
noncaloric beverage

*Open calorie suggestions:*

Add 1 cup milk to lunch or dinner and 2 ounces low-fat cookies to lunch or the afternoon snack.

## DAY 14

**ALL PROGRAMS** eight to ten minutes of warm-ups and cool-downs, including stretching exercises in Appendix B.

### WALKING

BLUE: 1.1 miles in 22 minutes (3.0 mph) for 86 calories.
GREEN: 1.3 miles in 25 minutes (3.0 mph) for 97 calories.
YELLOW: 1.7 miles in 33 minutes (3.0 mph) for 132 calories.
ORANGE: 1.9 miles in 33 minutes (3.5 mph) for 152 calories.
RED: 2.0 miles in 30 minutes (4.0 mph) for 175 calories.

### LIFECYCLE

PURPLE: Take the day off.
BLUE: level 2 for 12 minutes for 86 calories.
GREEN: level 4 for 12 minutes for 97 calories.
YELLOW: level 6 for 15 minutes (12 + 3) for 132 calories.
ORANGE: level 8 for 15 minutes (12 + 3) for 152 calories.
RED: level 10 for 15 minutes (12 + 3) for 175 calories.

### LIFESTEP

PURPLE: Day off.
BLUE: level 1 for 18 minutes for 73 calories.
GREEN: level 2 for 18 minutes for 101 calories.
YELLOW: level 4 for 18 minutes for 122 calories.
ORANGE: level 4 for 24 minutes for 163 calories.
RED: level 6 for 24 minutes for 189 calories.

**LIFECIRCUIT.** Take a rest.

**GENERIC/HOME STRENGTH TRAINING.** Take a rest.

**EXERCISE EXCHANGE.** Purple chooses two exchanges today. How about washing and waxing your car? Everyone else do one.

## D A Y  14

## 1,200-Calorie Meal Plan

| | |
|---|---|
| 4 meat | 3 fruit |
| 4 bread | 3 fat |
| 3 vegetable | 2 milk |

80 open calories

BREAKFAST
½ cup grapefruit juice
2 Blueberry Pancakes, page 293, topped with
    ½ cup nonfat fruited yogurt
coffee or tea (optional)

LUNCH
½ cup low-fat cottage cheese on lettuce leaves
1 cup carrot sticks
1¼ cups strawberries
noncaloric beverage

DINNER
1 serving Spinach Salad, page 308
2 ounces roast beef
1 serving Risotto with Radicchio and Peas, page 274
1 cup milk

SNACK
3 vanilla wafers
noncaloric beverage

*Open calorie suggestions:*

Add 1-ounce roll at lunch, or add 1⅓ cup honeydew melon for an
afternoon snack, or increase roast beef portion at dinner to 3 ounces,
or increase vanilla wafers to 6 and add ½ cup milk for evening snack.

# D A Y   14

## 1,500-Calorie Meal Plan

| | |
|---|---|
| 5 meat | 4 fruit |
| 5 bread | 3 fat |
| 3 vegetable | 2 milk |

200 open calories

BREAKFAST
½ cup grapefruit juice
2 Blueberry pancakes, page 293, topped with
    ½ cup nonfat fruited yogurt
coffee or tea (optional)

LUNCH
½ cup low-fat cottage cheese on lettuce leaves
1 cup carrot sticks
1 (1-ounce) roll
1¼ cup strawberries
noncaloric beverage

SNACK
1 cup honeydew melon
noncaloric beverage

DINNER
1 serving Spinach Salad, page 308
3 ounces roast beef
1 serving Risotto with Radicchio and Peas, page 274
1 cup milk

SNACK
3 vanilla wafers
noncaloric beverage

*Open calorie suggestions:*

Add 1 pancake at breakfast, and increase vanilla wafers to 6 and add 1
cup milk at evening snack.

# D A Y   14

## 1,800-Calorie Meal Plan

| | |
|---|---|
| 6 meat | 4 fruit |
| 6 bread | 4 fat |
| 4 vegetable | 2 milk |

300 open calories

BREAKFAST
½ cup grapefruit juice
2 Blueberry Pancakes, page 293, topped with
    ½ cup nonfat fruited yogurt
coffee or tea (optional)

LUNCH
½ cup low-fat cottage cheese on lettuce leaves
1½ cups carrot sticks and cherry tomatoes
1 (1-ounce) roll
1 teaspoon margarine
1¼ cups strawberries
noncaloric beverage

SNACK
1 cup honeydew melon
noncaloric beverage

DINNER
1 serving Spinach Salad, page 308, with
    ¼ cup croutons
4 ounces roast beef
1 serving Risotto with Radicchio and Peas, page 274
1 cup milk

SNACK
6 vanilla wafers
noncaloric beverage

*Open calorie suggestions:*

Increase grapefruit juice at breakfast to 1 cup, add 1 (1¼-ounce) muffin to afternoon snack, and add 1 cup milk to evening snack.

# DAY 15

ALL PROGRAMS eight to ten minutes of warm-ups and cool-downs, including stretching exercises in Appendix B.

## WALKING

BLUE: 1.4 miles in 27 minutes (3.0 mph) for 108 calories.
GREEN: 1.6 miles in 31 minutes (3.0 mph) for 121 calories.
YELLOW: 2.0 miles in 40 minutes (3.0 mph) for 159 calories.
ORANGE: 2.3 miles in 39 minutes (3.5 mph) for 183 calories.
RED: 2.4 miles in 36 minutes (4.0 mph) for 210 calories.

## LIFECYCLE

PURPLE: level 1 for 12 minutes for 83 calories.
BLUE: level 2 for 15 minutes (12 + 3) for 108 calories.
GREEN: level 4 for 15 minutes (12 + 3) for 121 calories.
YELLOW: level 6 for 18 minutes (12 + 6) for 159 calories.
ORANGE: level 8 for 18 minutes (12 + 6) for 183 calories.
RED: level 10 for 18 minutes (12 + 6) for 210 calories.

## LIFESTEP

PURPLE: level 1 for 18 minues for 73 calories.
BLUE: level 1 for 24 minutes (18 + 6) for 93 calories.
GREEN: level 3 for 18 minutes for 112 calories.
YELLOW: level 4 for 24 minutes (18 + 6) for 163 calories.
ORANGE: level 5 for 24 minutes for 176 calories.
RED: level 7 for 24 minutes for 204 calories.

LIFECIRCUIT. Time off.

GENERIC/HOME STRENGTH TRAINING. Time off.

EXERCISE EXCHANGE. One exchange for all colors.

## DAY 15

# 1,200-Calorie Meal Plan

| | |
|---|---|
| 4 meat | 3 fruit |
| 4 bread | 3 fat |
| 3 vegetable | 2 milk |

80 open calories

BREAKFAST
1 cup cantaloupe cubes
1 slice whole-wheat toast
1 teaspoon margarine
1 cup milk
coffee or tea (optional)

LUNCH
1 cup Rainbow Pasta Salad on salad greens, page 233
15 grapes
noncaloric beverage

DINNER
2 cups garden salad with 2 tablespoons low-calorie dressing (free
    food, see page 186)
1 serving Sweet 'n' Spicy Cornish Game Hens, page 240
1 small baked potato (3 oz.)
½ orange or ½ cup papaya, sliced
1 cup milk

SNACK
3 cups plain popcorn
noncaloric beverage

*Open calorie suggestions:*

Increase toast to 2 slices at breakfast, or add a 1-ounce roll at lunch, or
add 1 small glass wine or increase baked potato to 6 ounces at dinner,
or add 1 teaspoon margarine each to baked potato at dinner and
popcorn at snack.

## DAY  15

### 1,500-Calorie Meal Plan

| | |
|---|---|
| 5 meat | 4 fruit |
| 5 bread | 3 fat |
| 3 vegetable | 2 milk |

200 open calories

BREAKFAST
1 cup cantaloupe cubes
2 slices whole-wheat toast
1 teaspoon margarine
1 cup milk
coffee or tea (optional)

LUNCH
1 cup Rainbow Pasta Salad on salad greens, page 233
15 grapes
noncaloric beverage

SNACK
1 ounce string or low-fat cheese
1 small pear
noncaloric beverage

DINNER
2 cups garden salad with 2 tablespoons low-calorie dressing (free
    food, see page 186)
1 serving Sweet 'n' Spicy Cornish Game Hens, page 240
1 small baked potato (3 oz.)
½ orange or ½ cup papaya, sliced
1 cup milk

SNACK
3 cups plain popcorn
noncaloric beverage

*Open Calorie Suggestions:*

Add ½ tablespoon jelly at breakfast, add one 1-ounce roll at lunch,
increase potato to 5 ounces at dinner, and add 1 teaspoon margarine
to evening snack.

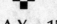

## DAY 15

## 1,800-Calorie Meal Plan

| | |
|---|---|
| 6 meat | 4 fruit |
| 6 bread | 4 fat |
| 4 vegetable | 2 milk |

300 open calories

BREAKFAST
1 cup cataloupe cubes
2 slices whole-wheat toast
1 teaspoon margarine
1 cup milk
coffee or tea (optional)

LUNCH
2 cups Rainbow Pasta Salad on salad greens, page 233
15 grapes
noncaloric beverage

SNACK
1½ ounces string or low-fat cheese
1 small pear
noncaloric beverage

DINNER
2 cups garden salad with 2 tablespoons low-calorie dressing (free
    food, see page 186)
1 serving Sweet 'n' Spicy Cornish Game Hens, page 240
1 small baked potato (3 oz.)
½ orange or ½ cup papaya, sliced
1 cup milk

SNACK
3 cups plain popcorn
noncaloric beverage

Open calorie suggestions:

Add 1 tablespoon jelly to breakfast, increase potato to 6 ounces and
add 1 ounce bread to dinner, and add 1 teaspoon margarine to both
dinner and evening snack.

# DAY 16

**ALL PROGRAMS** eight to 10 minutes of warm-ups and cool-downs, including stretching exercises in Appendix B.

**WALKING.** Enjoy a day off.

**LIFECYCLE.** Enjoy a day off.

**LIFESTEP.** Enjoy a day off.

## LIFECIRCUIT

BLUE: 1 set of 12 repetitions.
GREEN: 1 set of 12 repetitions.
YELLOW: 2 sets of 12 repetitions.
ORANGE: 2 sets of 12 repetitions.
RED: 3 sets of 12 repetitions.

## GENERIC/HOME STRENGTH TRAINING

BLUE: 1 set of 8 to 10 repetitions.
GREEN: 2 sets of 10 repetitions.
YELLOW: 2 sets of 12 repetitions.
ORANGE: 3 sets of 10 repetitions.
RED: 3 sets of 12 repetitions.

**EXERCISE EXCHANGE.** All colors choose two exchanges today. Remember, household tasks and errands—such as doing the wash—do count.

## DAY 16

# 1,200-Calorie Meal Plan

| | |
|---|---|
| 4 meat | 3 fruit |
| 4 bread | 3 fat |
| 3 vegetable | 2 milk |

80 open calories

BREAKFAST
½ grapefruit
¾ cup iron-fortified cold flake cereal
1 cup milk
coffee or tea (optional)

LUNCH
1 sandwich with
    1½ ounces lean ham
    2 slices whole-grain toast
    1 sliced tomato and lettuce leaves
    1 tablespoon reduced-calorie mayonnaise
½ small pear
1 cup milk

DINNER
1 serving Lettuce with Warm Sweet-Sour Sauce, page 231
2½ ounces broiled fish
½ cup Seasoned Wild Rice, page 278*
½ cup steamed carrots
1 teaspoon margarine or oil (for fish or carrots)
noncaloric beverage

*Prepare extra for tomorrow's luncheon salad, Chilled Wild Rice with Shrimp. To save even more time tomorrow, make the salad tonight and chill.

SNACK
1¼ cup strawberries
noncaloric beverage

*Open Calorie Suggestions:*

Increase cereal at breakfast to 1½ cups, or increase ham to 2 ounces and fruit to 1 whole medium pear at lunch, or add 2 tablespoons raisins for an afternoon snack, or add ¾ ounce low-fat crackers to evening snack (see page 176 for suggestions).

# DAY 16

## 1,500-Calorie Meal Plan

| | |
|---|---|
| 5 meat | 4 fruit |
| 5 bread | 3 fat |
| 3 vegetable | 2 milk |

200 open calories

BREAKFAST
½ grapefruit
1½ cups iron-fortified cold flake cereal
1 cup milk
coffee or tea (optional)

LUNCH
1 sandwich with
    2 ounces lean ham
    2 slices whole-grain toast
    1 sliced tomato and lettuce leaves
    1 tablespoon reduced-calorie mayonnaise
½ small pear
1 cup milk

SNACK
2 tablespoons raisins
noncaloric beverage

DINNER
1 serving Lettuce with Warm Sweet-Sour Sauce, page 231
3 ounces broiled fish
½ cup Seasoned Wild Rice, page 278*
½ cup steamed carrots
1 teaspoon margarine or oil (for fish or carrots)
noncaloric beverage

    *Prepare extra for tomorrow's luncheon salad, Chilled Wild Rice with Shrimp. To save time tomorrow, prepare salad this evening and chill.

SNACK
1¼ cup strawberries
noncaloric beverage

*Open calorie suggestions:*

And 2 Peanut Butter Cookies, page 296, at lunch and add 1 cup milk at dinner.

# D A Y   16

## 1,800-Calorie Meal Plan

| | |
|---|---|
| 6 meat | 4 fruit |
| 6 bread | 4 fat |
| 4 vegetable | 2 milk |

300 open calories

BREAKFAST
½ grapefruit
1½ cups iron-fortified cold flake cereal
1 cup milk
coffee or tea (optional)

LUNCH
1 sandwich with
    2 ounces lean ham
    2 slices whole-grain toast
    sliced tomato and lettuce leaves
    1 tablespoon reduced-calorie mayonnaise
1 cup jicama and green pepper strips
½ small pear
1 cup milk

SNACK
2 tablespoons raisins
noncaloric beverage

DINNER
1 serving Lettuce with Warm Sweet-Sour Sauce, page 231
4 ounces broiled fish
1 cup Seasoned Wild Rice, page 278*
½ cup steamed carrots
½ tablespoon margarine or oil (for fish or carrots)
noncaloric beverage

*Prepare extra for tomorrow's luncheon salad, Chilled Wild Rice with Shrimp. To save time tomorrow, prepare salad this evening and chill.

SNACK
1¼ cups strawberries
noncaloric beverage

*Open calorie suggestions:*

Add 2 Peanut Butter Cookies, page 296 anytime, and add ½ cup milk and ¼ cup granola to raisins for afternoon snack.

## DAY 17

**ALL PROGRAMS** eight to ten minutes of warm-ups and cool-downs, including stretching exercises in Appendix B.

### WALKING

BLUE: 1.4 miles in 27 minutes (3.0 mph) for 108 calories.
GREEN: 1.6 miles in 31 minutes (3.0 mph) for 121 calories.
YELLOW: 2.0 miles in 40 minutes (3.0 mph) for 159 calories.
ORANGE: 2.3 miles in 39 minutes (3.5 mph) for 183 calories.
RED: 2.4 miles in 36 minutes (4.0 mph) for 210 calories.

### LIFECYCLE

PURPLE: level 1 for 12 minutes for 83 calories.
BLUE: level 2 for 15 minutes (12 + 3) for 108 calories.
GREEN: level 4 for 15 minutes (12 + 3) for 121 calories.
YELLOW: level 6 for 18 minutes (12 + 6) for 159 calories.
ORANGE: level 8 for 18 minutes (12 + 6) for 183 calories.
RED: level 10 for 18 minutes (12 + 6) for 210 calories.

### LIFESTEP

PURPLE: level 1 for 18 minutes for 73 calories.
BLUE: level 1 for 24 minutes (18 + 6) for 93 calories.
GREEN: level 3 for 18 minutes for 112 calories.
YELLOW: level 4 for 24 minutes (18 + 6) for 163 calories.
ORANGE: level 5 for 24 minutes for 176 calories.
RED: level 7 for 24 minutes for 204 calories.

**LIFECIRCUIT.** Take a break.

**GENERIC/HOME STRENGTH TRAINING.** Take a break.

**EXERCISE EXCHANGE.** Choose one exchange today.

## DAY 17

# 1,200-Calorie Meal Plan

| | |
|---|---|
| 4 meat | 3 fruit |
| 4 bread | 3 fat |
| 3 vegetable | 2 milk |

80 open calories

BREAKFAST
¾ cups cold oat bran cereal
2 tablespoons raisins
1 cup milk
coffee or tea (optional)

LUNCH
½ cup cherry tomatoes with 1 tablespoon reduced-calorie salad
     dressing
1 serving Chilled Wild Rice with Shrimp, page 229
1 small apple, sliced
noncaloric beverage

DINNER
1 Vegetarian Omelette, page 307
1 serving Vegetable Medley with Honeyed Potatoes, page 281
1 cup fresh mixed strawberries, grapes, orange, and melon
noncaloric beverage

SNACK
½ cup nonfat fruited yogurt with 2 tablespoons granola
noncaloric beverage

*Open calorie suggestions:*

Increase cereal at breakfast to 1½ cups, or add 1 cup milk to dinner,
or add 1½ ounces lean ham to omelette at dinner.

# DAY 17

## 1,500-Calorie Meal Plan

| | |
|---|---|
| 5 meat | 4 fruit |
| 5 bread | 3 fat |
| 3 vegetable | 2 milk |

200 open calories

BREAKFAST
1½ cups cold oat bran cereal
2 tablespoons raisins
1 cup milk
coffee or tea (optional)

LUNCH
½ cup cherry tomatoes with 1 tablespoon reduced-calorie salad
    dressing
1 serving Chilled Wild Rice with Shrimp, page 229
1 small apple, sliced
noncaloric beverage

SNACK
1 cup honeydew melon
noncaloric beverage

DINNER
1 Omelette with 1 ounce lean ham or Canadian bacon, page 307
1 serving Vegetable Medley with Honeyed Potatoes, page 281
1 cup fresh mixed strawberries, grapes, orange, and melon
noncaloric beverage

SNACK
½ cup nonfat fruited yogurt with 2 tablespoons granola
noncaloric beverage

*Open calorie suggestions:*

Add 1 slice garlic bread (with 1 teaspoon margarine) and 1 cup milk
to dinner, or 2 Peanut Butter Cookies, page 296, to lunch and 1 cup
milk to dinner.

## D A Y  17

# 1,800-Calorie Meal Plan

6 meat                    4 fruit
6 bread                   4 fat
4 vegetable               2 milk
300 open calories

BREAKFAST
1½ cups cold oat bran cereal
2 tablespoons raisins
1 cup milk
noncaloric beverage

LUNCH
½ cup cherry tomatoes with 1 tablespoon reduced-calorie salad
    dressing
1 serving Chilled Wild Rice with Shrimp, page 229
1 small apple, sliced
noncaloric beverage

SNACK
1 cup honeydew melon
noncaloric beverage

DINNER
1 cup garden salad with seasoned vinegar
1 Omelette with 2 ounces lean ham or Canadian bacon, page 307
1 serving Vegetable Medley with Honeyed Potatoes, page 281
1 slice garlic bread with one teaspoon margarine
1 cup mixed fresh strawberries, grapes, orange, and melon
noncaloric beverage

SNACK
½ cup nonfat fruited yogurt with 2 tablespoons granola
noncaloric beverage

*Open calorie suggestions*

Increase Chilled Wild Rice with Shrimp to 1½ servings at lunch, add
¾ ounce low-fat crackers or pretzels to afternoon snack, and add 1
cup milk to dinner.

## DAY 18

**ALL PROGRAMS** eight to ten minutes of warm-ups and cool-downs, including stretching exercises in Appendix B.

### WALKING

BLUE: One day off.
GREEN: 1.6 miles in 31 minutes (3.0 mph) for 121 calories.
YELLOW: 2.0 miles in 40 minutes (3.0 mph) for 159 calories.
ORANGE: 2.3 miles in 39 minutes (3.5 mph) for 183 calories.
RED: 2.4 miles in 36 minutes (4.0 mph) for 210 calories.

### LIFECYCLE

PURPLE: One day off.
BLUE: One day off.
GREEN: level 4 for 15 minutes (12 + 3) for 121 calories.
YELLOW: level 6 for 18 minutes (12 + 6) for 159 calories.
ORANGE: level 8 for 18 minutes (12 + 6) for 183 calories.
RED: level 10 for 18 minutes (12 + 6) for 210 calories.

### LIFESTEP

PURPLE: Day off.
BLUE: Day off.
GREEN: level 3 for 18 minutes for 112 calories.
YELLOW: level 4 for 24 minutes (18 + 6) for 163 calories.
ORANGE: level 5 for 24 minutes for 176 calories.
RED: level 7 for 24 minutes for 204 calories.

**LIFECIRCUIT.** All colors take the day off.

**GENERIC/HOME STRENGTH TRAINING.** All colors take the day off.

**EXERCISE EXCHANGE.** Purple and Blue choose two exchanges. All other colors choose one.

# D A Y   18

## 1,200-Calorie Meal Plan

| | |
|---|---|
| 4 meat | 3 fruit |
| 4 bread | 3 fat |
| 3 vegetable | 2 milk |

80 open calories

BREAKFAST
1 cup honeydew melon
1 (1-ounce) bran muffin
1 cup nonfat plain yogurt
coffee or tea (optional)

LUNCH
½ 6-inch bread filled with
    1 ounce shredded low-fat cheese
    shredded lettuce
    tomato and onion slices
    grated carrot or radish
    1 tablespoon reduced-calorie mayonnaise
15 grapes
noncaloric beverage

DINNER
1 serving Lemon Chicken, page 238
⅓ cup rice
1 cup steamed broccoli and cauliflower
1 teaspoon margarine
noncaloric beverage

SNACK
1 serving sugar-free shake mix (Alba) with
    ⅓ banana blended in

*Open calorie suggestions:*

Increase pita to 1 whole pita bread at lunch, or increase cheese to 2
ounces and grapes to 22 at lunch, or increase rice to ⅔ cup at dinner,
or add 3 cups plain popcorn as a snack.

# D A Y   18

## 1,500-Calorie Meal Plan

5 meat          4 fruit
5 bread         3 fat
3 vegetable      2 milk

200 open calories

**BREAKFAST**
1 cup honeydew melon
1 (1-ounce) bran muffin
1 cup nonfat plain yogurt
coffee or tea (optional)

**LUNCH**
1 6-inch pita bread filled with
    2 ounces shredded low-fat cheese
    shredded lettuce
    tomato and onion slices
    grated carrot or radish
    1 tablespoon reduced-calorie mayonnaise
15 grapes
noncaloric beverage

**SNACK**
4 apricots or 1 cup papaya
noncaloric beverage

**DINNER**
1 serving Lemon Chicken, page 238
⅓ cup rice
1 cup steamed broccoli and cauliflower
1 teaspoon margarine
noncaloric beverage

**SNACK**
1 serving sugar-free shake mix (Alba) with
    ⅓ banana blended in

*Open calorie suggestions:*

Increase bran muffin at breakfast to 2 ounces and increase rice at dinner to ⅔ cup.

## DAY 18

### 1,800-Calorie Meal Plan

| | |
|---|---|
| 6 meat | 4 fruit |
| 6 bread | 4 fat |
| 4 vegetable | 2 milk |

300 open calories

BREAKFAST
1 cup honeydew melon
1 (1-ounce) bran muffin
1 cup nonfat plain yogurt
coffee or tea (optional)

LUNCH
1 6-inch bread filled with
    2 ounces shredded Swiss and/or jack cheese
    1 ounce turkey
    shredded lettuce
    tomato and onion slices
    grated carrot or radish
    1 tablespoon reduced-calorie mayonnaise
15 grapes
noncaloric beverage

SNACK
4 apricots or 1 cup papaya
noncaloric beverage

DINNER
1 sliced tomato with 1 teaspoon olive oil
1 serving Lemon Chicken, page 238
⅔ cup rice
1 cup steamed broccoli and cauliflower
1 teaspoon margarine
noncaloric beverage

SNACK
1 serving sugar-free shake mix (Alba) with
    ⅓ banana blended in

*Open calorie suggestions:*

Increase bran muffin at breakfast to 2 ounces, add 1 cup milk to dinner, and add ¾ ounce low-fat crackers for a snack.

## DAY 19

**ALL PROGRAMS** eight to ten minutes of warm-ups and cool-downs, including stretching exercises in Appendix B.

### WALKING

BLUE: 1.4 miles in 27 minutes (3.0 mph) for 108 calories.
GREEN: 1.6 miles in 31 minutes (3.0 mph) for 121 calories.
YELLOW: 2.0 miles in 40 minutes (3.0 mph) for 159 calories.
ORANGE: 2.3 miles in 39 minutes (3.5 mph) for 183 calories.
RED: 2.4 miles in 36 minutes (4.0 mph) for 210 calories.

### LIFECYCLE

PURPLE: level 1 for 12 minutes for 83 calories.
BLUE: level 2 for 15 minutes (12 + 3) for 108 calories.
GREEN: level 4 for 15 minutes (12 + 3) for 121 calories.
YELLOW: level 6 for 18 minutes (12 + 6) for 159 calories.
ORANGE: level 8 for 18 minutes (12 + 6) for 183 calories.
RED: level 10 for 18 minutes (12 + 6) for 210 calories.

### LIFESTEP

PURPLE: level 1 for 18 minutes for 73 calories.
BLUE: level 1 for 24 minutes (18 + 6) for 98 calories.
GREEN: level 3 for 18 minutes for 112 calories.
YELLOW: level 4 for 24 minutes (18 + 6) for 163 calories.
ORANGE: level 5 for 24 minutes for 176 calories.
RED: level 7 for 24 minutes for 204 calories.

### LIFECIRCUIT

BLUE: 1 set of 12 repetitions.
GREEN: 1 set of 12 repetitions.
YELLOW: 2 sets of 12 repetitions.

ORANGE: 2 sets of 12 repetitions.
RED: 3 sets of 12 repetitions.

## GENERIC/HOME STRENGTH TRAINING

BLUE: 1 set of 8 to 10 repetitions.
GREEN: 2 sets of 10 repetitions.
YELLOW: 2 sets of 12 repetitions.
ORANGE: 3 sets of 10 repetitions.
RED: 3 sets of 12 repetitions.

**EXERCISE EXCHANGE.** All colors choose one exchange.

# D A Y   19

## 1,200-Calorie Meal Plan

| | |
|---|---|
| 4 meat | 3 fruit |
| 4 bread | 3 fat |
| 3 vegetable | 2 milk |

80 open calories

BREAKFAST
½ cup oatmeal or oat bran with
    7 dried apricot halves, chopped
1 cup milk
coffee or tea (optional)

LUNCH
1 sandwich with
    1½ ounces chicken
    2 slices whole-wheat bread
    1 tomato, sliced
    lettuce leaves and mustard
1 orange
noncaloric beverage

DINNER
2 cups spinach salad with
    1 tablespoon slivered almonds
    2 tablespoons reduced-calorie herb vinaigrette dressing
2½ ounces seasoned pork tenderloin

¾ cup winter squash
1 teaspoon margarine or olive oil (for pork or squash)
noncaloric beverage

SNACK
1 cup sliced strawberries topped with ½ cup low-fat frozen yogurt
noncaloric beverage

*Open calorie suggestions:*

Increase oatmeal to 1 cup at breakfast, or add 1 cup milk to lunch, or add ½ cup potato or pasta to dinner, or increase frozen yogurt to 1 cup for evening snack.

## DAY 19

### 1,500-Calorie Meal Plan

| | |
|---|---|
| 5 meat | 4 fruit |
| 5 bread | 3 fat |
| 3 vegetable | 2 milk |

200 open calories

BREAKFAST
1 cup oatmeal or oat bran with
    1½ dried figs, chopped
1 cup milk
coffee or tea (optional)

LUNCH
1 sandwich with
    2 ounces chicken
    2 slices whole-wheat bread
    1 tomato, sliced
    lettuce leaves and mustard
1 orange
noncaloric beverage

SNACK
⅓ cantaloupe, sliced
noncaloric beverage

<u>DINNER</u>
2 cups spinach salad with
    1 tablespoon slivered almonds
    2 tablespoons reduced-calorie herb vinaigrette dressing
3 ounces seasoned pork tenderloin
¾ cup winter squash
1 teaspoon margarine or olive oil (for pork or squash)
noncaloric beverage

<u>SNACK</u>
1 cup sliced strawberries topped with ½ cup low-fat frozen yogurt
noncaloric beverage

*Open calorie suggestions:*

Add 1 cup milk and 1 cup assorted raw vegetables to lunch, and add
½ cup pasta to dinner.

## DAY 19

# 1,800-Calorie Meal Plan

| | |
|---|---|
| 6 meat | 4 fruit |
| 6 bread | 4 fat |
| 4 vegetable | 2 milk |

300 open calories

<u>BREAKFAST</u>
1 cup oatmeal or oat bran with
    1½ dried figs, chopped
1 cup milk
coffee or tea (optional)

<u>LUNCH</u>
1 cup assorted raw vegetables
1 sandwich with
    2 ounces chicken
    2 slices whole-wheat bread
    1 tomato, sliced
    lettuce leaves and mustard
1 tablespoon reduced-calorie mayonnaise
1 orange
noncaloric beverage

SNACK
⅓ cantaloupe, sliced
noncaloric beverage

DINNER
2 cups spinach salad with
    1 tablespoon slivered almonds
    2 tablespoons reduced-calorie herb vinaigrette dressing
4 ounces seasoned pork tenderloin
½ cup pasta
¾ cup winter squash
1 teaspoon margarine or olive oil (for pork, pasta, or squash)
noncaloric beverage

SNACK
1 cup sliced strawberries topped with ½ cup low-fat frozen yogurt
noncaloric beverage

*Open calorie suggestions:*

Add 1 cup milk to lunch, add 1 teaspoon margarine and 1 small glass
wine to dinner, and increase frozen yogurt to 1 cup at evening snack.

# DAY 20

**ALL PROGRAMS** eight to ten minutes of warm-ups and cool-downs,
including stretching exercises in Appendix B.

**WALKING.** Day off.

**LIFECYCLE.** Day off.

**LIFESTEP.** Day off.

**LIFECIRCUIT.** Day off.

**GENERIC/HOME STRENGTH TRAINING.** Day off.

**EXERCISE EXCHANGE.** All colors choose two exchanges. How about a
seasonal activity such as cross-country skiing or canoeing?

## DAY 20

## 1,200-Calorie Meal Plan

| | |
|---|---|
| 4 meat | 3 fruit |
| 4 bread | 3 fat |
| 3 vegetable | 2 milk |

80 open calories

---

BREAKFAST
½ cup orange juice
1 hard-cooked or poached egg
1 slice whole-wheat toast
1 cup milk
coffee or tea (optional)

LUNCH
1 cup low-fat fruited yogurt
1 (1-ounce) roll or 4 Ry-Krisp crackers
1 cup carrot and celery sticks
noncaloric beverage

DINNER
seafood salad with
    4½ ounces tuna or 6 ounces shrimp, crab, or lobster
    3 cups mixed vegetables and salad greens
    2 tablespoons reduced-calorie dressing, or vinegar and
        1 teaspoon oil
1 (1-ounce) whole-wheat roll
½ teaspoon margarine
noncaloric beverage

SNACK
3 cups plain popcorn
1 teaspoon margarine
noncaloric beverage

Open calorie suggestions:

Add 1 slice toast to breakfast, or increase orange juice to 1¼ cups at breakfast, or add 1 medium apple for a snack, or add 1 small glass wine at dinner.

# DAY 20

## 1,500-Calorie Meal Plan

| | |
|---|---|
| 5 meat | 4 fruit |
| 5 bread | 3 fat |
| 3 vegetable | 2 milk |

200 open calories

BREAKFAST
½ cup orange juice
1 English muffin
1 teaspoon margarine
1 cup milk
coffee or tea (optional)

LUNCH
2 ounces sliced turkey
½ cup potato, mashed or boiled
½ cup steamed vegetable
1 cup honeydew or watermelon cubes
1 cup milk
noncaloric beverage

SNACK
½ cup apple juice or cider

DINNER
seafood salad with
    4½ ounces tuna or 6 ounces shrimp, crab, or lobster
    3 cups mixed vegetables and salad greens
    2 tablespoons reduced-calorie dressing, or vinegar and 1
        teaspoon oil
1 (1-ounce) whole-wheat roll
noncaloric beverage
fresh fruit slices

SNACK
3 cups plain popcorn
1 teaspoon margarine
noncaloric beverage

*Open calorie suggestions:*

Add 1 tablespoon jelly to breakfast, increase orange juice to ¾ cup at breakfast, add 1 teaspoon margarine to lunch or dinner, and add ¾ ounce low-fat cookies to afternoon snack.

---

## D A Y  20

## 1,800-Calorie Meal Plan

| | |
|---|---|
| 6 meat | 4 fruit |
| 6 bread | 4 fat |
| 4 vegetable | 2 milk |

300 open calories

---

BREAKFAST
½ cup orange juice
1 English muffin
1 teaspoon margarine
1 cup milk
coffee or tea (optional)

LUNCH
1 cup carrot and celery sticks
3 ounces sliced turkey
½ cup potato, mashed or boiled
½ cup steamed vegetable
1 teaspoon margarine
1 cup honeydew or watermelon cubes
1 cup milk
noncaloric beverage

SNACK
½ cup apple juice or cider
¾ ounce low-fat cookies

DINNER
seafood salad with
    4½ ounces tuna or 6 ounces shrimp, crab, or lobster
    3 cups mixed vegetables and salad greens
    2 tablespoons reduced-calorie dressing, or vinegar and 1
        teaspoon oil
1 (1-ounce) whole-wheat roll

noncaloric beverage
fresh fruit slices

SNACK
3 cups plain popcorn
1 teaspoon margarine
noncaloric beverage

*Open calorie suggestions:*

Add 1 tablespoon jelly and increase orange juice to 1 cup at breakfast,
add 1 teaspoon margarine to dinner, and add ½ cup (1 scoop) ice
cream to lunch or dinner.

# DAY 21

**ALL PROGRAMS** eight to ten minutes of warm-ups and cool-downs,
including stretching exercises in Appendix B.

## WALKING

BLUE: 1.4 miles in 27 minutes (3.0 mph) for 108 calories.
GREEN: 1.6 miles in 31 minutes (3.0 mph) for 121 calories.
YELLOW: 2.0 miles in 40 minutes (3.0 mph) for 159 calories.
ORANGE: 2.3 miles in 39 minutes (3.5 mph) for 183 calories.
RED: 2.4 miles in 36 minutes (4.0 mph) for 210 calories.

## LIFECYCLE

PURPLE: level 1 for 12 minutes for 83 calories.
BLUE: level 2 for 15 minutes (12 + 3) for 108 calories
GREEN: level 4 for 15 minutes (12 + 3) for 121 calories.
YELLOW: level 6 for 18 minutes (12 + 6) for 159 calories.
ORANGE: level 8 for 18 minutes (12 + 6) for 183 calories.
RED: level 10 for 18 minutes (12 + 6) for 210 calories.

## LIFESTEP

PURPLE: level 1 for 18 minutes for 73 calories.
BLUE: level 1 for 24 minutes (18 + 6) for 98 calories.
GREEN: level 3 for 18 minutes for 112 calories.

YELLOW: level 4 for 24 minutes (18 + 6) for 163 calories.
ORANGE: level 5 for 24 minutes for 176 calories.
RED: level 7 for 24 minutes for 204 calories.

**LIFECIRCUIT.** All colors off.

**GENERIC/HOME STRENGTH TRAINING.** All colors off.

**EXERCISE EXCHANGE.** All colors choose one exchange today.

---

## D A Y   21

---

## 1,200-Calorie Meal Plan

| | |
|---|---|
| 4 meat | 3 fruit |
| 4 bread | 3 fat |
| 3 vegetable | 2 milk |
| 80 open calories | |

---

BREAKFAST
¾ cup bran flakes
½ banana
1 cup milk
coffee or tea (optional)

LUNCH
¼ cup low-fat cottage cheese on salad greens
1 (1-ounce) bran muffin
1 cup raw vegetables
1 cup cantaloupe
noncaloric beverage

DINNER
2 cups garden salad with 2 tablespoons low-calorie dressing (free
    food, see page 186)
1 Italian-Style Turkey Burger on lettuce leaves, page 256, with
    sliced tomato and onion
15 french fries
1 cup milk

SNACK
1 cup mixed fresh fruit
noncaloric beverage

*Open calorie suggestions:*

Add 1 slice toast at breakfast, or increase cottage cheese to ½ cup and
add ½ tablespoon cream cheese to muffin at lunch, or add ½ cup
nonfat frozen yogurt or ¾ ounce low-fat crackers for a snack (see page
176 for suggestions).

---

# D A Y  21

## 1,500-Calorie Meal Plan

| | |
|---|---|
| 5 meat | 4 fruit |
| 5 bread | 3 fat |
| 3 vegetable | 2 milk |

200 open calories

---

BREAKFAST
¾ cup bran flakes
½ banana
1 cup milk
coffee or tea (optional)

LUNCH
½ cup low-fat cottage cheese on salad greens
1 (1-ounce) bran muffin
1 cup raw vegetables
1 cup cantaloupe
noncaloric beverage

SNACK
1 peach
noncaloric beverage

DINNER
2 cups garden salad with 2 tablespoons low-calorie dressing (free
    food, see page 186)
1 open-faced Italian-Style Turkey Burger, page 256, with
    1 slice toasted Italian or sourdough bread
    sliced tomato and onion

15 french fries
1 cup milk

<u>SNACK</u>
1 cup mixed fresh fruit
noncaloric beverage

*Open calorie suggestions:*

Add 1 slice toast and ½ tablespoon jelly to breakfast, add ½ tablespoon cream cheese or 1 tablespoon low-cal dressing to lunch, and
add 1 slice toasted bread for burger at dinner.

## DAY  21

### 1,800-Calorie Meal Plan

| | |
|---|---|
| 6 meat | 4 fruit |
| 6 bread | 4 fat |
| 4 vegetable | 2 milk |

300 open calories

<u>BREAKFAST</u>
1 hard-cooked egg
1½ cups bran flakes
½ banana
1 cup milk
coffee or tea (optional)

<u>LUNCH</u>
½ cup low-fat cottage cheese on salad greens
1 (1-ounce) bran muffin
1 cup raw vegetables
1 cup cantaloupe
noncaloric beverage

<u>SNACK</u>
1 peach
noncaloric beverage

<u>DINNER</u>
2 cups garden salad with 2 tablespoons reduced-calorie dressing
1 open-face Italian-Style Turkey Burger, page 256, with
    1 slice toasted Italian or sourdough bread
    sliced tomato and onion

½ cup green beans
15 french fries
1 cup milk

SNACK
1 cup mixed fresh fruit
noncaloric beverage

*Open calorie suggestions:*

Increase muffin to 2 ounces and add 1 tablespoon cream cheese at
lunch, add 1 slice toasted bread for burger at dinner, and add ¼ cup
low-fat fruited yogurt to mixed fruit at evening snack.

---

# DAY 22

---

**ALL PROGRAMS** eight to ten minutes of warm-ups and cool-downs,
including stretching exercises in Appendix B.

## WALKING

BLUE: 1.4 miles in 27 minutes (3.0 mph) for 108 calories.
GREEN: 1.6 miles in 31 minutes (3.0 mph) for 121 calories.
YELLOW: 2.0 miles in 40 minutes (3.0 mph) for 159 calories.
ORANGE: 2.3 miles in 39 minutes (3.5 mph) for 183 calories.
RED: 2.4 miles in 36 minutes (4.0 mph) for 210 calories.

## LIFECYCLE

PURPLE: level 1 for 12 minutes for 83 calories.
BLUE: level 2 for 15 minutes (12 + 3) for 108 calories.
GREEN: level 4 for 15 minutes (12 + 3) for 121 calories.
YELLOW: level 6 for 18 minutes (12 + 6) for 159 calories.
ORANGE: level 8 for 18 minutes (12 + 6) for 183 calories.
RED: level 10 for 18 minutes (12 + 6) for 210 calories.

## LIFESTEP

PURPLE: level 1 for 18 minutes for 73 calories.
BLUE: level 1 for 24 minutes (18 + 6) for 98 calories.

GREEN: level 3 for 18 minutes for 112 calories.
YELLOW: level 4 for 24 minutes (18 + 6) for 163 calories.
ORANGE: level 5 for 24 minutes for 176 calories.
RED: level 7 for 24 minutes for 204 calories.

**LIFECIRCUIT** All colors take a rest.

**GENERIC/HOME STRENGTH TRAINING.** All colors take a rest.

**EXERCISE EXCHANGE.** All colors choose one exchange.

## D A Y   22

# 1,200-Calorie Meal Plan

| | |
|---|---|
| 4 meat | 3 fruit |
| 4 bread | 3 fat |
| 3 vegetable | 2 milk |
| 80 open calories | |

BREAKFAST
1 orange
½ cup shredded wheat
1 cup milk
coffee or tea (optional)

LUNCH
1 sandwich with
    1 small serving Tuna Salad, page 224
    2 slices whole-grain bread
    lettuce leaves
1 peach
1 cup milk

DINNER
1 cup salad greens with cherry tomatoes and flavored vinegar
2 ounces lean beef strips sautéed in 1 teaspoon olive oil on
    ½ cup fettuccine
½ cup zucchini and mushrooms mixed
1 teaspoon margarine

1 cup raspberries or 1 large kiwi, sliced
noncaloric beverage

SNACK
20 small peanuts
noncaloric beverage

*Open calorie suggestions:*

Increase shredded wheat to 1 cup at breakfast, or increase fettuccine
to 1 cup at dinner, or increase beef to 3 ounces at dinner and add 1
cup raw vegetables for a snack.

# D A Y   22

## 1,500-Calorie Meal Plan

| 5 meat | 4 fruit |
| --- | --- |
| 5 bread | 3 fat |
| 3 vegetable | 2 milk |

**200 open calories**

BREAKFAST
1 orange
1 cup shredded wheat
1 cup milk
coffee or tea (optional)

LUNCH
1 sandwich with
    1 small serving Tuna Salad, page 224
    2 slices whole-grain bread
    lettuce leaves
1 peach
1 cup milk

SNACK
1 small pear
noncaloric beverage

DINNER
1 cup salad greens with cherry tomatoes and flavored vinegar

3 ounces lean beef strips sautéed in 1 teaspoon olive oil on
  ½ cup fettuccine
½ cup zucchini and mushrooms mixed
1 teaspoon margarine
1 cup raspberries or 1 large kiwi, sliced
noncaloric beverage

SNACK
20 small peanuts
noncaloric beverage

*Open calorie suggestions:*

Increase afternoon snack to 1 medium pear, increase fettuccine at
dinner to 1 cup, and add ½ cup low-fat frozen yogurt to any meal or
snack.

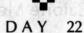

## D A Y  22

# 1,800-Calorie Meal Plan

| 6 meat | 4 fruit |
|--------|---------|
| 6 bread | 4 fat |
| 4 vegetable | 2 milk |

300 open calories

BREAKFAST
1 orange
1 cup shredded wheat
1 cup milk
coffee or tea (optional)

LUNCH
1 sandwich with
  1 large serving Tuna Salad, page 224
  2 slices whole-grain bread
  lettuce leaves
1 peach
1 cup milk

SNACK
1 small pear
noncaloric beverage

DINNER
1 cup salad greens with cherry tomatoes and flavored vinegar
3 ounces lean beef strips sautéed in 2 teaspoons olive oil on
    1 cup fettucine
¾ cup zucchini and mushrooms mixed
1 teaspoon margarine
1 cup raspberries or 1 large kiwi, sliced
noncaloric beverage

SNACK
20 small peanuts
noncaloric beverage

*Open calorie suggestions:*

Add ½ cup apple juice or cider for morning snack, increase afternoon snack to 1 large pear, and add 1 cup low-fat frozen yogurt to dinner or evening snack.

# DAY 23

ALL PROGRAMS eight to ten minutes of warm-ups and cool-downs, including stretching exercises in Appendix B.

WALKING. All colors take the day off.

LIFECYCLE. All colors take the day off.

LIFESTEP. All colors take the day off.

### LIFECIRCUIT

BLUE: 1 set of 12 repetitions.
GREEN: 1 set of 12 repetitions.
YELLOW: 2 sets of 12 repretitions.
ORANGE: 2 sets of 12 repetitions.
RED: 3 sets of 12 repetitions.

### GENERIC/HOME STRENGTH TRAINING

BLUE: 1 set of 8 to 10 repetitions.

GREEN: 2 sets of 10 repetitions.
YELLOW: 2 sets of 12 repetitions.
ORANGE: 3 sets of 10 repetitions.
RED: 3 sets of 12 repetitions.

**EXERCISE EXCHANGE.** All colors choose two exchanges. Is there an exchange category in Chapter 5 that you haven't tried yet?

## DAY 23

### 1,200-Calorie Meal Plan

| | |
|---|---|
| 4 meat | 3 fruit |
| 4 bread | 3 fat |
| 3 vegetable | 2 milk |

80 open calories

BREAKFAST
½ cup vegetable juice
1 slice whole-wheat toast
1 teaspoon margarine
2 plums
coffee or tea (optional)

LUNCH
1 cup plain low-fat yogurt with
    4 fresh sliced or ½ cup water-packed canned apricots
1 (1-ounce) muffin
noncaloric beverage

DINNER
2 cups garden salad with fresh lemon or seasoned rice vinegar
1 serving Really Easy Salmon Steaks, page 247
3 ounces boiled potato with parsley
½ cup asparagus
lemon wedges
1 teaspoon margarine
1 cup milk

SNACK
2 rice cakes
½ cup orange juice

*Open calorie suggestions:*

Increase toast at breakfast to 2 slices, or add 1 cup milk at breakfast, or increase potato to 6 ounces at dinner, or increase rice cakes to 3 and orange juice to ¾ cup for evening snack.

# D A Y   23

## 1,500-Calorie Meal Plan

| 5 meat | 4 fruit |
|---|---|
| 5 bread | 3 fat |
| 3 vegetable | 2 milk |

200 open calories

**BREAKFAST**
½ cup vegetable juice
2 slices whole-wheat toast
1 teaspoon margarine
2 plums
coffee or tea (optional)

**LUNCH**
1 cup plain low-fat yogurt with
    4 fresh sliced or ½ cup water-packed canned apricots
1 (1-ounce) muffin
noncaloric beverage

**SNACK**
1 cup cantaloupe cubes
noncaloric beverage

**DINNER**
2 cups garden salad with seasoned rice vinegar
1 serving Really Easy Salmon Steaks, page 247
3 ounces boiled potato with parsley
½ cup asparagus
1 teaspoon margarine
fresh lemon wedges
1 cup milk

**SNACK**
1 ounce low-fat soft cheese (such as low-cal Laughing Cow cheese)

2 rice cakes
½ cup orange juice

*Open calorie suggestions:*

Add ½ tablespoon jelly to breakfast, increase muffin to 2 ounces at lunch, and increase potato to 5 ounces at dinner.

---

# DAY 23

## 1,800-Calorie Meal Plan

| | |
|---|---|
| 6 meat | 4 fruit |
| 6 bread | 4 fat |
| 4 vegetable | 2 milk |

300 open calories

---

BREAKFAST
½ cup vegetable juice
1 ounce Canadian bacon
2 slices whole-wheat toast
1 teaspoon margarine
2 plums
coffee or tea (optional)

LUNCH
1 cup jicama and carrot strips
1 cup plain low-fat yogurt with
    4 fresh sliced or ½ cup water-packed canned apricots
1 (2-ounce) muffin
noncaloric beverage

SNACK
1 cup cantaloupe cubes
noncaloric beverage

DINNER
2 cups garden salad with seasoned rice vinegar
1 serving Really Easy Salmon Steaks, page 247
3 ounces boiled potato with parsley
½ cup asparagus
1 teaspoon margarine
fresh lemon wedges
1 cup milk

SNACK
1 ounce low-fat soft cheese (such as low-cal Laughing Cow cheese)
2 rice cakes
½ cup orange juice

*Open calorie suggestions:*

Add 1 tablespoon jelly to breakfast, add ⅓ cup low-fat cottage cheese
to cantaloupe at afternoon snack, and increase potato to 8 ounces and
margarine to 2 teaspoons at dinner.

# DAY 24

**ALL PROGRAMS** eight to ten minutes of warm-ups and cool-downs,
including stretching exercises in Appendix B.

## WALKING

BLUE: 1.4 miles in 27 minutes (3.0 mph) for 108 calories.
GREEN: 1.6 miles in 31 minutes (3.0 mph) for 121 calories.
YELLOW: 2.0 miles in 40 minutes (3.0 mph) for 159 calories.
ORANGE: 2.3 miles in 39 minutes (3.5 mph) for 183 calories.
RED: 2.4 miles in 36 minutes (4.0 mph) for 210 calories.

## LIFECYCLE

PURPLE: level 1 for 12 minutes for 83 calories.
BLUE: level 2 for 15 minutes (12 + 3) for 108 calories.
GREEN: level 4 for 15 minutes (12 + 3) for 121 calories.
YELLOW: level 6 for 18 minutes (12 + 6) for 159 calories
ORANGE: level 8 for 18 minutes (12 + 6) for 183 calories.
RED: level 10 for 18 minutes (12 + 6) for 210 calories.

## LIFESTEP

PURPLE: level 1 for 18 minutes for 73 calories.
BLUE: level 1 for 24 minutes (18 + 6) for 98 calories.
GREEN: level 3 for 18 minutes for 112 calories.
YELLOW: level 4 for 24 minutes for (18 + 6) for 163 calories.
ORANGE: level 5 for 24 minutes for 176 calories.
RED: level 7 for 24 minutes for 204 calories.

**LIFECIRCUIT.** Go ahead. Take a day off!

**GENERIC/HOME STRENGTH TRAINING.** Take the day off as well.

**EXERCISE EXCHANGE.** One exchange today for everyone.

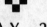

## D A Y   24

## 1,200-Calorie Meal Plan

| 4 meat | 3 fruit |
|---|---|
| 4 bread | 3 fat |
| 3 vegetable | 2 milk |

80 open calories

BREAKFAST
¾ cup iron-fortified cold flake cereal
½ grapefruit
1 cup milk
coffee or tea (optional)

LUNCH
1 6-inch pita bread filled with
    2 ounces shredded low-fat Cheddar cheese
    shredded lettuce and tomato slices
    grated green pepper
    1 tablespoon reduced-calorie mayonnaise
1¼ cups watermelon or 2 tangerines
noncaloric beverage

DINNER
1 serving Tofu-Vegetable Medley, page 270
⅓ cup rice
noncaloric beverage

SNACK
½ cup low-fat frozen yogurt
noncaloric beverage

*Open calorie suggestions:*

Add 1 slice toast at breakfast, or add 1 cup milk at dinner, or increase rice at dinner to ⅔ cup, or increase frozen yogurt to 1 cup in evening snack.

## D A Y   24

### 1,500-Calorie Meal Plan

| | |
|---|---|
| 5 meat | 4 fruit |
| 5 bread | 3 fat |
| 3 vegetable | 2 milk |

**200 open calories**

BREAKFAST
¾ cup iron-fortified cold flake cereal with
    1 tablespoon slivered almonds
½ grapefruit
1 cup milk
coffee or tea (optional)

LUNCH
1 Italian-style pita, heated, with
    1 ounce Canadian bacon or lean ham
    2 ounces shredded mozzarella or similar type cheese
    1 6-inch pita bread
    chopped tomato, onion, and green pepper
1¼ cup watermelon or 2 tangerines
noncaloric beverage

SNACK
1 small pear
noncaloric beverage

DINNER
1 serving Tofu-Vegetable Medley, page 270
⅔ cup rice
noncaloric beverage

SNACK
½ cup low-fat frozen yogurt
noncaloric beverage

*Open calorie suggestions:*

Add 1 cup milk to dinner and 2 Peanut Butter Cookies, page 296, to dinner or any snack.

## D A Y   24

### 1,800-Calorie Meal Plan

| | |
|---|---|
| 6 meat | 4 fruit |
| 6 bread | 4 fat |
| 4 vegetable | 2 milk |

300 open calories

BREAKFAST
1½ cups iron-fortified cold flake cereal with
    1 tablespoon slivered almonds
½ grapefruit
1 cup milk
coffee or tea (optional)

LUNCH
1 Italian-style pita, heated, with
    1 ounce Canadian bacon or lean ham
    2 ounces shredded mozzarella or similar type cheese
    1 6-inch pita bread
    chopped tomato, onion, and green pepper
    3 olives, sliced
1¼ cups watermelon or 2 tangerines
noncaloric beverage

SNACK
1 small pear
noncaloric beverage

DINNER
1½ servings Tofu-Vegetable Medley, page 270
⅔ cup rice
noncaloric beverage

SNACK
½ cup low-fat frozen yogurt
noncaloric beverage

*Open calorie suggestions:*

Add 1 cup milk and increase rice to 1 cup at dinner, and add 2 Peanut
Butter Cookies, page 296, to dinner or any snack.

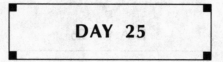

# DAY 25

**ALL PROGRAMS** eight to ten minutes of warm-ups and cool-downs, including stretching exercises in Appendix B.

## WALKING

BLUE: One day off.
GREEN: 1.6 miles in 31 minutes (3.0 mph) for 121 calories.
YELLOW: 2.0 miles in 40 minutes (3.0 mph) for 159 calories.
ORANGE: 2.3 miles in 39 minutes (3.5 mph) for 183 calories.
RED: 2.4 miles in 36 minutes (4.0 mph) for 210 calories.

## LIFECYCLE

PURPLE: One day off.
BLUE: One day off.
GREEN: level 4 for 15 minutes (12 + 3) for 121 calories.
YELLOW: level 6 for 18 minutes (12 + 6) for 159 calories.
ORANGE: level 8 for 18 minutes (12 + 6) for 183 calories.
RED: level 10 for 18 minutes (12 + 6) for 210 calories.

## LIFESTEP

PURPLE: One day off.
BLUE: One day off.
GREEN: level 3 for 18 minutes for 112 calories.
YELLOW: level 4 for 24 minutes (18 + 6) for 163 calories.
ORANGE: level 5 for 24 minutes for 176 calories.
RED: level 7 for 24 minutes for 204 calories.

**LIFECIRCUIT.** All colors take the day off.

**GENERIC/HOME STRENGTH TRAINING.** All colors take the day off.

**EXERCISE EXCHANGE.** Purple and Blue do two exchanges. Why not try some racquetball? Other colors need do only one exchange. Maybe shoot a little pool?

# D A Y   25

## 1,200-Calorie Meal Plan

4 meat                    3 fruit
4 bread                   3 fat
3 vegetable            2 milk
80 open calories

BREAKFAST
2 tablespoons raisins
¾ cup cold oat bran cereal
1 cup milk
coffee or tea (optional)

LUNCH
2 cups mixed vegetable salad with
    1 hard-cooked egg, sliced
    2 tablespoons reduced-calorie salad dressing
3 slices melba toast
1 small apple
noncaloric beverage

DINNER
1 serving Almond Snow Pea Salad, page 232
3 ounces roasted or broiled skinless chicken
1 small baked potato (3 ounces)
1 cup milk

SNACK
1 small pear
noncaloric beverage

*Open calorie suggestions:*

Add 1½ ounces chicken or lean ham to salad at lunch, or increase potato to 6 ounces at dinner, or add ¾ ounce low-fat (less than 30 percent) cookies for a snack.

# DAY 25

## 1,500-Calorie Meal Plan

| | |
|---|---|
| 5 meat | 4 fruit |
| 5 bread | 3 fat |
| 3 vegetable | 2 milk |

200 open calories

BREAKFAST
2 tablespoons raisins
1 cup cold oat bran cereal
1 cup milk
coffee or tea (optional)

LUNCH
2 cups mixed vegetable salad with
    1 hard-cooked egg, sliced
    1 ounce chicken
    2 tablespoons reduced-calorie salad dressing
5 slices melba toast
1 small apple
noncaloric beverage

SNACK
1 peach
noncaloric beverage

DINNER
1 serving Almond Snow Pea Salad, page 232
3 ounces roasted or broiled skinless chicken
1 (4-ounce) baked potato
1 cup milk

SNACK
1 small pear
noncaloric beverage

*Open calorie suggestions:*

Add 1 cup vegetable soup and 1 teaspoon margarine to dinner, and add ½ cup sugar-free pudding or fudge bar to dinner or snack.

# D A Y   25

## 1,800-Calorie Meal Plan

| | |
|---|---|
| 6 meat | 4 fruit |
| 6 bread | 4 fat |
| 4 vegetable | 2 milk |

300 open calories

BREAKFAST
2 tablespoons raisins
1½ cups cold oat bran cereal
1 cup milk
coffee or tea (optional)

LUNCH
2 cups mixed vegetable salad with
    1 hard-cooked egg, sliced
    1 ounce chicken
    2 tablespoons reduced-calorie salad dressing
1 ounce low-fat whole grain crackers
1 small apple
noncaloric beverage

SNACK
1 peach
noncaloric beverage

DINNER
1 serving Almond Snow Pea Salad, page 232
4 ounces roasted or broiled skinless chicken
1 (4-ounce) baked potato
½ cup Brussels sprouts or spinach or other greens
1 teaspoon margarine
1 cup milk

SNACK
1 small sliced pear
noncaloric beverage

*Open calorie suggestions:*

Increase apple at lunch to 1 large, add ¾ ounce low-fat crackers to afternoon snack, and add ¼ cup granola and ½ cup plain low-fat yogurt to sliced pear for evening snack.

# DAY 26

ALL PROGRAMS eight to ten minutes of warm-ups and cool-downs, including stretching exercises in Appendix B.

## WALKING

BLUE: 1.4 miles in 27 minutes (3.0 mph) for 108 calories.
GREEN: 1.6 miles in 31 minutes (3.0 mph) for 121 calories.
YELLOW: 2.0 miles in 40 minutes (3.0 mph) for 159 calories.
ORANGE: 2.3 miles in 39 minutes (3.5 mph) for 183 calories.
RED: 2.4 miles in 36 minutes (4.0 mph) for 210 calories.

## LIFECYCLE

PURPLE: level 1 for 12 minutes for 83 calories.
BLUE: level 2 for 15 minutes (12 + 3) for 108 calories.
GREEN: level 4 for 15 minutes (12 + 3) for 121 calories.
YELLOW: level 6 for 18 minutes (12 + 6) for 159 calories.
ORANGE: level 8 for 18 minutes (12 + 6) for 183 calories.
RED: level 10 for 18 minutes (12 + 6) for 210 calories.

## LIFESTEP

PURPLE: level 1 for 18 minutes for 73 calories.
BLUE: level 1 for 24 minutes (18 + 6) for 98 calories.
GREEN: level 3 for 18 minutes for 112 calories.
YELLOW: level 4 for 24 minutes (18 + 6) for 163 calories.
ORANGE: level 5 for 24 minutes for 178 calories.
RED: level 7 for 24 minutes for 204 calories.

## LIFECIRCUIT

BLUE: 1 set of 12 repetitions.
GREEN: 1 set of 12 repetitions.
YELLOW: 2 sets of 12 repretitions.
ORANGE: 2 sets of 12 repetitions.
RED: 3 sets of 12 repetitions.

## GENERIC/HOME STRENGTH TRAINING

BLUE: 1 set of 8 to 10 repetitions.

GREEN: 2 sets of 10 repetitions.
YELLOW: 2 sets of 12 repetitions.
ORANGE: 3 sets of 10 repetitions.
RED: 3 sets of 12 repetitions.

**EXERCISE EXCHANGE.** All colors do one exchange.

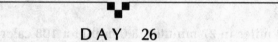

## D A Y  26

### 1,200-Calorie Meal Plan

| | |
|---|---|
| 4 meat | 3 fruit |
| 4 bread | 3 fat |
| 3 vegetable | 2 milk |

80 open calories

BREAKFAST
1 tablespoon peanut butter
1 (1-ounce) bagel
1 small banana, sliced
1 cup milk
coffee or tea (optional)

LUNCH
1 cup plain nonfat yogurt with
    1 cup sliced strawberries
1 ounce whole-wheat crackers
1 cup carrot sticks
noncaloric beverage

DINNER
2 cups garden salad with 2 tablespoons low-calorie dressing (free
    food, see page 186)
1 serving Marinated Skewered Shark, page 243
⅓ cup brown rice
noncaloric beverage

SNACK
3 cups plain popcorn
1 teaspoon margarine
noncaloric beverage

*Open calorie suggestions:*

Increase bagel at breakfast to 2 ounces, or increase brown rice at dinner to ⅔ cup, or add medium apple for a snack.

# D A Y   26

## 1,500-Calorie Meal Plain

| | |
|---|---|
| 5 meat | 4 fruit |
| 5 bread | 3 fat |
| 3 vegetable | 2 milk |

200 open calories

BREAKFAST
2 tablespoons peanut butter
1 (2-ounce) bagel
1 small banana, sliced
1 cup milk
coffee or tea (optional)

LUNCH
1 cup plain nonfat yogurt with
    1 cup sliced strawberries
¾ ounce low-fat, whole-wheat crackers
1 cup carrot sticks
noncaloric beverage

SNACK
1¼ cups watermelon or 2 tangerines
noncaloric beverage

DINNER
2 cups garden salad with 2 tablespoons low-calorie dressing (free
    food, see page 186)
1 serving Marinated Skewered Shark, page 243
⅓ cup brown rice
noncaloric beverage

SNACK
3 cups plain popcorn
1 teaspoon margarine
noncaloric beverage

*Open calorie suggestions:*

Increase crackers at lunch to 2 ounces and increase brown rice at dinner to ⅔ cup.

## DAY 26

## 1,800-Calorie Meal Plan

| | |
|---|---|
| 6 meat | 4 fruit |
| 6 bread | 4 fat |
| 4 vegetable | 2 milk |

300 open calories

### BREAKFAST
2 tablespoons peanut butter
1 (2-ounce) bagel
1 small banana, sliced
1 cup milk
coffee or tea (optional)

### LUNCH
1 cup plain nonfat yogurt with 1 cup sliced strawberries
¾ ounce low-fat, whole-wheat crackers
1 cup carrot sticks
noncaloric beverage

### SNACK
1 ounce Cheddar cheese
1¼ cups watermelon or 2 tangerines
noncaloric beverage

### DINNER
2 cups garden salad with 2 tablespoons low-calorie dressing (free food, see page 186)
1 serving Marinated Skewered Shark, page 243, on shredded cabbage
⅔ cup brown rice
noncaloric beverage

### SNACK
3 cups plain popcorn
1 teaspoon margarine
noncaloric beverage

*Open calorie suggestions:*

Increase crackers at lunch to 2 ounces, increase brown rice at dinner to 1 cup, and increase popcorn to 5 cups and margarine to 2 teaspoons at evening snack.

# DAY 27

**ALL PROGRAMS** eight to ten minutes of warm-ups and cool-downs, including stretching exercises in Appendix B.

**WALKING.** A day off.

**LIFECYCLE.** A day off.

**LIFESTEP.** A day off.

**LIFECIRCUIT.** A day off.

**GENERIC/HOME STRENGTH TRAINING.** A day off here, too.

**EXERCISE EXCHANGE.** All colors choose two exchanges. Why not try a new recreational sport?

## DAY 27

### 1,200-Calorie Meal Plan

| | |
|---|---|
| 4 meat | 3 fruit |
| 4 bread | 3 fat |
| 3 vegetable | 2 milk |

80 open calories

BREAKFAST
1 cup cantaloupe cubes
1 (1-ounce) bran muffin
1 cup milk
coffee or tea (optional)

LUNCH
½ sandwich with
    1 ounce chicken
    1 slice whole-wheat bread
    tomato and onion slices
    lettuce leaves
1 cup nonfat plain yogurt with 1 cup raspberries
noncaloric beverage

DINNER
1 serving Broiled Lamb Chops with Mint Dressing, page 262
2 to 4 small new potatoes (3 ounces), boiled or broiled
⅔ cup peas and carrots
1 teaspoon margarine
noncaloric beverage

SNACK
1 small apple
noncaloric beverage

Open calorie suggestions:

Increase potatoes at dinner to 6 ounces, or add ½ cup sugar-free
pudding at dinner for dessert, or add snack of ¾ ounce pretzels, or
have a large apple for evening snack.

## D A Y   27

## 1,500-Calorie Meal Plan

| 5 meat | 4 fruit |
| --- | --- |
| 5 bread | 3 fat |
| 3 vegetable | 2 milk |

200 open calories

BREAKFAST
1 cup cantaloupe cubes
1 (1-ounce) bran muffin
1 cup milk
coffee or tea (optional)

LUNCH
1 sandwich with
    2 ounces chicken
    2 slices whole-wheat bread
    tomato and onion slices
    lettuce leaves
1 cup nonfat plain yogurt with 1 cup raspberries
noncaloric beverage

SNACK
1 peach or 2 plums
noncaloric beverage

DINNER
1 serving Broiled Lamb Chops with Mint Dressing, page 262
2 to 4 small new potatoes (3 ounces), boiled or broiled
⅔ cup peas and carrots
1 teaspoon margarine
noncaloric beverage

SNACK
1 small apple
noncaloric beverage

*Open calorie suggestions:*

Increase bran muffin at breakfast to 2 ounces, and add ¾ ounce
pretzels to evening snack.

## D A Y  27

### 1,800-Calorie Meal Plan

| | |
|---|---|
| 6 meat | 4 fruit |
| 6 bread | 4 fat |
| 4 vegetable | 2 milk |

300 open calories

BREAKFAST
1 cup cantaloupe cubes
1 (2-ounce) bran muffin with
    1 ounce low-fat soft cheese (such as low-cal Laughing Cow
      cheese)
1 cup milk
coffee or tea (optional)

LUNCH
1 sandwich with
    2 ounces chicken
    2 slices whole-wheat bread
    tomato and onion slices
    lettuce leaves
1 cup nonfat plain yogurt with 1 cup raspberries
noncaloric beverage

SNACK
1 peach or 2 plums
noncaloric beverage

DINNER
1 serving Broiled Lamb Chops with Mint Dressing, page 262
2 to 4 small new potatoes (3 ounces), boiled or broiled
⅔ cup peas and carrots
1 teaspoon margarine
noncaloric beverage

SNACK
1 small apple, sliced
1 cup celery sticks
noncaloric beverage

*Open calorie suggestions:*

Add 1 ounce low-fat crackers to afternoon snack, 1 cup milk to
dinner, and 1 tablespoon peanut butter to evening snack.

# DAY 28

**ALL PROGRAMS** eight to ten minutes of warm-ups and cool-downs, including stretching exercises in Appendix B.

## WALKING

BLUE: 1.4 miles in 27 minutes (3.0 mph) for 108 calories.
GREEN: 1.6 miles in 31 minutes (3.0 mph) for 121 calories.
YELLOW: 2.0 miles in 40 minutes (3.0 mph) for 159 calories.
ORANGE: 2.3 miles in 39 minutes (3.5 mph) for 183 calories.
RED: 2.4 miles in 36 minutes (4.0 mph) for 210 calories.

## LIFECYCLE

PURPLE: level 1 for 12 minutes for 83 calories.
BLUE: level 2 for 15 minutes (12 + 3) for 108 calories.
GREEN: level 4 for 15 minutes (12 + 3) for 121 calories.
YELLOW: level 6 for 18 minutes (12 + 6) for 159 calories.
ORANGE: level 8 for 18 minutes (12 + 6) for 183 calories.
RED: level 10 for 18 minutes (12 + 6) for 210 calories.

## LIFESTEP

PURPLE: level 1 for 18 minutes for 73 calories.
BLUE: level 1 for 24 minutes (18 + 6) for 98 calories.
GREEN: level 3 for 18 minutes for 112 calories.
YELLOW: level 4 for 24 minutes (18 + 6) for 163 calories.
ORANGE: level 5 for 24 minutes for 178 calories.
RED: level 7 for 24 minutes for 204 calories.

**LIFECIRCUIT.** A day off.

**GENERIC/HOME STRENGTH TRAINING.** Another day off.

**EXERCISE EXCHANGE.** All you need is just one exchange today. Pick something fun. Take along a friend.

## DAY 28

### 1,200-Calorie Meal Plan

| | |
|---|---|
| 4 meat | 3 fruit |
| 4 bread | 3 fat |
| 3 vegetable | 2 milk |

80 open calories

BREAKFAST
½ grapefruit
1 slice whole-grain toast
1 teaspoon margarine
1 cup milk

LUNCH
grilled open-face small hamburger (or ½ of commercial ⅓-pound
hamburger) with 2 ounces ground beef and
    ½ hamburger bun
    fresh tomato and onion slices
    lettuce leaves
fresh fruit slices
noncaloric beverage

DINNER
garden salad with fresh lemon or seasoned vinegar
soft-shell chicken tacos with
    2 ounces cooked chicken
    2 6-inch corn tortillas
    shredded lettuce
    tomato slices
    2 tablespoons sour cream or guacamole
    fresh salsa
noncaloric beverage

SNACK
1 cup berries with ½ cup nonfat frozen yogurt
noncaloric beverage

*Open calorie suggestions:*

Add 1 slice toast at breakfast, *or* add ½ hamburger bun at lunch, *or*
add ½ ounce tortilla chips at dinner, *or* add 1 medium pear for a
snack.

# DAY 28

## 1,500-Calorie Meal Plan

| | |
|---|---|
| 5 meat | 4 fruit |
| 5 bread | 3 fat |
| 3 vegetable | 2 milk |

200 open calories

BREAKFAST
½ grapefruit
2 slices whole-grain toast
1 teaspoon margarine
1 cup milk

LUNCH
grilled open-face, small hamburger (or ½ of a commercial ⅓-pound hamburger) with 2 ounces ground beef and
    ½ hamburger bun
    fresh tomato and onion slices
    lettuce leaves
fresh fruit slices
noncaloric beverage

SNACK
1 cup fresh mixed fruit
noncaloric beverage

DINNER
garden salad with fresh lemon or seasoned vinegar
soft-shell chicken tacos with
    3 ounces cooked chicken
    2 6-inch corn tortillas
    shredded lettuce and tomato slices
    2 tablespoons sour cream or guacamole
    fresh salsa
noncaloric beverage

SNACK
1 cup berries with ½ cup nonfat frozen yogurt
noncaloric beverage

*Open calorie suggestions:*

Add ½ tablespoon jelly at breakfast, ½ cup coleslaw at lunch, and 1 small glass wine or ½ ounce tortilla chips at dinner.

## DAY 28

### 1,800-Calorie Meal Plan

| | |
|---|---|
| 6 meat | 4 fruit |
| 6 bread | 4 fat |
| 4 vegetable | 2 milk |

300 open calories

BREAKFAST
½ cup vegetable juice
½ grapefruit
2 slices whole-grain toast
½ tablespoon (1 pat) margarine
1 cup milk

LUNCH
grilled small hamburger of 3 ounces ground beef
    1 hamburger bun
    fresh tomato and onion slices
    lettuce leaves
fresh fruit slices
noncaloric beverage

SNACK
1 cup fresh mixed fruit
noncaloric beverage

DINNER
garden salad with fresh lemon or seasoned vinegar
soft-shell chicken tacos with
    3 ounces cooked chicken
    2 6-inch corn tortillas
    shredded lettuce and tomato slices
    2 tablespoons sour cream or guacamole
    fresh salsa
noncaloric beverage

SNACK
1 cup berries with ½ cup nonfat frozen yogurt
noncaloric beverage

*Open calorie suggestions:*

Add ½ cup coleslaw at lunch and 1½ ounces tortilla chips at dinner.

## DAY 29

ALL PROGRAMS eight to ten minutes of warm-ups and cool-downs, including stretching exercises in Appendix B.

### WALKING

BLUE: 1.4 miles in 26 minutes (3.25 mph) for 113 calories.
GREEN: 1.6 miles in 28 minutes (3.5 mph) for 131 calories.
YELLOW: 2.0 miles in 37 minutes (3.25 mph) for 159 calories.
ORANGE: 2.2 miles in 35 minutes (3.75 mph) for 183 calories.
RED: 2.2 miles in 29 minutes (4.5 mph) for 210 calories.

### LIFECYCLE

PURPLE: level 1 for 15 minutes (12 + 3) for 104 calories.
BLUE: level 3 for 15 minutes (12 + 3) for 113 calories.
GREEN: level 5 for 16 minutes (12 + 4) for 131 calories.
YELLOW: level 6 for 18 minutes for 159 calories.
ORANGE: level 8 for 18 minutes for 183 calories.
RED: level 10 for 18 minutes for 210 calories.

### LIFESTEP

PURPLE: level 1 for 24 minutes (18 + 6) for 98 calories.
BLUE: level 2 for 18 minutes for 101 calories.
GREEN: level 3 for 24 minutes (18 + 6) for 149 calories.
YELLOW: level 4 for 24 minutes for 163 calories.
ORANGE: level 6 for 24 minutes for 189 calories.
RED: level 8 for 24 minutes for 222 calories.

LIFECIRCUIT. A day of rest for all colors.

GENERIC/HOME STRENGTH TRAINING. A day of rest for all colors.

EXERCISE EXCHANGE. All of you do one exchange today.

## D A Y   29

## 1,200-Calorie Meal Plan

| | |
|---|---|
| 4 meat | 3 fruit |
| 4 bread | 3 fat |
| 3 vegetable | 2 milk |

80 open calories

<u>BREAKFAST</u>
1 serving sugar-free shake mix (Alba) with
    ½ banana blended in
coffee or tea (optional)

<u>LUNCH</u>
1 cup Fruit Spritzer with ½ cup orange juice, page 309
1 serving Eggplant Frittata, page 252
1 Sun-Kissed Muffin, page 290
½ cup fresh melon salad
noncaloric beverage

<u>DINNER</u>
2 cups mixed green salad with 2 tablespoons reduced-calorie
    dressing
1 serving Scallop Pesto Capellini, page 250
noncaloric beverage

<u>SNACK</u>
3 vanilla wafers
1 cup milk

*Open calorie suggestions:*

Have ¾ cup cold flake cereal with a cup milk and ½ banana instead
of sugar-free shake mix at breakfast, or add 1 (1-ounce) slice bread at
dinner, or add 1 small glass wine at lunch or dinner, or omit wafers
and add 1 Sun-Kissed Muffin to evening snack.

## DAY 29

# 1,500-Calorie Meal Plan

| | |
|---|---|
| 5 meat | 4 fruit |
| 5 bread | 3 fat |
| 3 vegetable | 2 milk |

200 open calories

BREAKFAST
¾ cup cold flake cereal with
    ½ banana, sliced
1 cup milk
coffee or tea (optional)

LUNCH
1 cup Fruit Spritzer with ½ cup orange juice, page 309
1 serving Eggplant Frittata, page 252
1 ounce low-fat soft cheese on
    1 Sun-Kissed Muffin, page 290
½ cup fresh melon salad
noncaloric beverage

DINNER
2 cups mixed green salad with 2 tablespoons reduced-calorie
    dressing
1 serving Scallop Pesto Capellini, page 250
1 cup berries
noncaloric beverage

SNACK
3 vanilla wafers
1 cup milk

*Open calorie suggestions:*

Add 1 slice Cheese Bread, page 309, to dinner, or add 1 small glass
wine to lunch or dinner and 1 (1-ounce) slice bread and 1 teaspoon
margarine to dinner.

## DAY 29

## 1,800-Calorie Meal Plan

| | |
|---|---|
| 6 meat | 4 fruit |
| 6 bread | 4 fat |
| 4 vegetable | 2 milk |

300 open calories

BREAKFAST
¾ cup cold flake cereal with
    ½ banana, sliced
1 cup milk
coffee or tea (optional)

LUNCH
1 cup Fruit Spritzer with ½ cup orange juice, page 309
1 serving Eggplant Frittata, page 252
1 ounce low-fat soft cheese on
    1 Sun-Kissed Muffin, page 290
½ cup fresh melon salad
noncaloric beverage

DINNER
2 cups mixed green salad with 2 tablespoons reduced-calorie
    dressing
1 serving Scallop Pesto Capellini, page 250
½ cup green beans
1 slice Cheese Bread, page 309
1 cup berries
noncaloric beverage

SNACK
3 vanilla wafers
1 cup milk

*Open calorie suggestions:*

Increase cereal to 1½ cups at breakfast, increase muffin at lunch to 2,
and add 1 small glass wine to lunch or dinner.

# DAY 30

**ALL PROGRAMS** eight to ten minutes of warm-ups and cool-downs including stretching exercises in Appendix B.

**WALKING.** All colors take a well-deserved break.

**LIFECYCLE.** All colors take a well-deserved break.

### LIFECIRCUIT

BLUE: 1 set of 12 repetitions.
GREEN: 2 sets of 12 repetitions.
YELLOW: 2 sets of 12 repetitions.
ORANGE: 3 sets of 12 repetitions.
RED: 3 sets of 12 repetitions.

### GENERIC/HOME STRENGTH TRAINING

BLUE: 1 set of 10 repetitions.
GREEN: 2 sets of 10 repetitions.
YELLOW: 2 sets of 12 repetitions.
ORANGE: 3 sets of 10 repetitions.
RED: 3 sets of 12 repetitions.

**EXERCISE EXCHANGE.** All colors pick two challenging exchanges.

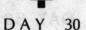

## D A Y   30

# 1,200-Calorie Meal Plan

| | |
|---|---|
| 4 meat | 3 fruit |
| 4 bread | 3 fat |
| 3 vegetable | 2 milk |

80 open calories

BREAKFAST
½ cup shredded wheat
2 fresh or 1½ dried figs, sliced
1 cup milk
coffee or tea (optional)

LUNCH
2 cups garden salad with
    2 ounces lean ham
    2 tablespoons reduced-calorie salad dressing
3 slices melba toast
1 orange, sliced
noncaloric beverage

DINNER
1 cup assorted raw vegetables
1 serving Blue Buffalo Calzone, page 255
2 plums
noncaloric beverage

SNACK
½ cup low-fat frozen yogurt
noncaloric beverage

*Open calorie suggestions:*

Increase cereal to 1 cup or add 1 slice toast at breakfast, or omit melba toast and add 1 (1-ounce) roll and 1 teaspoon margarine at lunch, or increase frozen yogurt in evening snack to 1 cup.

# DAY 30

## 1,500-Calorie Meal Plan

| | |
|---|---|
| 5 meat | 4 fruit |
| 5 bread | 3 fat |
| 3 vegetable | 2 milk |

200 open calories

BREAKFAST
1 cup shredded wheat
2 fresh or 1½ dried figs, sliced
1 cup milk
coffee or tea (optional)

LUNCH
2 cups garden salad with
    3 ounces lean ham
    2 tablespoons reduced-calorie salad dressing
3 slices melba toast
1 orange, sliced
noncaloric beverage

SNACK
2 plums
noncaloric beverage

DINNER
1 cup assorted raw vegetables
1 serving Blue Buffalo Calzone, page 255
1 orange, sliced
noncaloric beverage

SNACK
½ cup low-fat frozen yogurt
noncaloric beverage

*Open Calorie Suggestions:*

Omit melba toast and add 1 (1-ounce) roll and 1 teaspoon margarine to lunch, add 1 cup milk to lunch or dinner, and increase frozen yogurt in evening snack to ⅔ cup.

## D A Y   30

# 1,800-Calorie Meal Plan

| | |
|---|---|
| 6 meat | 4 fruit |
| 6 bread | 4 fat |
| 4 vegetable | 2 milk |

300 open calories

<u>BREAKFAST</u>
1¼ cups shredded wheat
2 fresh or 1½ dried figs, sliced
1 cup milk
coffee or tea (optional)

<u>LUNCH</u>
2 cups garden salad with
    3 ounces lean ham
    2 tablespoons reduced-calorie salad dressing
1 (1-ounce) roll
1 teaspoon margarine
1 orange, sliced
noncaloric beverage

<u>SNACK</u>
2 plums
noncaloric beverage

<u>DINNER</u>
1 serving Tomato Salad, page 308
1 serving Blue Buffalo Calzone, page 255
½ cup steamed zucchini
1 orange, sliced
noncaloric beverage

<u>SNACK</u>
½ cup low-fat frozen yogurt
noncaloric beverage

*Open calorie suggestions:*

Add ½ cup juice at breakfast, add ½ sandwich, with 1 slice bread, 1
ounce chicken, lettuce, and mustard to afternoon snack, and increase
frozen yogurt in evening snack to 1 cup.

# 4

# THE TWENTY-WEEK PROGRAM

Time and commitment. You'll need both to succeed with this program.

If you've ever tried to change a habit and failed, chances are you didn't stick with your new way long enough. Research in my laboratory and others has shown that it takes a good six months to lock in a new habit, especially if that habit is a departure for you, as exercise and low-fat eating are for many people.

That's why, in this chapter, we have provided twenty-week programs for walking, for the Lifecycle, for the Lifestep, for Lifecircuit strength training, for generic strength training using other types of equipment, and for home strength training.

All you do from now on is continue what you began with the Thirty-Day Eating and Exercise Starter Plan.

To eat well, repeat the thirty-day eating plan if you like. Or use the recipes in the recipe section, which begins on page 202, to design your own eating plan.

To exercise well, you'll need to start with the fifth week of your particular program, as you've already completed the first four weeks.

The Twenty-Week Walking Program chart tells you the mileage you need to cover, how fast you need to walk (pace), how long it should take, the number of calories you will burn with each workout, and how many days a week you need to walk.

The Twenty-Week Lifecycle and Lifestep program charts tell you at which level to exercise, the time you need to exercise, the number of calories you will burn with each workout, and how many times each week you need to cycle or stair-step.

The 20-Week Lifecircuit Program chart tells you how many repetitions ("reps") to do with each machine, how many sets (groups of reps) to do, and how many times a week to strength-train.

The Twenty-Week Generic/Home Strength Training Program chart can be used with most other brands of strength training equipment you will find in a health club or recreational facility. You can also use this chart if you've been strength-training at home using the exercises in Appendix F. It gives you the number of reps and sets as well as the number of times per week you need to strength-train.

As you proceed with this program, don't neglect the exercise and food exchanges listed in Chapters 5 and 6. The idea behind them, as we've told you, is to enable you to blend healthful eating and activity into your day. If you allow yourself to be creative, the exchanges will add fun to your program. The more you like your program, the more likely it is that you'll stick with it.

To check your progress, be sure to retake the *Rockport Fitness Walking Test*, the *Lifecycle FIT Test*, or the *Lifestep Electronic FIT Test* at weeks ten and twenty.

At the same time, remeasure the circumferences of your waist, abdomen, buttocks, and midthigh to see how many "inches" you lost, and record all results in Appendix G. I'll bet you'll be thrilled when you see the difference!

If keeping track on a daily basis will motivate you, use the walking log in Appendix C, the Lifecycle log in Appendix D, or the Lifestep log in Appendix E. Strength-training logs can be found in Appendix F.

Best of luck in your journey. And remember, if you hit a snag, turn to Chapter 7 for help.

## Twenty-Week Walking Program*

Completed the Thirty-Day Plan? Start here. →

| Program | Weeks | 1 | 2 | 3-4 | 5-6 | 7-8 | 9-10 | 11-12 | 13-14 | 15-16 | 17-18 | 19-20 | Progression or Maintenance |
|---|---|---|---|---|---|---|---|---|---|---|---|---|---|
| **BLUE** | Pace | 3.0 | 3.0 | 3.0 | 3.25 | 3.5 | 3.5 | 3.75 | 3.75 | 3.75 | 4.0 | 4.0 | Go to Green, week 15 |
| | Minutes | 22.0 | 22.0 | 27.0 | 26.0 | 29.0 | 29.0 | 28.0 | 28.0 | 34.0 | 34.0 | 34.0 | |
| | Mileage | 1.1 | 1.1 | 1.4 | 1.4 | 1.7 | 1.7 | 1.8 | 1.8 | 2.1 | 2.2 | 2.2 | |
| | Calories | 86.0 | 86.0 | 108.0 | 113.0 | 136.0 | 136.0 | 145.0 | 145.0 | 177.0 | 196.0 | 196.0 | |
| | Days/week | 3 | 4 | 4 | 5 | 5 | 5 | 5 | 5 | 5 | 5 | 5 | |
| **GREEN** | Pace | 3.0 | 3.0 | 3.0 | 3.5 | 3.5 | 3.5 | 3.5 | 4.0 | 4.0 | 4.0 | 4.0 | Go to Yellow, week 17, or add hills, light hand weights |
| | Minutes | 25.0 | 25.0 | 31.0 | 28.0 | 31.0 | 31.0 | 34.0 | 27.0 | 33.0 | 39.0 | 39.0 | |
| | Mileage | 1.3 | 1.3 | 1.6 | 1.6 | 1.8 | 1.8 | 2.0 | 1.8 | 2.2 | 2.6 | 2.6 | |
| | Calories | 97.0 | 97.0 | 121.0 | 131.0 | 147.0 | 147.0 | 159.0 | 159.0 | 194.0 | 227.0 | 227.0 | |
| | Days/week | 4 | 4 | 5 | 5 | 5 | 5 | 5 | 5 | 5 | 5 | 5 | |
| **YELLOW** | Pace | 3.0 | 3.0 | 3.0 | 3.25 | 3.5 | 3.5 | 4.0 | 4.0 | 4.0 | 4.5 | 4.5 | Go to Orange, week 19, or add hills, light hand weights |
| | Minutes | 27.0 | 33.0 | 40.0 | 37.0 | 37.0 | 37.0 | 29.0 | 32.0 | 38.0 | 33.0 | 36.0 | |
| | Mileage | 1.4 | 1.7 | 2.0 | 2.0 | 2.1 | 2.1 | 1.9 | 2.1 | 2.5 | 2.5 | 2.7 | |
| | Calories | 106.0 | 132.0 | 159.0 | 159.0 | 171.0 | 171.0 | 171.0 | 183.0 | 223.0 | 240.0 | 262.0 | |
| | Days/week | 4 | 5 | 5 | 5 | 5 | 5 | 5 | 5 | 5 | 5 | 5 | |
| **ORANGE** | Pace | 3.5 | 3.5 | 3.5 | 3.75 | 4.0 | 4.0 | 4.0 | 4.0 | 4.5 | 4.5 | 4.5 | Go to Red, week 19, or add hills, light hand weights |
| | Minutes | 26.0 | 33.0 | 39.0 | 35.0 | 34.0 | 34.0 | 34.0 | 36.0 | 29.0 | 31.0 | 42.0 | |
| | Mileage | 1.5 | 1.9 | 2.3 | 2.2 | 2.2 | 2.2 | 2.2 | 2.4 | 2.2 | 2.3 | 3.1 | |
| | Calories | 122.0 | 152.0 | 183.0 | 183.0 | 197.0 | 197.0 | 197.0 | 210.0 | 210.0 | 224.0 | 298.0 | |
| | Days/week | 5 | 5 | 5 | 5 | 5 | 5 | 5 | 5 | 4-5 | 4-5 | 4-5 | |
| **RED** | Pace | 4.0 | 4.0 | 4.0 | 4.5 | 4.5 | 4.5 | 4.5 | 4.5 | 4.5 | 4.5 | 4.5 | Add hills, light hand weights |
| | Minutes | 24.0 | 30.0 | 36.0 | 29.0 | 31.0 | 31.0 | 31.0 | 21.0 | 31.0 | 32.0 | 43.0 | |
| | Mileage | 1.6 | 2.0 | 2.4 | 2.2 | 2.3 | 2.3 | 2.3 | 2.3 | 2.3 | 2.4 | 3.2 | |
| | Calories | 140.0 | 175.0 | 210.0 | 210.0 | 224.0 | 224.0 | 224.0 | 224.0 | 224.0 | 235.0 | 313.0 | |
| | Days/week | 5 | 5 | 5 | 5 | 5 | 5 | 4-5 | 4-5 | 4-5 | 3-5 | 3-6 | |

*Adapted from James M. Rippe and Ann Ward. "Rockport's Guide to Fitness Walking," p. 221, Dr. James M. Rippe's Complete Book of Fitness Walking (New York: Prentice Hall Press, 1989), p. 25-41.

HEART RATE RANGE, ALL GROUPS: Weeks 1-10, 60-70 percent maximum; weeks 11-20, 70-80 percent maximum caloric expenditure based on 154 pound person. To determine your caloric expenditure, add or subtract 10 percent for every 15 pounds above or below 154 pounds. If you are in between, round to the nearer weight range.

Example: If you weigh 169 lbs. and are beginning the Blue level, multiply 86 calories by 10 percent (86 × .10 = 8.6) and add 8.6 to 86 (86 + 8.6 = 94.6). Your caloric expenditure for weeks 1-2, Blue, would be approximately 95 calories.

## Twenty-Week Lifecycle Program (Hill Profile)*

Completed the Thirty-Day Plan? Start here. →

| Program | Weeks | 1 | 2 | 3–4 | 5–6 | 7–8 | 9–10 | 11–12 | 13–14 | 15–16 | 17–18 | 19–20 | Progression or Maintenance |
|---|---|---|---|---|---|---|---|---|---|---|---|---|---|
| PURPLE | Level | 1 | 1 | 1 | 1 | 2 | 2 | 2 | 2 | 2 | 2 | 3 | Go to Blue, week 15 |
| | Minutes | 4+4+4 | 6+6 | 12 | 12+3 | 12+3 | 12+6 | 18 | 18+3 | 18+6 | 24 | 12+12 | |
| | Calories | 83 | 83 | 83 | 104 | 104 | 129 | 129 | 151 | 173 | 173 | 181 | |
| | Days/week | 3 | 3 | 4 | 4 | 5 | 5 | 5 | 5 | 5 | 5 | 5 | |
| BLUE | Level | 2 | 2 | 2 | 2 | 3 | 3 | 4 | 4 | 4 | 5 | 5 | Go to Green, week 15 |
| | Minutes | 12 | 12 | 12+3 | 12+3 | 12+6 | 18 | 12+6 | 18 | 18+4 | 12+12 | 24 | |
| | Calories | 86 | 86 | 108 | 113 | 136 | 136 | 145 | 145 | 177 | 196 | 196 | |
| | Days/week | 3 | 4 | 4 | 5 | 5 | 5 | 5 | 5 | 5 | 5 | 5 | |
| GREEN | Level | 4 | 4 | 4 | 5 | 5 | 5 | 6 | 6 | 6 | 7 | 7 | Go to Yellow, week 15 |
| | Minutes | 12 | 12 | 12+3 | 12+4 | 12+6 | 18 | 12+6 | 18 | 18+4 | 12+12 | 24 | |
| | Calories | 97 | 97 | 121 | 131 | 147 | 147 | 159 | 159 | 194 | 227 | 227 | |
| | Days/week | 4 | 4 | 5 | 5 | 5 | 5 | 5 | 5 | 5 | 5 | 5 | |
| YELLOW | Level | 6 | 6 | 6 | 6 | 7 | 7 | 7 | 8 | 8 | 9 | 9 | Maintain or go to Orange, week 15 |
| | Minutes | 12 | 12+3 | 12+6 | 18 | 12+6 | 18 | 18 | 12+6 | 18+4 | 18+4 | 18+6 | |
| | Calories | 106 | 132 | 159 | 159 | 171 | 171 | 171 | 183 | 223 | 240 | 262 | |
| | Days/week | 4 | 4 | 5 | 5 | 5 | 5 | 5 | 5 | 5 | 5 | 5 | |
| ORANGE | Level | 8 | 8 | 8 | 8 | 9 | 9 | 9 | 10 | 10 | 11 | 11 | Maintain or go to Red, week 15 |
| | Minutes | 12 | 12+3 | 12+6 | 18 | 12+6 | 18 | 18 | 12+6 | 18 | 18 | 18+6 | |
| | Calories | 122 | 152 | 183 | 183 | 197 | 197 | 197 | 210 | 210 | 224 | 298 | |
| | Days/week | 5 | 5 | 5 | 5 | 5 | 5 | 5 | 5 | 4–5 | 4–5 | 4–5 | |
| RED | Level | 10 | 10 | 10 | 10 | 11 | 11 | 11 | 11 | 12 | 12 | 12 | Maintain or cross-train |
| | Minutes | 12 | 12+3 | 12+6 | 18 | 12+6 | 12+6 | 18 | 18 | 12+6 | 18 | 18+6 | |
| | Calories | 140 | 175 | 210 | 210 | 224 | 224 | 224 | 224 | 235 | 235 | 313 | |
| | Days/week | 5 | 5 | 5 | 5 | 5 | 4–5 | 4–5 | 4–5 | 4–5 | 3–5 | 3–5 | |

*Adapted from Rippe, James, and Ward, Ann, *Starting and Staying with Exercise*, brochure by Life Fitness, Inc., 1989.
HEART RATE RANGE, ALL GROUPS: Weeks 1–10, 60–70 percent maximum; weeks 11–20, 70–80 percent maximum. To determine your caloric expenditure, add or subtract 10 percent for every 15 pounds above or below 154 pounds. If you are in between, round to the nearer weight range. Caloric expenditure based on 154-pound person. Example: if you weigh 169 pounds and are beginning the purple level, multiply 83 calories by 10 percent (83 × .10 = 8.3) and add 8.3 to 83 (83 + 8.3 = 91.3). Your caloric expenditure for weeks 1–4, Purple, and level 1, would be approximately 91 calories.

## Twenty-Week Lifestep Program (Hill Profile)*

Completed the Thirty-Day Plan? Start here. →

| Program | Weeks | 1 | 2 | 3–4 | 5–6 | 7–8 | 9–10 | 11–12 | 13–14 | 15–16 | 17–18 | 19–20 | Progression or Maintenance |
|---|---|---|---|---|---|---|---|---|---|---|---|---|---|
| PURPLE | Level | 1 | 1 | 1 | 1 | 1 | 2 | 2 | 2 | 3 | 3 | 3 | Go to Blue, week 15 |
| | Minutes | 6+6+6 | 12+6 | 18 | 18+6 | 24 | 12+12 | 24 | 24+4 | 24+4 | 24+4 | 18+12 | |
| | Calories | 73 | 73 | 73 | 98 | 98 | 134 | 134 | 157 | 174 | 174 | 186 | |
| | Days/week | 3 | 3 | 4 | 4 | 5 | 5 | 5 | 5 | 5 | 5 | 5 | |
| BLUE | Level | 1 | 1 | 1 | 2 | 2 | 2 | 3 | 3 | 3 | 3 | 4 | Go to Green, week 15 |
| | Minutes | 12+6 | 18 | 18+6 | 18 | 18+6 | 24 | 12+12 | 18+6 | 18+12 | 24+6 | 18+12 | |
| | Calories | 73 | 73 | 98 | 101 | 134 | 134 | 149 | 149 | 186 | 186 | 204 | |
| | Days/week | 3 | 4 | 4 | 5 | 5 | 5 | 5 | 5 | 5 | 5 | 5 | |
| GREEN | Level | 2 | 2 | 3 | 3 | 3 | 4 | 4 | 4 | 5 | 5 | 6 | Go to Yellow, week 15 |
| | Minutes | 12+6 | 18 | 18 | 18+6 | 24 | 12+12 | 18+6 | 24 | 12+12 | 18+12 | 18+12 | |
| | Calories | 101 | 101 | 112 | 149 | 149 | 149 | 163 | 163 | 176 | 220 | 236 | |
| | Days/week | 4 | 4 | 5 | 5 | 5 | 5 | 5 | 5 | 5 | 5 | 5 | |
| YELLOW | Level | 3 | 4 | 4 | 4 | 5 | 5 | 5 | 6 | 7 | 8 | 8 | Maintain or go to Orange, week 15 |
| | Minutes | 12+6 | 18 | 18+6 | 24 | 12+12 | 18+6 | 24 | 12+12 | 12+12 | 12+12 | 18+12 | |
| | Calories | 112 | 122 | 163 | 163 | 176 | 176 | 176 | 189 | 204 | 222 | 278 | |
| | Days/week | 4 | 5 | 5 | 5 | 5 | 5 | 5 | 5 | 5 | 5 | 5 | |
| ORANGE | Level | 4 | 4 | 5 | 6 | 7 | 7 | 8 | 8 | 8 | 9 | 9 | Maintain or go to Red, week 15 |
| | Minutes | 18 | 24 | 24 | 24 | 24 | 24 | 18+4 | 18+6 | 24 | 24 | 18+12 | |
| | Calories | 122 | 163 | 176 | 189 | 204 | 204 | 204 | 222 | 222 | 238 | 298 | |
| | Days/week | 5 | 5 | 5 | 5 | 5 | 5 | 5 | 5 | 5 | 4–5 | 4–5 | |
| RED | Level | 6 | 6 | 7 | 8 | 9 | 10 | 10 | 11 | 11 | 12 | 12 | Maintain or cross-train |
| | Minutes | 18 | 24 | 24 | 24 | 24 | 12+12 | 24 | 12+12 | 24 | 12+12 | 24 | |
| | Calories | 142 | 189 | 204 | 222 | 238 | 254 | 254 | 272 | 272 | 288 | 288 | |
| | Days/week | 5 | 5 | 5 | 5 | 5 | 5 | 4–5 | 4–5 | 4–5 | 3–5 | 3–5 | |

*Adapted from Rippe, James, and Ward, Ann, Starting and Staying with Exercise, brochure by Life Fitness, Inc., 1989. HEART RATE RANGE, ALL GROUPS: Weeks 1–10, 60–70 percent maximum; weeks 11–20, 70–80 percent maximum caloric expenditure based on 154 pound person. To determine your caloric expenditure, add or subtract 10 percent for every 15 pounds -above or below 154 pounds. If you are in between, round to the nearer weight range. Example: if you weigh 169 pounds and are beginning the purple Level, multiply 73 calories by 10 percent (73 x .10 = 7.3) and add 7.3 to 73 (73 + 7.3 = 81.3). Your caloric expenditure for weeks 1–4, Purple, and Level 1, would be approximately 80 calories.

## Twenty-Week Lifecircuit Program*

**Completed the Thirty-Day Plan? Start here.**

| | Week | 1 | 2 | 3–4 | 5–20 | Progression or Maintenance |
|---|---|---|---|---|---|---|
| | **Program** | | | | | |
| **BLUE** | Reps | 12 | 12 | 12 | 12 | |
| | Sets | 1 | 1 | 1 | 1 | Go to Green, week 5 |
| | Days/week | 2 | 2 | 2 | 2 | |
| **GREEN** | Reps | 12 | 12 | 12 | 12 | |
| | Sets | 1 | 1 | 1 | 2 | Go to Orange, week 3 |
| | Days/week | 2 | 2 | 2 | 2 | |
| **YELLOW** | Reps | 12 | 12 | 12 | 12 | |
| | Sets | 1 | 1 | 2 | 2 | Go to Orange, week 5 |
| | Days/week | 2 | 2 | 2 | 2 | |
| **ORANGE** | Reps | 12 | 12 | 12 | 12 | |
| | Sets | 2 | 2 | 2 | 3 | Go to Red, week 5 |
| | Days/week | 2 | 2 | 2 | 2 | |
| **RED** | Reps | 12 | 12 | 12 | 12 | Maintain; add different/more stations; |
| | Sets | 2 | 2–3 | 3 | 3 | try exercising each limb *separately;* try |
| | Days/week | 2 | 2 | 2 | 2 | "regular" mode for variety. |

*Although 1 set of 12 reps of Lifecircuit provides an adequate training stimulus for all fitness levels, some may want to use this equipment in a more standard training fashion. The progression of sets was designed with that in mind.

With Lifecircuit, it is expected that a setup test will be done prior to *each* workout per station, this eliminates the need for 1 RM testing every 2 weeks. Follow instructions as illustrated on the equipment and per your club trainer.

## Twenty-Week Generic/Home Strength Training Program*

**Completed the Thirty-Day Plan? Start here. →** (5-6)

| Program | | Weeks | 1† | 2 | 3-4† | 5-6 | 7-8† | 9-10 | 11-12† | 13-14 | 15-16† | 17-18 | 19-20† | Progression or Maintenance |
|---|---|---|---|---|---|---|---|---|---|---|---|---|---|---|
| BLUE | Reps | | 8-10 | 8-10 | 8-10 | 10 | 10 | 10 | 10 | 10 | 10 | 10 | 10 | Go to Green, Week 9 |
| | Sets | | 1 | 1 | 2 | 1 | 1 | 1 | 1 | 1 | 1 | 1 | 1 | |
| | Days/week | | 2 | 2 | 2 | 2 | 2 | 2 | 2 | 2 | 2 | 2 | 2 | |
| GREEN | Reps | | 10 | 10 | 10 | 10 | 10 | 10 | 10 | 10 | 10 | 10 | 10 | Go to Yellow, Week 9 |
| | Sets | | 1 | 1 | 2 | 2 | 2 | 2 | 2 | 2 | 2 | 2 | 2 | |
| | Days/week | | 2 | 2 | 2 | 2 | 2 | 2 | 2 | 2 | 2 | 2 | 2 | |
| YELLOW | Reps | | 12 | 12 | 12 | 12 | 12 | 12 | 12 | 12 | 12 | 12 | 12 | Go to Orange, Week 9 |
| | Sets | | 1 | 1 | 2 | 2 | 2 | 2 | 2 | 2 | 2 | 2 | 2 | |
| | Days/week | | 2 | 2 | 2 | 2 | 2 | 2 | 2 | 2 | 2 | 2 | 2 | |
| ORANGE | Reps | | 10 | 10 | 10 | 10 | 10 | 10 | 10 | 10 | 10 | 10 | 10 | Go to Red, Week 9 |
| | Sets | | 3 | 3 | 3 | 3 | 3 | 3 | 3 | 3 | 3 | 3 | 3 | |
| | Days/week | | 2 | 2 | 2 | 2 | 2 | 2 | 2 | 2 | 2 | 2 | 2 | |
| RED | Reps | | 12 | 12 | 12 | 12 | 12 | 12 | 12 | 12 | 12 | 12 | 12 | Add more Weight Stations; Try new Equipment |
| | Sets | | 3 | 3 | 3 | 3 | 3 | 3 | 3 | 3 | 3 | 3 | 3 | |
| | Days/week | | 2 | 2 | 2 | 2 | 2 | 2 | 2 | 2 | 2 | 2 | 2 | |

*For use on other strength training equipment if Lifecircuit is not available.
†Time for a 1 RM test to evaluate your progress; ask a staff member at your health club for assistance.

# 5

# THE EXERCISE EXCHANGES

Activity. That, in a word, is the key to *The Exercise Exchange Program*. If you can stay active, you'll have won half the battle. The 200 calories or more that you burn per workout add up to pounds *lost* when you're consistent. And the lean muscle you maintain through exercise will keep your metabolism humming.

But if you stop, those unburned calories and the muscle you lose can—and will—add up to pounds *gained*. And feelings of discouragement.

How important is activity, *really*? Let's say you exercise six times a week and burn 200 calories with each workout. If you were to stop, and your diet remained the same, you could, theoretically *regain* eighteen pounds or more in a year's time, *even if you were eating properly*. And that's not even taking into account the mental benefits you'd sacrifice by stopping your activity.

Exercise gives you a feeling of accomplishment, of moving forward. It reduces stress and improves your mood. And that kind of ammunition is so essential to making changes in your life—especially one as challenging as weight loss.

Those positive feelings, as far as I'm concerned, are just too precious to give up.

# CATEGORY 1: OUTDOOR WORK*

### 1 AEROBIC EXCHANGE
(100 Calories)

| Activity | Minutes of Activity Needed | |
| --- | --- | --- |
| | Women | Men |
| Car | | |
| Repairing | 28 | 24 |
| Wash and wax (by hand) | 29 | 25 |
| Chopping wood | 16 | 13 |
| Construction (general) | 21 | 18 |
| Gardening | | |
| Digging | 14 | 11 |
| Hedging | 22 | 19 |
| Planting | 16 | 13 |
| Weeding | 24 | 20 |
| Mowing lawn | | |
| Pushing hand mower | 15 | 13 |
| Pushing power mower | 26 | 21 |
| Painting house | 22 | 19 |
| Raking leaves | 32 | 26 |
| Shoveling snow | 15 | 12 |
| Stacking firewood | 20 | 16 |
| Sweeping | 30 | 26 |
| Window cleaning | 29 | 25 |

*Calculations are based on 154-pound man and 128-pound woman. However, the heavier you are, the less time you will have to spend doing your activity to burn the calories you want. The lighter you are, the more time it will take to burn those calories.

To figure the calories burned subtract 10 percent from the minutes needed for every 15 pounds you are *over* the reference weight; add 10 percent to the minutes needed for every 15 pounds you are *under* the reference weight. For example:

It takes 32 minutes for a 128-pound woman to burn 100 calories raking leaves. Women A weighs 143 pounds.

Multiply $32 \times 10\%$:    $32 \times .10 = 3.2$
Subtract 3.2 from 32:    $32 - 3.2 = 28.8$

It would take Woman A approximately 29 minutes to burn 100 calories raking leaves.

It takes 26 minutes for a 154-pound man to burn 100 calories raking leaves. Man B weighs 139 pounds.

Multiply $26 \times 10\%$:    $26 \times .10 = 2.6$
Subtract 2.6 from 32:    $26 + 2.6 = 28.6$

It would take Man B approximately 29 minutes to burn 100 calories raking leaves.

Above calculation formula modified from *Physiological Fitness and Weight Control* by B. J. Sharkey. Mountain Press Publishing Company. Additional references can be found in the "Further Reading" section.

As you use the exchanges in this chapter, keep the following tips in mind:

- Concentrate on duration, not intensity.
- Get the equipment you need.
- Remind yourself to exercise.
- Exercise when you don't feel like it.
- Set up a reward system.
- When you try something new, give it time.
- Remember to relax.
- Find support when you need it.
- Attend to the details.
- Make up your mind to do whatever it takes to accomplish your goal.

## CATEGORY 2: INDOOR WORK

### 1 AEROBIC EXCHANGE
### (100 Calories)

| Activity | Minutes of Activity Needed | |
|---|---|---|
| | Women | Men |
| Carpentry | 22 | 17 |
| Cleaning | 28 | 25 |
| Grocery shopping | 28 | 25 |
| Mopping floor | 28 | 25 |
| Musicianship (vigorous) | 26 | 21 |
| Painting walls | 51 | 42 |
| Plastering walls | 22 | 18 |
| Polishing furniture | 52 | 43 |
| Scraping paint from walls | 27 | 23 |
| Scrubbing floor | 16 | 13 |
| Standing (cashier/artist) | 48 | 40 |
| Stocking shelves | 32 | 26 |
| Sweeping floor | 30 | 26 |
| Tailoring | 38 | 32 |
| Vacuuming | 38 | 30 |
| Wall papering | 36 | 30 |
| Washing/drying clothes | | |
|    Automated | 38 | 32 |
|    Hand washing small items | 41 | 34 |
|    Hanging clothes to dry | 29 | 25 |
| Woodworking (light) | 34 | 29 |

## CATEGORY 3: LEISURE ACTIVITIES

### 1 AEROBIC EXCHANGE
(100 Calories)

| Activity | Minutes of Activity Needed | |
|---|---|---|
| | Women | Men |
| Archery | 26 | 22 |
| Badminton | 18 | 15 |
| Billiards (shooting pool) | 41 | 34 |
| Bowling | 34 | 29 |
| Canoeing (slow) | 39 | 32 |
| Croquet | 39 | 32 |
| Cycling (5.5 mph) | 27 | 22 |
| (total miles) | (2.4 mi.) | (2.0 mi.) |
| Dancing | | |
|   Ballroom | 34 | 28 |
|   Modern rock | 10 | 9 |
|   Square or folk | 15 | 13 |
| Fishing | 28 | 23 |
| Hiking (no load) | 14 | 12 |
| Horse grooming | 13 | 11 |
| Horseback riding | 23 | 19 |
| Horseshoes | 31 | 26 |
| Ping-Pong | 24 | 20 |
| Rowing (slow) | 24 | 20 |
| Sailing | 26 | 21 |
| Scuba diving | 8 | 7 |
| Shuffleboard | 34 | 29 |
| Skating | 15 | 12 |
| Skiing (slow) | 16 | 15 |
| Sledding | 17 | 14 |
| Snowshoeing | 10 | 9 |
| Swimming (slow) | 20 | 17 |
| Water skiing | 15 | 13 |

## CATEGORY 4: RECREATIONAL SPORTS

1 AEROBIC EXCHANGE
(100 Calories)

| Activity | Minutes of Activity Needed | |
|---|---|---|
| | Women | Men |
| Baseball (not pitcher) | 25 | 21 |
| Basketball | 13 | 10 |
| Boxing | 10 | 8 |
| Canoe racing | 17 | 14 |
| Cricket | 20 | 16 |
| Cycle racing | 10 | 9 |
| Fencing | 11 | 10 |
| Field hockey | 13 | 11 |
| Football (touch) | 13 | 11 |
| Golf (walking with hand-pulled cart for clubs) | 20 | 17 |
| Gymnastics | 26 | 22 |
| Handball | | |
|   Light/moderate | 13 | 11 |
|   Vigorous | 9 | 7 |
| Horse Racing | 13 | 10 |
| Ice Hockey | 13 | 11 |
| Judo | 9 | 7 |
| Karate | 9 | 8 |
| Mountain Climbing | | |
|   (25-pound load) | 12 | 10 |
| Racquetball | | |
|   Light/moderate | 13 | 11 |
|   Vigorous | 10 | 8 |
| Skiing | | |
|   Downhill, moderate | 13 | 11 |
|   Downhill, racing | 7 | 6 |
| Rowing/crew racing | 8 | 7 |
| Soccer | 13 | 11 |
| Squash | | |
|   Light/moderate | 13 | 11 |
|   Vigorous | 8 | 7 |
| Table tennis | 25 | 21 |
| Tennis | | |
|   Doubles | 21 | 17 |
|   Singles | 15 | 12 |
| Volleyball | 34 | 19 |

## CATEGORY 5: CARDIOVASCULAR FITNESS

1 AEROBIC EXCHANGE
(100 Calories)

| Activity | Minutes of Activity Needed | |
|---|---|---|
| | Women | Men |
| Aerobic dance | | |
| Light-impact/moderate | 17 | 14 |
| Heavy-impact | 13 | 11 |
| Bench stepping | | |
| 11-inch bench, 18 steps/minute | 20 | 16 |
| 11-inch bench, 30 steps/minute | 12 | 10 |
| 16-inch bench, 18 steps/minute | 15 | 13 |
| 16-inch bench, 30 steps/minute | 9 | 8 |
| Cycling (outdoor), 9.4 mph | 17 | 14 |
| (total miles) | (2.7 mi.) | (2.2 mi.) |
| Cycling (stationary bicycle ergometer, pedal speed 50–60 rpm) | | |
| 300 kgm (1.0 KP) | 22 | 27 |
| 450 kgm (1.5 KP) | 17 | 20 |
| 600 kgm (2.0 KP) | 13 | 16 |
| 750 kgm (2.5 KP) | 11 | 14 |
| 900 kgm (3.0 KP) | 10 | 12 |
| Cycling, Lifecycle—see Category 6 | | |
| Jumping rope | | |
| 70 jumps/minute | 11 | 9 |
| 80 jumps/minute | 10 | 9 |
| 125 jumps/minute | 10 | 8 |
| 145 jumps/minute | 9 | 7 |
| Running | | |
| Cross-country | 11 | 9 |
| 12-minute mile (5 mph) | 12 | 10 |
| 8-minute mile (7.5 mph) | 8 | 7 |
| 6-minute mile (10 mph) | 6 | 5 |
| 5-minute mile (12 mph) | 5 | 4 |
| Skiing, cross-country | | |
| 3 mph | 13 | 11 |
| (total miles) | (0.7 mi.) | (0.6 mi.) |
| 8 mph | 7 | 6 |
| (total miles) | (0.9 mi.) | (0.8 mi.) |
| Stair climbing | 17 | 14 |
| Stair climbing, Lifestep—see Category 7 | | |
| Swimming | | |
| 20 yard/minute | 26 | 21 |
| (total yards) | (520 yd.) | (420 yd.) |

| Activity | Minutes of Activity Needed | |
| --- | --- | --- |
| | Women | Men |
| 25 yards/minute | 20 | 17 |
| (total yards) | (500 yd.) | (425 yd.) |
| 50 yards/minute | 9 | 8 |
| (total yards) | (450 yd.) | (400 yd.) |
| Walking | | |
| Track/treadmill | | |
| 3.0 mph | 30 | 25 |
| (total miles) | (1.5 mi.) | (1.3 mi.) |
| 3.5 mph | 26 | 21 |
| (total miles) | (1.6 mi.) | (1.3 mi.) |
| 4.0 mph | 21 | 17 |
| (total miles) | (1.4 mi.) | (1.2 mi.) |
| 4.5 mph | 16 | 14 |
| (total miles) | (1.2 mi.) | (1.0 mi.) |
| Road, 3.5 mph | 21 | 18 |
| (total miles) | (1.3 mi.) | (1.1 mi.) |
| Field, 3.5 mph | 17 | 14 |
| (total miles) | (1.0 mi.) | (0.8 mi.) |
| Snow, 3.0 mph | 8 | 7 |
| (total miles) | (0.4 mi.) | (0.4 mi.) |

# CATEGORY 6: LIFECYCLE FITNESS
### (a subdivision of cardiovascular fitness)

**Caloric Expenditure for the Lifecycle**

### 1 AEROBIC EXCHANGE
### (100 Calories)

*Hill Profile*

| Intensity Level | Minutes of Activity Needed | |
| --- | --- | --- |
| | Women | Men |
| 1 | 17.0 | 15.0 |
| 2 | 16.0 | 14.0 |
| 3 | 15.0 | 13.0 |
| 4 | 14.5 | 12.5 |
| 5 | 14.0 | 12.3 |
| 6 | 13.0 | 11.0 |
| 7 | 12.0 | 10.5 |
| 8 | 11.5 | 10.0 |
| 9 | 10.5 | 9.3 |

| Intensity Level | Minutes of Activity Needed | |
|---|---|---|
| | Women | Men |
| 10 | 10.0 | 8.5 |
| 11 | 9.0 | 8.0 |
| 12 | 8.5 | 7.5 |

### Manual Program

| | Women | Men |
|---|---|---|
| 1 | 15.0 | 13.0 |
| 2 | 13.0 | 11.0 |
| 3 | 10.0 | 9.0 |
| 4 | 9.0 | 8.0 |
| 5 | 8.5 | 7.5 |
| 6 | 8.0 | 7.0 |
| 7 | 7.0 | 6.0 |
| 8 | 6.5 | 5.5 |
| 9 | 6.0 | 5.3 |
| 10 | 5.8 | 5.0 |
| 11 | 5.5 | 4.8 |
| 12 | 5.0 | 4.5 |

## CATEGORY 7: LIFESTEP FITNESS
### (a subdivision of cardiovascular fitness)

### Caloric Expenditure for the Lifestep

### 1 AEROBIC EXCHANGE
#### (100 Calories)

| Intensity Level | Minutes of Activity Needed | |
|---|---|---|
| | Women | Men |
| 1 | 27.0 | 23.0 |
| 2 | 19.0 | 16.0 |
| 3 | 18.0 | 15.0 |
| 4 | 17.0 | 14.0 |
| 5 | 15.0 | 13.0 |
| 6 | 14.5 | 12.0 |
| 7 | 13.0 | 11.0 |
| 8 | 12.0 | 10.0 |
| 9 | 11.0 | 9.0 |
| 10 | 10.0 | 8.0 |
| 11 | 9.0 | 7.5 |
| 12 | 8.0 | 7.0 |

# 6

# THE FOOD
# EXCHANGES

Order, consistency, and control. They're all fundamental to permanent weight loss.

You now know how *The Exercise Exchange Program* helps to remove much of the clutter, chaos, and feelings of powerlessness that result from unbalanced eating and exercise habits.

The trick is to stick with your newly formed good habits once you're on your own—and fend off the chaos.

You may, for example, choose to repeat the Thirty-Day Eating Starter Plan many more times, or to follow it loosely with your own modifications. Or you may want to go it on your own completely.

Whatever path you choose, keep these thoughts in mind:

■ Check up on yourself periodically by using Your Daily Meal Plan checklist (Table 2), or by filling out the food diary in Appendix A.

■ Plan what you are going to eat on special occasions.

■ Don't eat out at both lunch and dinner if you can help it.

■ Consume most of your calories when you need them—in the first half of the day.

■ Adjust your food intake to your hunger, making sure you don't skip any meals.

## TABLE 2: YOUR DAILY MEAL PLAN

Date _____

_____CALORIES

| List | Food Exchange | Daily | Breakfast | Snack | Lunch | Snack | Dinner | Snack |
|------|---------------|-------|-----------|-------|-------|-------|--------|-------|
| 1 | Starch/bread | | | | | | | |
| 2 | Meat/protein | | | | | | | |
| 3 | Vegetable | | | | | | | |
| 4 | Fruit | | | | | | | |
| 5 | Milk | | | | | | | |
| 6 | Fat | | | | | | | |

Open calories:

■ Concentrate on keeping the amount of fat you're consuming to 30 percent or less.

■ Don't let yourself get too hungry while you're away from home.

And be sure to make daily use of the exchange lists in this chapter. The system breaks lifestyle into bite-size pieces, so the task of staying with your new lifestyle doesn't have to be difficult. (Should you find yourself straying off course, read the next chapter for suggestions to get back on track.)

As you already know, the beauty of the exchanges is that they allow you to substitute one food serving in a particular category for another in the same category and still get the nutrients you need for that day, so you won't ever have to count calories compulsively or deprive yourself of all of the foods you like. You can be extremely flexible in your food choices and still maintain your weight.

Where did such a practical system come from? Here's some background:

The *Exercise Exchange Program* has incorporated the American Heart Association guidelines with the American Diabetes Association/American Dietetic Association Exchange Lists for Meal Planning.* The 1,200-, the 1,500-, and the 1,800-calorie meal plans in the

---

*The exchange lists are the bases of a meal-planning system designed by a committee of the American Diabetes Association and American Dietetic Association. While designed primarily for people with diabetes and others who must follow special diets, the exchange lists are based on principles of good nutrition that apply to everyone. Copyright © 1986 American Diabetes Association, American Dietetic Association.

Thirty-Day Eating Starter Plan provide no more than 30 percent fat. While we make no specific recommendations for sodium and fiber, the ADA/ADA exchange lists do include guidelines for these nutrients, so this information has been included for readers who would like to decrease the sodium and increase the fiber in their diets. Foods high in sodium or fiber have been highlighted throughout the exchange lists.

Following the exchange lists, you will find an additional list that our nutritionists have developed to add further variety to your diet.

## The Six Exchange Lists

The foods listed within each category have approximately the same amount of protein, fat, carbohydrate, and calories per serving. *Every food is listed with a serving size that equals one exchange.*

### STARCH/BREAD LIST

Each item in this list contains approximately 15 grams of carbohydrates, 3 grams of protein, a trace of fat, and 80 calories. Whole-grain products average about 2 grams of fiber per exchange. Some foods are higher in fiber. Those foods that contain 3 or more grams of fiber per exchange are footnoted.

You can choose your starch exchanges from any of the items on this list. If you want to eat a starch food that is not on this list, the general rule is that:

- ½ cup of cereal, grain, or pasta is one exchange
- 1 ounce of a bread product is one exchange

---

### CEREALS/GRAINS/PASTA

| | |
|---|---|
| Bran cereals,* concentrated (such as Bran Buds, All Bran) | ⅓ cup |
| Bran cereals,* flaked | ½ cup |
| Bulgur (cooked) | ½ cup |
| Cooked cereals | ½ cup |
| Cornmeal (dry) | 2½ tbsp |
| Grape-Nuts | 3 tbsp. |
| Grits (cooked) | ½ cup |
| Other ready-to-eat unsweetened cereals | ¾ cup |
| Pasta (cooked) | ½ cup |
| Puffed cereal | 1½ cups |
| Rice, white or brown (cooked) | ⅓ cup |

| | |
|---|---|
| Shredded wheat | ½ cup |
| Wheat germ* | 3 tbsp. |

*3 g. or more of fiber per exchange.

## DRIED BEANS/PEAS/LENTILS

| | |
|---|---|
| Beans* and peas* (cooked),<br>   such as kidney, white, split, black-eyed | ⅓ cup |
| Lentils* (cooked) | ⅓ cup |
| Baked beans* | ¼ cup |

*3 g. or more of fiber per exchange.

## STARCHY VEGETABLES

| | |
|---|---|
| Corn* | ½ cup |
| Corn on cob,* 6 in. long | 1 |
| Lima beans* | ½ cup |
| Peas, green* (canned or frozen) | ½ cup |
| Plantain* | ½ cup |
| Potato, baked | 1 small (3 oz.) |
| Potato, mashed | ½ cup |
| Squash, winter* (acorn, butternut) | ¾ cup |
| Yam, sweet potato, plain | ⅓ cup |

*3 g. or more of fiber per exchange.

## BREAD

| | |
|---|---|
| Bagel | ½ (1 oz.) |
| Breadsticks, crisp, 4 in. long × ½ in. | 2 (⅔ oz.) |
| Croutons, low-fat | 1 cup |
| English muffin | ½ |
| Frankfurter or hamburger bun | ½ (1 oz.) |
| Pita, 6 in. across | ½ |
| Plain roll, small | 1 (1 oz.) |
| Raisin, unfrosted | 1 slice (1 oz.) |
| Rye, pumpernickel | 1 slice (1 oz.) |
| Tortilla, 6 in. across | 1 |

| | |
|---|---|
| White (including French, Italian) | 1 slice (1 oz.) |
| Whole wheat | 1 slice (1 oz.) |

## CRACKERS/SNACKS

| | |
|---|---|
| Animal crackers | 8 |
| Graham crackers, 2½ in. square | 3 |
| Matzoh | ¾ oz. |
| Melba toast | 5 slices |
| Oyster crackers | 24 |
| Popcorn (popped, no fat added) | 3 cups |
| Pretzels | ¾ oz. |
| Ry-Krisp,* 2 in. × 3½ in. | 4 |
| Saltine-type crackers | 6 |
| Whole-wheat crackers,* no fat added (crisp breads, such as Finn, Kavli, Wasa) | 2–4 slices (¾ oz.) |

*3 g. or more of fiber per exchange.

## STARCH FOODS PREPARED WITH FAT

### COUNT AS 1 STARCH/BREAD EXCHANGE, PLUS 1 FAT EXCHANGE

| | |
|---|---|
| Biscuit, 2½ in. across | 1 |
| Chow mein noodles | ½ cup |
| Corn bread, 2-in. cube | 1 (2 oz.) |
| Cracker, round butter type | 6 |
| French-fried potatoes, 2 in. to 3½ in. long | 10 (1½ oz.) |
| Muffin, plain, small | 1 |
| Pancake, 4 in. across | 2 |
| Stuffing, bread (prepared) | ¼ cup |
| Taco shell, 6 in. across | 2 |
| Waffle, 4½ in. square | 1 |
| Whole-wheat crackers,* fat added (such as Triscuit) | 4–6 (1 oz.) |

*3 g. or more of fiber per exchange.

## MEAT LIST

Each serving of meat and substitutes in this list contains about 7 grams of protein. The amount of fat and number of calories varies, depending on what kind of meat or substitute you choose. The list is divided into three parts based on the amount of fat and calories: lean meat, medium-fat meat, and high-fat meat. One ounce (one meat exchange) of each of these includes:

| | Carbohydrate (Grams) | Protein (Grams) | Fat (Grams) | Calories |
|---|---|---|---|---|
| Lean | 0 | 7 | 3 | 55 |
| Medium-fat | 0 | 7 | 5 | 75 |
| High-fat | 0 | 7 | 8 | 100 |

You are encouraged to use lean meat, poultry, and fish in your meal plan. This will help decrease your fat intake, which may help decrease your risk of heart disease. The items from the high-fat group are high in saturated fat, cholesterol, and calories. Meat and substitutes do not contribute any fiber to your meal plan.

Meats and meat substitutes that have 400 milligrams or more of sodium per exchange are footnoted.

Meats and meat substitutes that have 400 milligrams or more of sodium if two or more exchanges are eaten are footnoted.

## TIPS

- Bake, roast, broil, grill, or boil these foods rather than frying them with added fat.
- Use a nonstick pan spray or a nonstick pan to brown or fry these foods.
- Trim off visible fat before and after cooking.
- Do not add flour, bread crumbs, coating mixes, or fat to these foods when preparing them.
- Weigh meat after removing bones and fat, and after cooking. Three ounces of cooked meat is about equal to 4 ounces of raw meat. Some examples of meat portions are:

  2 ounces meat (2 meat exchanges) =
  1 small chicken leg or thigh
  ½ cup cottage cheese or tuna
  3 ounces meat (3 meat exchanges) =
  1 medium pork chop
  1 small hamburger
  ½ whole chicken breast
  1 unbreaded fish fillet
  cooked meat, about the size of a deck of cards
- Restaurants usually serve prime cuts of meat, which are high in fat and calories.

## LEAN MEAT AND SUBSTITUTES

One exchange is equal to any one of the following items:

| | | |
|---|---|---|
| Beef | USDA Select or Choice grades of lean beef, such as round, sirloin, and flank steak; tenderloin; and chipped beef* | 1 oz. |
| Pork | Lean pork, such as fresh ham; canned, cured, or boiled ham,* Canadian bacon,* tenderloin | 1 oz. |
| Veal | All cuts are lean except for veal cutlets (ground or cubed); examples of lean veal are chops and roasts | 1 oz. |
| Poultry | Chicken, turkey, Cornish hen (without skin) | 1 oz. |
| Fish | All fresh and frozen fish | 1 oz. |
| | Crab, lobster, scallops, shrimp, clams (fresh or canned in water) | 2 oz. |
| | Oysters | 6 medium |
| | Tuna† (canned in water) | ¼ cup |
| | Herring† (uncreamed or smoked) | 1 oz. |
| | Sardines (canned) | 2 medium |
| Wild game | Venison, rabbit, squirrel | 1 oz. |
| | Pheasant, duck, goose (without skin) | 1 oz. |
| Cheese | Any cottage cheese† | ¼ cup |
| | Grated Parmesan | 2 tbsp. |
| | Diet cheeses* (with less than 55 calories per ounce) | 1 oz. |
| Other | 95 percent fat-free luncheon meat* | 1 oz. |
| | Egg whites | 3 whites |
| | Egg substitutes with less than 55 calories per cup | ¼ cup |

*400 mg. or more of sodium per exchange.
†400 mg. or more of sodium if two or more exchanges are eaten.

## MEDIUM-FAT MEAT AND SUBSTITUTES

One exchange is equal to any one of the following items:

| | | |
|---|---|---|
| Beef | Most beef products fall into this category, such as all ground beef, roast (rib, chuck, rump), steak (cubed, porterhouse, T-bone), and meat loaf | 1 oz. |
| Pork | Most pork products fall into this category, such as chops, loin roast, Boston butt and cutlets | 1 oz. |
| Lamb | Most lamb products fall into this category, such as chops, leg, and roast | 1 oz. |
| Veal | Cutlet (ground or cubed, unbreaded) | 1 oz. |

| Poultry | Chicken (with skin), domestic duck or goose (well drained of fat), ground turkey | 1 oz. |
| Fish | Tuna* (canned in oil and drained) | ¼ cup |
| | Salmon* (canned) | ¼ cup |
| Cheese | Skim or part-skim milk cheeses, such as | |
| |    Ricotta | ¼ cup |
| |    Mozzarella | 1 oz. |
| |    Diet cheeses (with 56–80 calories per ounce) | 1 oz. |
| Other | 86 percent fat-free luncheon meat* | 1 oz. |
| | Egg (high in cholesterol, limit to 3 per week) | 1 |
| | Egg substitutes with 56–80 calories per ¼ cup | ¼ cup |
| | Tofu (2½ in. × 2¾ in. × 1 in.) | 4 oz. |
| | Liver, heart, kidney, sweetbreads (high in cholesterol) | 1 oz. |

*400 mg. or more of sodium if two or more exchanges are eaten.
†400 mg. or more of sodium per exchange.

## HIGH-FAT MEAT AND SUBSTITUTES

Remember, these items are high in saturated fat, cholesterol, and calories. One exchange is equal to any one of the following items.

| Beef | Most USDA prime cuts of beef, such as ribs, corned beef* | 1 oz. |
| Pork | Spareribs, ground pork, pork sausage† (patty or link) | 1 oz. |
| Lamb | Patties (ground lamb) | 1 oz. |
| Fish: | Any fried fish product | 1 oz. |
| Cheese | All regular cheeses, such as American,† Blue,† Cheddar,† Monterey Jack,† Swiss | 1 oz. |
| Other | Luncheon meat such as bologna, salami, pimento loaf† | 1 oz. |
| | Sausage,† such as Polish, Italian smoked | 1 oz. |
| | Knockwurst† | 1 oz. |
| | Bratwurst* | 1 oz. |
| | Frankfurter† (turkey or chicken) | 1 frank (10/lb.) |
| | Peanut butter (contains unsaturated fat) | 1 tbsp. |

Count as one high-fat meat plus one fat exchange
Frankfurter† (beef, pork, or combination)                              1 frank (10/lb.)

*400 mg. or more of sodium if two or more exchanges are eaten.
†400 mg. or more of sodium per exchange.

## VEGETABLE LIST

Each vegetable serving in this list contains about 5 grams of carbohydrates, 2 grams of protein, and 25 calories. Vegetables contain 2 to 3 grams of dietary fiber. Vegetables that contain 400 milligrams or more of sodium per exchange are footnoted.

Vegetables are good sources of vitamins and minerals. Fresh and frozen vegetables have more vitamins and less added salt. Rinsing canned vegetables will remove much of the salt.

Unless otherwise noted, the serving size for vegetables (one vegetable exchange) is:

- ½ cup of cooked vegetables or vegetable juice
- 1 cup of raw vegetables

Starchy vegetables such as corn, peas, and potatoes are in the starch/bread list.

Artichoke (½ medium)
Asparagus
Beans (green, wax, Italian)
Bean sprouts
Beets
Broccoli
Brussels sprouts
Cabbage, cooked
Carrots
Cauliflower
Eggplant
Greens (collard, mustard, turnip)
Kohlrabi
Leeks

Mushrooms, cooked
Okra
Onions
Pea pods
Peppers (green)
Rutabaga
Sauerkraut*
Spinach, cooked
Summer squash (crookneck)
Tomato (one large)
Tomato/vegetable juice*
Turnips
Water chestnuts
Zucchini, cooked

*400 mg. or more of sodium per exchange.

## FRUIT LIST

Each item in this list contains about 15 grams of carbohydrates and 60 calories. Fresh, frozen, and dried fruits have about 2 grams of fiber per exchange. Fruits that have 3 or more grams of fiber per exchange are footnoted.

The carbohydrate and calorie contents for a fruit exchange are based on the usual serving of the most commonly eaten fruits. Use fresh fruits or fruits frozen or canned without sugar added. Whole fruit is more filling than fruit juice and may be a better choice for those who are trying to lose weight. Unless otherwise noted, the serving size for one fruit exchange is:

- ½ cup of fresh fruit or fruit juice
- ¼ cup of dried fruit

## FRESH, FROZEN, AND UNSWEETENED CANNED FRUIT

| | |
|---|---|
| Apple (raw, 2 in. across) | 1 apple |
| Applesauce (unsweetened) | ½ cup |
| Apricots (medium, raw) | 4 apricots |
| Apricots (canned) | ½ cup, or 4 halves |
| Banana (9 in. long) | ½ banana |
| Blackberries* (raw) | ¾ cup |
| Blueberries* (raw) | ¾ cup |
| Cantaloupe (5 in. across) | ⅓ melon |
| (cubes) | 1 cup |
| Cherries (large, raw) | 12 cherries |
| Cherries (canned) | ½ cup |
| Figs (raw, 2 in. across) | 2 figs |
| Fruit cocktail (canned) | ½ cup |
| Grapefruit (medium) | ½ grapefruit |
| Grapefruit (segments) | ¾ cup |
| Grapes (small) | 15 grapes |
| Honeydew melon (medium) | ⅛ melon |
| (cubes) | 1 cup |
| Kiwi (large) | 1 kiwi |
| Mandarin oranges | ¾ cup |
| Mango (small) | ½ mango |
| Nectarine* (2½ in. across) | 1 nectarine |
| Orange (2½ in. across) | 1 orange |
| Papaya | 1 cup |
| Peach (2¾ in. across) | 1 peach, or ¾ cup |
| Peaches (canned) | ½ cup, or 2 halves |
| Pear | ½ large, or 1 small |
| Pears (canned) | ½ cup, or 2 halves |
| Persimmon (medium, native) | 2 persimmons |
| Pineapple (raw) | ¾ cup |
| Pineapple (canned) | ⅓ cup |
| Plum (raw, 2 in. across) | 2 plums |
| Pomegranate* | ½ pomegranate |
| Raspberries* (raw) | 1 cup |
| Strawberries* (raw, whole) | 1¼ cup |
| Tangerine* (2½ in. across) | 2 tangerines |
| Watermelon (cubes) | 1¼ cup |

3 g. or more of fiber per exchange.

## DRIED FRUIT

| | |
|---|---|
| Apples* | 4 rings |
| Apricots* | 7 halves |
| Dates | 2½ medium |
| Figs* | 1½ |
| Prunes* | 3 medium |
| Raisins | 2 tbsp. |

3 g. or more of fiber per exchange.

## FRUIT JUICE

| | |
|---|---|
| Apple juice/cider | ½ cup |
| Cranberry juice cocktail | ⅓ cup |
| Grapefruit juice | ½ cup |
| Grape juice | ⅓ cup |
| Orange juice | ½ cup |
| Pineapple juice | ½ cup |
| Prune juice | ⅓ cup |

## MILK LIST

Each serving of milk or milk products in this list contains about 12 grams of carbohydrates and 8 grams of protein. The amount of fat in milk is measured in percent of butterfat. The calories vary, depending on what kind of milk you choose. The list is divided into three parts, based on the amount of fat and calories: skim/very low-fat milk, low-fat milk, and whole milk. One serving (one milk exchange) of each of these includes:

| | Carbohydrate (grams) | Protein (Grams) | Fat (Grams) | Calories |
|---|---|---|---|---|
| Skim/very low-fat | 12 | 8 | trace | 90 |
| Low-fat | 12 | 8 | 5 | 120 |
| Whole | 12 | 8 | 8 | 150 |

Milk is the body's main source of calcium, the mineral needed for growth and repair of bones. Yogurt is also a good source of calcium. Yogurt and many dry or powdered milk products have different amounts of fat. If you have questions about a particular item, read the label to find out the fat and calorie content.

Milk is good to drink, but it can also be added to cereal and to other foods.

## SKIM AND VERY LOW-FAT MILK

| | |
|---|---|
| Skim milk | 1 cup |
| ½ percent milk | 1 cup |
| 1 percent milk | 1 cup |
| Low-fat buttermilk | 1 cup |
| Evaporated skim milk | ½ cup |
| Dry nonfat milk | ⅓ cup |
| Plain nonfat yogurt | 8 oz. |

## LOW-FAT MILK

| | |
|---|---|
| 2 percent milk | 1 cup fluid |
| Plain low-fat yogurt (with added nonfat milk solids) | 8 oz. |

## WHOLE MILK

The whole milk group has much more fat per serving than the skim and lowfat groups. Whole milk has more than 3¼ percent butterfat. Try to limit your choices from the whole milk group as much as possible.

| | |
|---|---|
| Whole milk | 1 cup |
| Evaporated whole milk | ½ cup |
| Whole plain yogurt | 8 oz. |

## FAT LIST

Each serving in this list contains about 5 grams of fat and 45 calories.

The foods in this list contain mostly fat, although some items may also contain a small amount of protein. All fats are high in calories and should be carefully measured. Everyone should modify fat intake by eating unsaturated fats instead of saturated fats.

## UNSATURATED FATS

| | |
|---|---|
| Avocado | ⅛ medium |
| Margarine | 1 tsp. |
| Margarine* diet | 1 tbsp. |
| Mayonnaise | 1 tsp. |
| Mayonnaise* reduced-calorie | 1 tbsp. |
| Nuts and seeds: | |
|    Almonds, dry roasted | 6 whole |
|    Cashews, dry roasted | 1 tbsp. |
|    Pecans | 2 whole |
|    Peanuts | 20 small or 10 large |
|    Walnuts | 2 whole |
|    Other nuts | 1 tbsp. |
|    Seeds, pine nuts, sunflower (without shells) | 1 tbsp. |
|    Pumpkin seeds | 2 tsp. |
| Oil (corn, cottonseed, safflower, soybean, sunflower, olive, peanut) | 1 tsp. |
| Olives* | 10 small or 5 large |
| Salad dressing, mayonnaise-type | 2 tsp. |
| Salad dressing, mayonnaise-type, reduced-calorie | 1 tbsp. |
| Salad dressing* (oil varieties) | 1 tbsp. |
| Salad dressing,† reduced-calorie | 2 tbsp. |

*400 mg. or more of sodium if two or more exchanges are eaten.
†400 mg. or more of sodium per exchange.

## SATURATED FATS

| | |
|---|---|
| Butter | 1 tsp. |
| Bacon* | 1 slice |
| Chitterlings | ½ ounce |
| Coconut, shredded | 2 tbsp. |
| Coffee whitener, liquid | 2 tbsp. |
| Coffee whitener, powder | 4 tsp. |
| Cream (light, coffee, table) | 2 tbsp. |
| Cream, sour | 2 tbsp. |
| Cream (heavy, whipping) | 1 tbsp. |
| Cream cheese | 1 tbsp. |
| Salt pork* | ¼ ounce |

*400 mg. or more of sodium if two or more exchanges are eaten.

## FREE FOODS

A free food is any food or drink that contains less than 20 calories per serving. You can eat as much as you want of those items that have no serving size specified. You may eat two or three servings per day of those items that have a specific serving size. Be sure to spread them out through the day.

---

### DRINKS

Bouillon, or broth without fat*
Bouillon, low-sodium
Carbonated drinks, sugar-free
Carbonated water
Club soda

Cocoa powder, unsweetened (1 tbsp.)
Coffee/tea
Drink mixes, sugar-free
Tonic water, sugar-free

---

*400 mg. or more of sodium per exchange.

---

### NONSTICK PAN SPRAY

---

### FRUIT

Cranberries, unsweetened (½ cup)     Rhubarb, unsweetened (½ cup)

---

### VEGETABLES (raw, 1 cup)

Cabbage
Celery
Chinese cabbage*
Cucumber
Green onion

Hot peppers
Mushrooms
Radishes
Zucchini*

---

*3 g. or more of fiber per exchange.

---

### SALAD GREENS

Endive
Escarole
Lettuce

Romaine
Spinach

---

## SWEET SUBSTITUTES

Candy, hard, sugar-free
Gelatin, sugar-free
Gum, sugar-free
Jam/jelly, sugar-free
   (less than 20 cal./2 tsp.)

Pancake syrup, sugar-free (1–2 tbsp.)
Sugar substitutes (saccharin, aspartame)
Whipped topping (2 tbsp.)

## CONDIMENTS

Ketchup (1 tbsp.)
Horseradish
Mustard
Pickles,* dill, unsweetened

Salad dressing,† low-calorie (2 tbsp.)
Taco sauce (1 tbsp.)
Vinegar

---

*400 mg. or more of sodium per exchange.
†The nutritionists who developed the diet for *The Rockport Walking Program* suggest that only those salad dressings with 10 calories or less per tablespoon be considered "free foods."

Seasonings (see the following material) can be very helpful in making food taste better. Be careful of how much sodium you use. Read the label, and choose those seasonings that do not contain sodium or salt.

## SEASONINGS

Basil (fresh)
Celery seeds
Chili powder
Chives
Cinnamon
Curry
Dill
Flavoring extracts (vanilla, almond, walnut,
   peppermint, butter, lemon, etc.)
Garlic
Garlic powder
Herbs
Hot pepper sauce
Lemon
Lemon juice

Lemon pepper
Lime
Lime juice
Mint
Onion powder
Oregano
Paprika
Pepper
Pimento
Spices
Soy sauce*
Soy sauce,* low-sodium ("lite")
Wine, used in cooking (¼ cup)
Worcestershire sauce

---

*400 mg. or more of sodium per exchange.

## COMBINATION FOODS

Much of the food we eat is mixed in various combinations. These combination foods do not fit into only one exchange list. It can be quite hard to tell what is in a certain casserole dish or baked food item. This is a list of average values for some typical combination foods. This list will help you fit these foods into your meal plans.

| Food | Amount | Exchanges |
| --- | --- | --- |
| Casseroles, homemade | 1 cup (8 oz.) | 2 starch, 2 medium-fat meat, 1 fat |
| Cheese pizza,* thin crust | ¼ of 15 oz., or ¼ of 10″ | 2 starch, 1 medium-fat meat, 1 fat |
| Chili with beans*† (commercial) | 1 cup (8 oz.) | 2 starch, 2 medium-fat meat, 2 fat |
| Chow mein* (without noodles or rice) | 2 cups (16 oz.) | 1 starch, 2 vegetable, 2 lean meat |
| Macaroni and cheese* | 1 cup (8 oz.) | 2 starch, 1 medium-fat meat, 2 fat |
| **Soup** | | |
| Bean*† | 1 cup (8 oz.) | 1 starch, 1 vegetable, 1 lean meat |
| Chunky, all varieties* | 10¾ oz. can | 1 starch, 1 vegetable, 1 medium-fat meat |
| Cream* (made with water) | 1 cup (8 oz.) | 1 starch, 1 fat |
| Vegetable* or broth-type* | 1 cup (8 oz.) | 1 starch |
| Spaghetti and meatballs* (canned) | 1 cup (8 oz.) | 2 starch, 1 medium-fat meat, 1 fat |
| **If beans are used as a meat substitute** | | |
| Dried beans,† peas,† lentils | 1 cup (cooked) | 2 starch, 1 lean meat |

*400 mg. or more of sodium per exchange.
†3 g. or more of fiber per exchange.

## THE EXERCISE EXCHANGE PROGRAM ADDITIONAL EXCHANGE LIST*

*Starch/Bread List*

| | |
|---|---|
| Bread, low-calorie (40 calories per slice) | 2 slices |
| Bread crumbs, dried | 3 tbsp. |
| Rice cakes | 2 |
| Zwieback cookies | 2 |
| Arrowroot cookies | 4 |
| Vanilla wafers | 5 |
| Gingersnaps | 3 |
| Flour | 3 tbsp. |
| Cornstarch | 3 tbsp. |
| Lowfat cookies | ¾ oz. |

*Vegetable List*

| | |
|---|---|
| Mixed vegetables (frozen) | ⅓ cup |
| Peas and carrots (frozen) | ⅓ cup |

*Fat List*

| | |
|---|---|
| Tartar sauce | 2 tsp. |

*Milk List*

| | |
|---|---|
| Sugar-free hot cocoa (40 calories) | 2 packets |
| Sugar-free pudding made with skim milk | ½ cup |
| Sugar-free shake mix (70 calories) | 1 packet |
| Fruited yogurt, nonfat, any flavor | ½ cup |
| Frozen yogurt, low-fat, any flavor | ½ cup |
| Frozen yogurt bar, low-fat | 1 bar |
| Fudge bar, Fudgsicle, etc.† | 1 bar |
| Ice milk (no more than 110 calories per serving) | ½ cup |

*Additional Combination Foods*

| | | |
|---|---|---|
| Refried beans | ⅓ cup | 1 starch, 1 fat |
| Fruited yogurt, Any flavor, low-fat | 1 cup | 1 milk, 2 fruit, ½ fat |
| Granola | ¼ cup | 1 starch, 1 fat |
| Granola bar | 1 small | 1 starch, 1 fat |
| Snack chips | 1 ounce | 1 starch, 2 fat |
| Microwave popcorn | 3½ cups (or ⅓ of a 10-cup bag) | 1 starch, 1 fat |

*Adapted with permission from *The Rockport Walking Program* (New York: Prentice Hall, 1989).
†There are many low-calorie frozen desserts on the market today. Many of them are made with low-fat milk and have less than 100 calories. These may be included in the diet and counted as one milk exchange.

---

## ADDITIONAL FREE FOODS*

*Seasonings*
Flavored crystals (Butter Buds, Molly McButter, etc.)
Crystal Light Bars (14 calories/bar)
Tabasco
Salsa
Teriyaki
Salt
Celery salt
Garlic salt
Onion salt
All spices and herbs
Ginger, fresh or powder
Tenderizers
No-oil salad dressing

---

*Adapted with permission from *The Rockport Walking Program*. New York: Prentice Hall, 1989.

## Alcohol

We've designed *The Exercise Exchange Program* to be a practical, flexible plan that you'll want to stick with for the long term. And because we recognize that having a glass of wine or a beer with dinner is appropriate for many people, we're including information on alcoholic beverages in reasonable amounts.

We stress moderation here, not only because of the obvious physical and psychological dangers of too much alcohol but also because alcohol provides calories and not much else in the way of nutrition. And with seven calories per gram, alcohol nearly matches fat's nine calories per gram.

| Type | Amount | Exchange |
|------|--------|----------|
| Table wine | 4 oz. | 2 fats |
| Beer | 12 oz. | 1 starch, 2 fats |
| Beer, light | 12 oz. | 2 fats |
| Whiskey, gin, vodka, Scotch, etc. | 1.5 oz. (1 shot) | 2 fats |

# 7

# THE MIND-SET

Attitude. It can make you or break you when it comes to lifestyle change.

You can choose to encourage yourself to achieve success. Or you can choose to worry and stress yourself out of reaching your goal. It's really that simple.

How do you keep a positive outlook? I'll say it again: *Exercise*. In one of the experiments we did on the relationship between exercise and mood in my laboratory at the University of Massachusetts Medical School, we measured the mental processes of thirty-six people who walked at slow, medium, fast, and self-selected speeds on a treadmill.

The results: immediate and significant reductions in anxiety and tension, and improvement in overall mood—at all speeds.

In this chapter you'll find a list of the ten most common mental roadblocks you may encounter at various points in the program, along with practical suggestions for getting past these blocks. This information was supplied by my staff, including Judy Fredal Pang, M.P.H., R.D., our chief nutritionist; and Bonita Marks, Ph.D., our consulting exercise physiologist. Our research subjects shared their very real experiences with these issues as well.

Refer to this chapter whenever you have a question. Reread it if you're feeling discouraged. If you like, copy the tips you find most helpful on index cards and carry them with you. Or have your spouse or a friend read them back to you periodically to keep you on track.

## BLOCK 1: Change Is Too Hard

*Learning this eating plan is just too much. And the exercise is too tiring. I'll never make it through this.*

Changing both your eating and exercise habits is putting a tremendous demand on both your body and your mind.

To make things easier:

■ *Acknowledge and accept your feelings of fatigue or of being overwhelmed and do it anyway.* What you're feeling is completely normal, and the best thing to do is to admit you have the feelings without dwelling on them. Just make sure you eat well and exercise on a day like this. You'll feel better for having stuck with it. By all means, don't criticize yourself for not feeling 100 percent.

Paula Schofield remembers feeling discouraged—but determined—in the beginning: "I had expected to feel better right away, and I thought, where is all the 'better' I'm supposed to be feeling. . . . I guess it takes your body time to adjust, and mine did. But it took a good two months before I started to feel better about it. I was just determined to stick with it."

As you start this program, make sure you're getting enough sleep, and relish that good sleep. You've earned it. Paula, who used to have trouble sleeping through the night, sleeps more soundly than ever: "Now I find that I have to go to bed about ten at night, and I sleep—I'm in a coma. But I can get up at five or six A.M. and have energy."

■ *Break your long-term goal into many, smaller "minigoals."* You might tell yourself, "For three weeks, I'll concentrate on understanding this system rather than on losing weight." Maybe you've started eating breakfast or stopped eating fatty snacks at night. Or you take the stairs at work for extra exercise. All of these small steps will eventually lead to weight loss.

■ *Give yourself time to master the program.* The food exchange system may seem awkward or cumbersome at first, but follow it. If you stay with it, you'll catch on soon. Keeping to the appropriate number of exchanges and measuring portions are key. In a few weeks you'll have the exchanges memorized, and your eyes will be trained to judge portion sizes without measuring.

Mastering the exchange system didn't take Ann Marie Nelson long. And, once mastered, the system made food choices easier. Says Ann Marie: "It took about two weeks. A good two weeks of solid effort, really practicing it, watching it," she remembers. "Then I knew what my lunch would be, what my breakfast would be. Once I got dinner squared away, it was 'a piece of cake.' "

■ *Set up a reward system.* Here, too, think short-term and long-term. How about a nice, hot bath if you exercise at home? Or time in the whirlpool after your workout if you exercise at a health club? For the long term, you may want to put aside fifty cents or a dollar for every 10 minutes of exercise you do, and save it for that special coat or set of golf clubs you've had your eyes on.

Helene Freed rewarded herself in that way. Note this passage from her journal: "March 1. A few new clothes if down five to ten more pounds. When I get to 150 pounds, I'll buy a new coat."

■ *Encourage positive self-talk and imagery.* We all have conversations with ourselves. Learn to support rather than sabotage your efforts with your thoughts.

You may, for example, be feeling nervous for fear of failure, especially if you've been on lots of diets before. Listen to your own mind. Are you saying, "This will never work," rather than, "I can do it. I'm going to do whatever it takes to reach my goal"?

Remember: This program is different. There's no time pressure. No cheating or "good" or "bad" eating. You do it on your own personal schedule, whatever that is.

If negative thoughts are a nagging problem, try this exercise: Sit down with pencil and paper and write down something you did successfully. Now analyze why you were successful. Did you have a lot of knowledge in that area which helped you? Did you have support from others? If so, you're already halfway there. This program will give you the knowledge and much of the support you'll need to be successful. It's up to you to find the additional support you need from others.

A little positive imagery can help when it comes to exercise as well. Imagine yourself wearing that size 8 dress or those size 33 pants in your closet. Stand in front of the mirror and see the fat melting away like wax, revealing a trimmer, happier you. While they may sound simple, mind exercises like these can be very effective.

## BLOCK 2: Cravings

*I want sugar. I want fat. I'm afraid I'll binge. Besides that, I'm finding it so hard to exercise.*

It may be tedious, but keeping a record of your eating and exercise habits is one of the best things you can do to improve your relationship with food and exercise.

As you write down your feelings, ask yourself:

■ *Have you tailored this program to fit your own needs?* It may take you a month or so to realize how the exercise you're doing may be changing your nutritional needs, and to adjust your eating accordingly so you don't get overly hungry.

If you exercise in the morning, you may need a healthy snack in the late morning so you don't feel starved. Under this plan, eating four or five times a day is okay, even encouraged, as long as you stay within your meal plan guidelines. It's normal to be hungry every three or four hours. Try to forget the notion that eating is bad and that snacking is something to be ashamed of. Snacking, in fact, is a smart practice to stave off feelings of deprivation as long as you make smart choices, and are eating because you're truly hungry, rather than out of habit.

■ *Are you tempted to eat for emotional reasons?* Think back to your childhood eating experiences. These memories can shed a lot of light on your eating habits today. They'll also explain why certain situations trigger the urge to eat.

Write down one thing from childhood that currently affects your eating habits. Is it cleaning your plate? Getting dessert as a reward for eating food you really don't want? Grabbing a bowl of ice cream to console yourself when you're feeling down?

Paula Schofield remembers: "I went to a boarding school for women run by nuns. And you cleaned your plate, or you would answer to the top one about why you hadn't done so. So you figure, for eighteen years you are programmed to clean that plate. I used to clean my kid's plate. Now I throw the food out."

She adds: "Maybe there was just something missing in my life. I can't figure out what it was, but there was plenty of satisfaction in food. Right now there is so much satisfaction in knowing that I *don't* need food to feel good."

■ *Are you eating to avoid doing an unpleasant task?* Is your stomach empty, or are you bored or stressed with your work? Write down what you're feeling. Rating your hunger level from "0" to "5" may help.

If you're tempted to eat because you're bored, make a list of things you'd like to be doing, then visualize yourself doing them. If you're lonely, call a friend. Boredom and loneliness are legitimate feelings. Accept them. Don't try to satisfy them—or numb them—with food.

Molly Woodbury, a caseworker who deals with sick or developmentally disabled children, admitted to herself that she was eating after dinner to avoid doing paperwork because it reminded her of some of the sad situations she had to deal with. Her solution? Molly realized she was overworking. Now she tries to do her paperwork during office hours so she has her evenings free.

## BLOCK 3: Progress Is Too Slow

*I'm following the eating plan. I've learned the exchanges, and they're a snap. I manage to exercise three times a week or more, even when I don't feel like it. And yet I'm not losing enough. What am I doing wrong?*

Probably nothing. You just need to face the fact that fat loss takes time to show up. Remember:

■ *Your body is not a machine.* Your eating and exercise success for today will not be reflected on the scale for several days. While it is important to monitor your weight, weigh yourself no more often than once every two weeks. Weighing yourself every day will only discourage you.

■ *Fluctuations in your weight are natural.* Initially, as you change your eating habits, your body may shed water—from two to ten pounds' worth. Don't be fooled into thinking that you'll lose that much consistently. Fat comes off more safely at the rate of about one-half pound per week for women and one to two pounds per week for men.

Should you find you've gained a pound, *do not* cut back on your calories. That pound may be due to the amount of sodium or carbohydrates or fiber you've eaten. Or, if you're a woman, it might be due to your menstrual cycle. Cutting back may make your body think it's starving, causing it to store fat.

■ *Don't cut back on the liquids you're consuming, either.* One of our research subjects did just that and became so constipated she was tempted to abandon the program. But once she began drinking the appropriate amount of fluids—between six and eight eight-ounce glasses of water per day—her problem was solved, and she went on to achieve her weight loss goal.

## BLOCK 4: Sabotage

*I'm frustrated. People don't understand how hard this is. My husband bought me chocolates for Valentine's Day. Somebody at work keeps offering me snacks. My daughter is nagging me about my "diet." And yet, when she bakes brownies, the aroma nearly drives me crazy. Why are they doing this?*

Maybe because they don't understand how to support you. Keep in mind:

■ *It's your responsibility to ask for the kind of support you need.* Tell them you'd like to reduce the amount of junk food in the house, or move it to a shelf that's less accessible. If food shopping tempts you, see if someone else can do it for you.

Helene Freed, who enjoys going out to dinner several nights a week with her husband, has asked for and now gets his support in choosing better restaurants: "My husband is more cooperative in reference to going out. I'll say, 'Gee, Larry. This restaurant really doesn't have anything for me.' He'll say, 'Fine. Okay. We'll go someplace that does.'"

■ *Keep in mind that sabotage can be unintentional.* You also need to recognize that others may not really know how to support you. Your daughter may feel her constant reminders to you are helpful; to you, it feels like nagging. And she may not be aware how much the smell of those brownies bothers you. Your husband may give you chocolates thinking you need a "treat" because you've been working too hard.

This may be unintended sabotage. In this society, we offer food to people we care about. They may be completely unaware how difficult they are making it for you. Tell those around you *exactly* the kind of support you need. Expressing your goal as a health need may help.

■ *Learn not to sabotage yourself.* Maybe this thought crossed your mind: "I'll eat this bag of Doritos now and exercise later." Don't do it. It's using exercise as a punishment for eating. Or, "I'll eat these Doritos now, and fast tomorrow." That's expecting the impossible. Set yourself up to win, not to lose.

Instead, take note of what Helen Morin does to support herself: "I'll have a little bowl of pretzels around or I'll have a whole bunch of vegetables cut up in the refrigerator all the time. If I eat some, it will take the edge off and I'll be okay. They're a safety precaution in case I'm having company and I have some high-calorie foods around."

## BLOCK 5: Overemphasizing Weight Loss

*Okay, I've lost some weight. But it's not enough. Is all this effort worth it?*

It's very much worth it if you look at what you've accomplished in total. Weight loss is only one part of this program. The overall objective is improved well-being and better health. Don't overlook these factors when evaluating your success:

■ *The reasonableness of your goal.* Though weight loss varies greatly among individuals, you can expect to have lost five to ten pounds after five weeks in the program. If you haven't reached your goal, it may not have been a practical one.

Are you still holding on to the old-fashioned quick-loss-by-starvation notion of a diet?

Regardless of what the fad diet "experts" tell you, from a medical standpoint five or ten pounds is respectable. To get a clear idea of just how much that is, pick up a ten-pound sack of flour the next time you're at the grocery store. Think about the extra load that weight was putting on your heart and on your joints and limbs with every step you took. Now pretend it's a ten-pound lump of bacon grease. Get the idea?

■ *Improvements in aerobic capacity and strength.* Retest your strength with the sit-up and push-up tests we've given you in Appendix F, and aerobic capacity with either the *Rockport Fitness Walking*

Test in Appendix C, the *Lifecycle FIT Test* in Appendix D, or the *Lifestep Electronic FIT Test* in Appendix E.

Can you walk a mile faster and more easily, climb more floors on the Lifestep, or ride the Lifecycle at a higher level? Are you stronger than you were when you started? You are? That's great!

I understand that weight loss is important to you. But don't let yourself get overly focused on weight. Give yourself a lot of credit for making progress in these other areas, too.

■ *Lost "inches."* As we've said, one of your goals is to lose fat and preserve or gain lean muscle. But because of the nature of your body—the muscle you have weighs more than the fat you have—that kind of shift won't show up quickly on the scale. But you will see the change when you measure your girth. Have you lost inches in your waist, abdomen, or thighs? If you have, you've toned up and lost fat. "People tell me appearancewise it looks like I've lost forty to forty-five pounds, which is the range I was hoping for," says Paula Schofield, whose actual loss was a total of thirty pounds.

■ *The total picture.* Look in the mirror. Do you look healthier? Thinner? Does your skin glow? Do you have more energy? Are you more relaxed? All of these things will show up in your facial expressions and how you carry yourself. If you think you look better, others will, too. And they'll be attracted to your smile and your energy. "I hoped that, when I lost weight, I would look good," says Paula. "But I didn't realize that the improvement would be reflected so much in my face and expressions."

## BLOCK 6: Expecting Too Much During Holidays and Vacations

*We're going on vacation and will be eating out a lot. I don't want to negate all of my effort so far. But how will I ever lose weight?*

You're still thinking like a dieter, which means thinking in extremes. Moderation is the key here, though it's often the hardest to achieve. Here's how to take the middle road:

■ *Be happy with holding the line.* Expecting weight loss in every circumstance isn't practical. For example, if you've always gained weight during the holidays or on vacation, make it your goal to *maintain* your weight, rather than lose. Is it really reasonable to expect to keep to the letter of your meal plan during high-pressure, supersocial holidays, when you're attending a lot of parties? Think of it this way: Not gaining the weight is a little like losing the weight you would have gained otherwise. You're that far ahead.

■ *Plan a strategy ahead of time.* Paula Schofield has learned that, with a little discipline and forethought, she can thoroughly enjoy special occasions while neither overeating nor depriving herself. "A friend of mind had a nice Italian dinner—stuffed manicotti, home-made spaghetti sauce, homemade meatballs, and cheesecake. I had a small portion of everything, and I found that I could not finish the meal, which surprised me. That was a good feeling—that I could leave food on the plate."

Why was Paula successful? Rather than eating at will, she pre-pared herself for the occasion by deciding ahead of time how she would handle the dinner. As a result, she was able to enjoy the food, but in moderation.

■ *Develop your own system.* Breakfast can easily be the most calorie-laden, fattening meal you can get in a restaurant. And yet Helene Freed and her husband enjoy a restaurant breakfast several mornings a week. She does it with a "system" she's developed.

For starters, Helene chooses better restaurants, where she can exert some control over how her food is made, rather than "greasy breakfast joints." She'll often order a low-fat, low-cholesterol meal such as oatmeal with a banana and low-fat milk. Once in a while she'll have coffee and two fried eggs, with the yolk removed from one of the eggs, and dry toast with jam or with a "shave" of cream cheese.

Whenever Helene is in a restaurant, she asks the server to remove complimentary predinner snacks or appetizers she didn't order. She also asks that side orders of french fries, potato chips, or other foods she doesn't want be left off her plate, and sees that her plate is taken away as soon as she's finished.

## BLOCK 7: Confusing Lapses with Relapses

*I'm so ashamed. I had five cookies yesterday. I've blown it, I know it. All these weeks of effort wasted.*

Relax. The problem may not be as big as you think. It may be a matter of adjusting your outlook.

For example:

■ *You still have the "diet mentality."* Do you see potato chips as a food you must kiss good-bye forever? Try not to do that. That's an all-or-nothing mentality, which tends to lead to feelings of deprivation. Remember, you can have potato chips once in a while, if you eat them in moderation and cut out some fat elsewhere. You'll be surprised—having or not having potato chips will become less important.

■ *You're short on patience.* If you stay with *The Exercise Ex-change Program* long enough, your tastes will begin to change, and you'll want high-fat foods less often. That's what happened to Helen Morin. Her diet used to consist of more than 60 percent fat; now it's down to 20 percent fat or less. And she doesn't miss the fat one bit: "Now I have a hard time with greasy foods. If I eat something and it's really fatty, it sits kind of hard in my stomach. I don't enjoy it as much as I used to. I don't even think I enjoyed it before. I think I just ate it."

■ *You don't know the difference between a "lapse" and a "relapse."* Remember: One piece of cake does not a failure make.

A lapse is when you have five cookies—once—and you continue the next day with your meal plan. On the other hand, if you've started snacking on cookies every night in front of the television because you think you've "blown the diet," that's a relapse. You haven't taken a break; you've given up on yourself.

Paula, for one, learned to keep believing in herself even when she lapsed: "I did have cravings, and, once in a while, I would satisfy them—maybe more than I should have. I just made up for it the rest of the week. I said, okay, I did it today, but that doesn't mean I've blown it for the rest of my life. You get back on track, and get back to where you left off, and keep on going. I found that with this attitude I didn't punish myself."

Give yourself permission to be imperfect, as Paula has. If you're too self-critical, you will relapse.

## BLOCK 8: Slacking Off

*I've been slacking off a little bit on the exercise. I know it's important, but I can't seem to fit it in the way I had been. Why am I so lazy?*

Maybe you're not as lazy as you think. Any of these situations may easily affect your exercise:

■ *You haven't adapted your workout to a change in the weather.* If you can't seem to stay with your walking program during very cold or very hot weather, maybe you need to dress more appropriately, find an indoor track to use, or choose an alternate activity that you can do instead.

When it's cold, dress in light layers of cotton, wool or breathable synthetics that you can remove as your body heats up. Cover your head, ears, and hands. Protect yourself from the wind and light rain with a jacket made of one of the newer breathable, water-resistant fabrics.

When the weather's just too lousy for outdoor exercise, call your local American Heart or Lung associations to get the names of indoor shopping malls where you can walk. Some have even calculated and posted the mileage for you. Contact colleges, high schools, or recreational facilities in your area to find indoor tracks you can use.

When it's hot, walk during the early morning or late evening, which are the coolest times of the day. Make sure you're wearing loose clothing and sunblock on the portion of your skin that's exposed. Drink six to eight ounces of water before you start. And consider bringing a plastic water bottle with you so you can refresh yourself along the way. But keep water, not high-calorie soft drinks, in your bottle.

A change in the seasons may also be the time to think about purchasing a Lifecycle or other piece of equipment to give you an alternative activity to pursue at home.

It's also a good time to look for *exercise exchanges* that you can do indoors—washing and waxing the car in the garage, or giving the house a top-to-bottom cleaning. See Chapter 5 for ideas.

■ *It's a busy season, and you're expecting too much.* While consistency in exercise is important, you need to realize that some times of the year will be busier than others, and you may not always exercise as often as you would like.

Helene Freed has learned to keep that in perspective. While she tries to exercise at the gym or walk a total of five times a week, she doesn't get upset if that doesn't happen during the summer. And she knows how to give herself credit for what she does do. "The summertime has been more erratic, because my children are out of school. I'm a little less consistent. But I still walk or exercise three times a week. I've gotten up and out by six-thirty A.M., and signed in at the gym at six-forty. In a trillion years, I wouldn't have done that in the past."

■ *You really don't like what you're doing.* Just because you started with one exercise, you don't have to stick with it. If you find something you like better, you'll be more successful at it.

Paula Schofield, for example, now cycles and swims with her husband on weekends in the summer, and enjoys cross-country skiing with him in the winter.

Ann Marie Nelson has gone back to running. Recently she completed a three-mile run, which delighted her teenage daughter. Says Ann Marie: "She'd been tempting me for weeks to go with her. So one day I did, and she was so amazed. She said, 'Mom, I can't believe you're doing this!'"

■ *You're too isolated.* If you're exercising alone and don't enjoy it, maybe you're asking too much of yourself. Maybe you need the reinforcement of exercising with a partner or with a group at a recreational facility or health club. If that's the way you are, don't expect to "tough it out alone." It won't work. Just be yourself.

■ *You don't know how to motivate yourself.* Could it be you need a new challenge? Add some hills to your walking route. Switch from the Lifecycle to the Lifestep at your club. Add some rowing or try the treadmill. Changing your routine can help a lot.

Helene Freed disliked exercise and never dreamed that she'd learn to appreciate it. But she learned to use positive self-talk to motivate herself in small—but effective—ways: "While I was on the Lifecycle, I could set small goals. I played mind games the whole time. The music would be on, I would ride to the end of a song, then to the end of the news. When I got there, I'd think, 'I feel pretty good. I'll go a little farther.'"

Mastering the Lifecycle encouraged Helene to look around her gym for new challenges. She's gone on to using the rowing machine and the Lifestep. "My big goal was the stair climber, because everyone said it was 'the killer.' So I said, 'That is where I'm going to go first.'" Helen started with five flights and has now mastered forty-five. Her goal is fifty.

## BLOCK 9: Plateau

*I think I've hit a plateau. I haven't lost any weight in a week. I've even gained a pound. Have I done something wrong?*

Don't panic. Here's what to do:

■ *Overall, stick with the plan for at least three weeks before making any changes.* You will probably start losing again. But whatever you do, do not drop your calorie level. Doing this will sabotage your weight loss effort. A drop in calories will convince your body that you're starving, and your metabolism will come down to compensate.

■ *Pull out your food diary and write down what you're eating.* Are your portions the right size? Are you getting most of your exchanges? Count your exchanges for a few days to make sure you're on target. If you're consistent with both eating and exercise, you should start losing again within a few weeks—barring any medical problems.

■ *Study your exercise log.* Have you been slacking off? If so, that's probably the problem.

If not, maybe you need to burn more calories. Think about burning 50 to 100 more a day by exercising a little longer at each workout, or by adding more activities to your day. But build up gradually. Use the exercise exchange lists in Chapter 5 to find something you like.

Whatever you do, continue what you've been doing for two to four weeks before making any major changes. Then reevaluate if you're still at the same level.

## BLOCK 10: Program End

*I can't believe I've really done it! I've made it to twenty weeks. What do I do now?*

Congratulate yourself, reward yourself. Celebrate. Give yourself a major pat on the back. But by all means, stay with the program.

This is only the beginning. The worst thing you could do is let out all the stops and go back to your old habits.

The best way to keep your momentum is to set more goals, complete with attractive rewards.

The goals you set now will, of course, depend on precisely where you are. If you still have more weight to lose, you'll be taking a different path than if you've already reached your goal weight and just need to maintain.

Let's look at both scenarios:

■ *You need to lose more.* Now is the time to set new goals, so grab your food diary and exercise log, sit down, reflect on the past five months, and write what you plan to do now.

Set some general short-term and long-term weight-loss goals, and put time limits on them. Set goals for next week, next month, and the next six months.

Now think of specific minigoals. How about choosing better snacks? Or learning to show more restraint at parties without feeling deprived? Or finding a way to eat moderately during the holidays while keeping up with your exercise?

New goals helped Helene Freed lose an additional 10 pounds after she reached the end of the twenty-week *Exercise Exchange Program* study. Here's a passage from her journal: "After the U-Mass program is completed, continue to exercise three times a week. Maintain 1,200 to 1,400 calories per day with 30 percent fat content."

■ *You need to maintain.* You must be thrilled that you've reached your ideal weight. But you still must *plan* to maintain that weight. Planning will keep you from going back to haphazard eating and inconsistent exercise. Haphazard behavior, even for a week, can make you feel like you've lost control, which, in turn, can lead to weight gain.

Since the eating and exercise plan you've been using is designed for weight loss, you'll need to *add* some calories to maintain your weight. Obviously you'll need to add them in moderation.

If you've been losing one-half pound per week, add 250 calories to your daily eating plan. If you've been losing one pound per week, add 500 calories per day.

But keep your diet low in fat. And exercise at least three times per week.

As I've said before, don't be too strict with yourself. Give yourself a five-pound range to allow for normal fluctuations in weight. Should you find yourself gaining more than that, look to your old, loyal friends—your food diary and your exercise log—to find out why.

Above all, remember: *The Exercise Exchange Program* is a lifestyle plan you can always turn to. It's your safety net. Take advantage of it whenever you need it!

# 8

# THE RECIPES

## 101 Recipes

If you're convinced that healthy, low-fat, low-calorie cooking has to be dull, just taste a few of the recipes in this section, developed by *Exercise Exchange Program* chief nutritionist Judy Fredal Pang.

Does "Curly Endive with Warm Goat Cheese," "Marinated Skewered Shark," "Chilled Wild Rice with Shrimp," or "Scallop Pesto Capellini" sound dull to you?

You'll find the recipes in this section easy to make, attractive to look at, and satisfying to eat. Best of all, you'll feel good when you've finished. For each one, there are fat, calorie, and cholesterol analyses, and an exchange breakdown per serving, so you can easily stay within the guidelines of your daily meal plan.

And, if you're the type who would rather eat than cook, there's a section for you, too—"Recipes for Kitchen Phobics." You'll find it after the main recipe section.

Make these dishes for yourself. Treat your family. Surprise your guests. Share the dishes with friends. But above all, enjoy each and every one of them. And as you do, keep these points in mind:

■ The letter "M" that appears after some of the recipes indicates that a microwave may be called for in preparation. Cooking times listed for microwave cooking are meant as guidelines only. Actual cooking time depends on the size and shape of the dish you're using, the amount of food to be cooked, the arrangement and size of the food pieces, the desired doneness, and the wattage of the oven itself. If you are uncertain about the cooking time, start with the shorter time, check the dish for doneness, then add time in small increments until cooked. Once you know how much time is needed, make a note of it so you'll know the next time you prepare the recipe.

In this book, "low wattage" refers to ovens with 500 to 550 watts of power; "high wattage" refers to ovens with 720 to 750 watts. For ovens with 550 to 720 watts, the best cooking time will fall between the shortest time and the longest time listed.

■ Some of the recipes call for special utensils or specialty food items that are available from many health food stores, international food markets, or the international section of most larger grocery stores. We suggest you read each recipe well before you make it so you have time to buy these items.

■ Some of the recipes call for defatted chicken broth. Canned chicken broth can be easily defatted by storing it in the refrigerator overnight and skimming the fat from the surface just before using.

■ Many of the recipes call for extra-light olive oil, which is better to use than many other oils because it's high in monounsaturated fats. And because extra-light olive oil has no distinctive flavor (as virgin olive oil does), it can be used with any recipe. However, should you run out, you can use canola oil instead. Remember, though, like any other fat, these oils are high in calories—with nine calories per gram—so use them sparingly.

■ Preparation time tells you how long it will take to prepare the recipe, from start to finish. It does not include cooling, refrigeration, or freezing time, unless otherwise noted.

# Appetizers and Beverages

## VERY BERRY COOLER

Smooth and not too sweet, the invigorating berry flavor comes through.

YIELD: 2 servings

PREPARATION TIME: 15 minutes

1 cup mashed ripe strawberries (or frozen, thawed)
1½ cups strawberry-flavored frozen yogurt
2 cups chilled cherry-flavored sparkling mineral water
2 strawberries for garnish

Gently fold strawberries into frozen yogurt. Divide this mixture into two tall glasses. Pour half of the water into each glass slowly, while stirring to blend in some of the melted yogurt. Place a strawberry on the rim of each glass. Serve with a straw and a long spoon.

EXCHANGES

1½ fruit; 1 milk per serving; 185 calories; 1.8 grams fat; 0.0 milligram cholesterol

# Favorite Mock Champagne
•

Perfect for a brunch or afternoon gathering.

YIELD: 25 (½-cup) servings

PREPARATION TIME: 5 minutes

### *Special utensil*
1 punch bowl

2 liters sparkling, nonalcoholic grape juice (available in wine stores and some
    supermarkets)
1 liter dry ginger ale
1 lime, thinly sliced
ice cubes

Combine all ingredients in punch bowl; stir.

---

E X C H A N G E S

> 1 fruit per serving; 67 calories; 0.1 gram fat; 0.0 milligram cholesterol

# Sangria
•

Serve at your next south-of-the-border-style gathering.

YIELD: 6 (1-cup) servings

PREPARATION TIME: 10 minutes

### *Special utensils*
2½-quart pitcher

1 (750-milliliter) bottle dry red wine, chilled
¼ cup lemon juice
½ cup orange juice
⅓ cup sugar
¼ cup brandy
12 ounces strawberry- or orange-flavored sparkling mineral water, chilled
1 small lemon, sliced
1 small orange, sliced
1 tray ice cubes

Combine wine, lemon and orange juices, sugar, and brandy in 2½ quart pitcher. Stir contents until sugar dissolves. Add mineral water and ice cubes. Garnish with lemon and orange slices and serve.

EXCHANGES

> 1 fruit; 2 fats per serving (alcohol is counted in fat exchanges); 179 calories; 0.1 gram fat; 0.0 milligram cholesterol

## GOLDEN STUFFED WON TON
▪

Superb for a large party. You can make these up to 24 hours ahead, filling the won tons, covering them with plastic wrap, and refrigerating them until ready to bake.

YIELD:  about 80 won tons

PREPARATION TIME: 1 hour, 25 minutes

½ pound ground turkey
½ pound finely diced cooked lean ham
1 egg white
1 small onion, finely chopped
¼ cup minced cilantro
¼ cup finely chopped Chinese or Napa cabbage
1 clove garlic, minced
1 slice fresh ginger, minced, or ¼ teaspoon ground ginger
1 tablespoon soy sauce
2 (12-ounce) packages 3¾-inch-square won ton wrappers (about 80 wrappers), available in produce section of larger markets or from an Oriental market.

Combine all ingredients except won ton wrappers. Place a teaspoonful of mixture into the center of each wrapper. Wet fingertips and moisten edges of won ton. Press opposite corners together tightly. Fold other corners to center and press tightly all along edges to seal.

Make as many won tons as you have filling. Lay won tons on lightly greased cookie sheets in single layer ½ inch apart. Spray lightly with water. Bake in hot 325-degree oven until browned, about 10 minutes, or 3 to 5 minutes longer if won tons were cold to start. Serve with sweet and sour sauce and hot mustard.

E X C H A N G E S

> ½ bread; ½ meat per 3 won tons; 60 calories; 1.6 grams fat; 9.5 milligrams cholesterol

# LIVELY CRAB DIP

■

This dip will liven up any party! Serve with low-fat crispbread or bagel chips, or with tender lettuce, endive, or radicchio leaves.

YIELD: about 2¼ cups

PREPARATION TIME: 15 minutes

⅓ cup reduced-calorie mayonnaise
¼ cup plain nonfat yogurt
1 (7-ounce) can crabmeat, rinsed and drained
1 teaspoon fresh lemon juice
⅓ cup finely chopped green onion (including tops)
⅓ cup blanched, chopped sun-dried tomato (or seeded, chopped and drained fresh tomato)
⅛ teaspoon red pepper sauce (or to taste)
2 teaspoons prepared horseradish
dash Worcestershire sauce

Combine mayonnaise and yogurt in small bowl until smooth. Remove cartilage and shell bits from crabmeat. Place in medium bowl, top with lemon juice, and break up with a fork. Add green onion, tomato, red pepper sauce, horseradish, Worcestershire sauce, and mayonnaise-yogurt mixture, and mix well. Cover and chill for several hours before serving.

E X C H A N G E S

> ½ meat; ½ fat per 3 tablespoon serving; 41 calories; 2.1 grams fat; 16.8 milligrams cholesterol

# SALMON PATÉ ON JICAMA
■

This smooth salmon paté is made with low-fat cheese and served on crunchy jicama rounds.

YIELD: about 1¼ cups

PREPARATION TIME: 10 minutes

1 pound slender jicama
1 (7½-ounce) can salmon, trimmed of bone and skin and drained
2 ounces Laughing Cow Lowfat Soft Cheese Spread (packaged in a bar similar
    to cream cheese)
2 tablespoons chopped green onion
½ tablespoon lemon juice
⅛ teaspoon sugar
⅛ teaspoon salt
⅛ teaspoon pepper
⅛ teaspoon dill weed
1 tablespoon capers, drained
fresh dill for garnish

Peel jicama. Slice crosswise into ½-inch rounds. If rounds are too large, cut into wedges. In blender or food processor, whirl salmon, cheese spread, green onion, lemon juice, sugar, salt, pepper, and dill weed until smooth. Add capers and chop coarsely, using the "pulse" setting. Transfer mixture to bowl, cover, and refrigerate until chilled, at least 2 hours. Top jicama rounds with paté; sprinkle lightly with fresh dill.

---

EXCHANGES

1 meat; 1 vegetable per 2 tablespoons; 73 calories; 3.1 grams fat; 9.7 milligrams cholesterol

# Shrimp-Stuffed Artichoke

■

A low-fat appetizer alternative to chips and guacamole, fried vegetables, and other traditionally high-fat fare. This dish can also be served as a luncheon entrée along with Lentil Bread, page 288, or Sun-Kissed Muffins, page 290.

YIELD: 4 appetizer or 2 main-dish
servings                                   PREPARATION TIME: 35 minutes

## Special utensils
cocktail forks

6 ounces (about 1⅛ cups) cooked small cocktail shrimp or imitation crabmeat
1 large artichoke, cooked
⅓ cup finely chopped cucumber, drained
1 tablespoon minced green onion
2 teaspoons lemon juice
3 tablespoons nonfat plain yogurt
3 tablespoons reduced-calorie mayonnaise
1 teaspoon fresh dill or ¼ teaspoon dill weed
dash hot pepper sauce
salt and pepper to taste
lemon wedges and fresh dill for garnish (optional)

Toss shrimp or imitation crabmeat, cucumber, green onion, and lemon juice. In small cup blend yogurt with mayonnaise until smooth. Mix in dill weed, hot pepper sauce, salt, and pepper. Add to shrimp or imitation crabmeat mixture; mix well. Remove center petals and choke from cooled artichoke. Spoon shrimp mixture into artichoke center; sprinkle fresh dill on top. Garnish with lemon wedges. Serve with cocktail forks.

EXCHANGES

| | |
|---|---|
| **with 4 servings:** | 1½ meat; 1 vegetable per serving; 108 calories; 3.8 grams fat; 86.4 milligrams cholesterol |
| **with 2 servings:** | 2 meat; 2 vegetable; 1 fat per serving; 216 calories; 7.6 grams fat; 172.8 milligrams cholesterol |

## Cajun Stuffed Mushrooms

■

Serve this party favorite at your next gathering. Your guests will never know they're low in fat!

YIELD: about 20

PREPARATION TIME: 1 hour

1¼ pounds or about 20 extra-large mushrooms suitable for stuffing
1 large or 2 small shallots, minced
1 small onion, finely chopped
1 medium bell pepper, finely chopped
1 celery rib, finely chopped
2 tablespoons margarine
1 pound uncooked crab or imitation crabmeat
¾ cup defatted chicken broth or bouillon
¼ cup plus 1 tablespoon lemon juice
2 tablespoons chopped green onion
¼ cup finely chopped parsley, divided
1 cup seasoned bread crumbs
½ teaspoon salt
¼ teaspoon ground red pepper
¼ teaspoon black pepper
1 teaspoon Worcestershire sauce
1 teaspoon Tabasco sauce
½ tablespoon vermouth

Remove stems from mushrooms; discard or save for another recipe. Wash and pat dry. Melt 1 tablespoon margarine in nonstick skillet over medium-high heat. Add shallots, onion, pepper, and celery, and sauté until tender. Stir in crabmeat, ½ cup of chicken broth or bouillon, and ¼ cup of lemon juice. Bring to boil, then reduce heat and simmer for 10 minutes, breaking up crabmeat with spatula. Add green onion, half of parsley, bread crumbs, salt, red pepper, and black pepper. Cook for 4 to 5 more minutes, stirring often. Set aside to cool.

Stuff mushroom caps generously with dressing; arrange in single layer in shallow, ovenproof pan. Melt remaining margarine; add remaining chicken broth or bouillon, 1 tablespoon lemon juice, Worcestershire sauce, Tabasco sauce, and vermouth. Simmer for 1 minute. Spoon about 1 teaspoon of sauce onto each mushroom. Bake in preheated 350-degree oven for 15 minutes, or broil at 450 degrees for 5 minutes. Sprinkle with remaining parsley and serve.

# JAPANESE-STYLE TOFU

■

Try this simple recipe if you've never had tofu. It will surprise you.

YIELD: **4 servings**

PREPARATION TIME: **7 minutes**

1 (14-ounce) block medium tofu
1 green onion, finely chopped
1 teaspoon grated fresh ginger
2 tablespoons soy sauce
1 teaspoon peanut oil

Gently squeeze excess water from tofu; cut into ¾-inch to 1-inch
cubes. Place in small serving bowl or dish. Toss gently with green
onions, ginger, soy sauce, and peanut oil.

# TUNA ROLLS

■

Served as an appetizer or a light main dish, these sushi-style rolls are as easy to make and as nutritionally balanced as they are appealing. To make traditional sushi, substitute the nori (seaweed wrapper) for the lettuce.

YIELD: 12 appetizer or 4 main
       dish servings          PREPARATION TIME: 45 minutes

## Special utensils
bamboo sushi mat if nori is used

1½ cups cooked short- or medium-grain stick-style rice, or
    ¾ cup uncooked rice and ¾ cup water
2 tablespoons seasoned rice vinegar,
    or 2 tablespoons rice vinegar and 2 teaspoons sugar
1 (6-ounce) can water-packed white tuna, drained and flaked
¼ cup cucumber cut into 1-inch-long matchstick strips, drained
1 small carrot cut into 1-inch-long matchstick strips
1 teaspoon grated lemon peel
2 tablespoons reduced-calorie mayonnaise
12 large romaine or green leaf lettuce leaves, or 1 package (six sheets) seasoned,
    roasted seaweed (Ajitsuke Nori)
tomato slices for garnish
low-sodium soy sauce
wasabi (Japanese horseradish paste available in Japanese markets or the
    Oriental section of large supermarkets) if desired

If using uncooked rice, combine rice and water in 2-quart pan. Bring to a boil over high heat; cover and simmer until liquid is absorbed, about 15 minutes. Remove from heat; let set for about 10 minutes. Uncover, fluff with a fork, and let cool. Stir seasoned rice vinegar into rice. Mix in tuna, cucumber, carrot, lemon peel, and mayonnaise.

Cut thick core end from lettuce leaves; discard. Spoon rice mixture onto lettuce leaf in a row, packing with fingers. Fold lettuce around rice and roll tightly into a tube shape. Line the lettuce edge with a small amount of wasabi, if desired, and seal the roll shut. Cut into 1-inch to 1½-inch pieces, discarding uneven edges. (To make cutting easier, chill rolls for 30 to 60 minutes before slicing.) Lay pieces on a plate, or stand them up in a row. Garnish with tomato slices and serve with soy sauce.

EXCHANGES

> **with 12 servings:**  ¼ meat; ¼ bread; 1 vegetable per serving; 64 calories;
> 0.9 gram fat; 3.3 milligrams cholesterol
>
> **with 4 servings:**  1½ meat; 1 bread; 1 vegetable per serving; 193 calories;
> 2.6 grams fat; 9.9 milligrams cholesterol

# HUMMUS
■

An easy, popular Middle Eastern dip traditionally eaten with pita bread. The main ingredient, chickpeas (garbanzo beans), is high in protein and a good source of cholesterol-lowering fiber.

YIELD: about 1½ cups

PREPARATION TIME: 15 minutes

1 (15-ounce) can chickpeas, drained
5 tablespoons lemon juice
¼ cup tahini* (see page 236)
1 tablespoon water
1 teaspoon sesame oil
1 teaspoon olive oil
1 very large or 3 small cloves garlic
1 teaspoon salt
2 teaspoons sugar
2 green onions, finely chopped (optional)
2 tablespoons fresh, finely chopped parsley (optional)

Place chickpeas in blender or bowl of food processor and blend until smooth. Add other ingredients except green onions and parsley and blend thoroughly. Remove dip to small bowl or container. Stir in green onions and parsley. Cover and refrigerate until ready to serve.

EXCHANGES

> ⅓ meat; ½ bread; ½ fat per 2 tablespoons; 86 calories; 3.6 grams; 0.0 milligram cholesterol

*Tahini can also be purchased in Middle Eastern markets and health food stores.

# Soups

## SEAFOOD BISQUE

•

A mild-flavored soup made creamy with the help of puréed potato.

YIELD: 6 main-dish servings
(about 10 cups)          PREPARATION TIME: 30 minutes

1 large white potato, peeled and cubed
1 bay leaf
2 cups clam juice
1 pound white meat fish fillets
1 tablespoon margarine
1 tablespoon olive oil
¼ cup minced shallots
1 (12-ounce) can evaporated nonfat milk
3 cups nonfat milk
1½ tablespoons cornstarch
1 (10-ounce) can whole baby clams, drained
salt and pepper to taste
¼ cup minced chives

Boil potato and bay leaf in clam juice until tender, about 10 minutes.
Cut fish into 1-inch cubes; set aside.

Heat margarine and olive oil in large, heavy pot. Sauté shallots
until tender; remove with slotted spoon and reserve. Add evaporated
nonfat milk, nonfat milk, and cornstarch to pot and stir. Remove bay
leaf from clam juice; discard. Purée potato and clam juice in blender
or food processor until smooth; add to milk mixture. Cook and stir

over medium heat until liquid is hot but not boiling. Reduce heat to low; stir in fish and shallots. Simmer, stirring frequently, until fish is cooked, 5 to 10 minutes. Add clams, salt, and pepper; heat through. Serve, topped with minced chives.

EXCHANGES

2½ meat; 1½ milk; ½ bread per serving; 301 calories; 6.1 grams fat; 71.2 milligrams cholesterol

# WONG'S WON TON SOUP
■

Don't let the won tons scare you away—they're very easy to make.

YIELD: **6 servings**

PREPARATION TIME: **25 minutes**

Won tons
½ pound ground turkey
½ (8-ounce) can water chestnuts, chopped
1 egg white
1 teaspoon soy sauce
¼ teaspoon salt
⅛ teaspoon pepper
2 green onions, chopped
24 (3¾-inch) square won ton wrappers
boiling salted water

Soup
6 cups defatted chicken broth or stock
1 cup chopped Napa (Chinese) cabbage
2 tablespoons soy sauce
pepper to taste
2 tablespoons chopped green onions (optional)

To make won tons, combine turkey, water chestnuts, egg white, soy sauce, salt, pepper, and green onions in medium bowl. Place 1 rounded teaspoon of the mixture on won ton skin, slightly off-center. Fold over one corner to the opposite corner, forming a triangle; seal on both sides with wet fingertips. Place won ton on wax paper. Continue to fill won ton wrappers until all the turkey mixture has been used.

Immerse won tons in boiling water and cook until they float to the surface, about 1 to 2 minutes. Remove with slotted spoon; drain on clean towels.

Heat chicken broth or stock to boiling. Add cabbage, soy sauce, and pepper, and simmer just until cabbage is tender. Place 4 won tons in each individual serving bowl. Spoon broth into bowls. Top with green onion, if desired; serve.

---

EXCHANGES

2 bread; 1 meat; 1 vegetable; ½ fat per serving; 273 calories; 6.6 grams fat; 24.3 milligrams cholesterol

## WATERCRESS SOUP WITH SHRIMP AND TOFU
▪

Easy, tasty, and filling.

YIELD: 8 (1-cup) servings

PREPARATION TIME: 20 minutes

7 cups defatted chicken broth
1 teaspoon grated lemon zest
1 thin slice fresh ginger, slivered
⅛ teaspoon white pepper
1 (14-ounce) package firm tofu, cubed
¾ pound medium-size shrimp, shelled and deveined
3 cups hot cooked rice
2 cups watercress, rinsed and drained
1 tablespoon tarragon vinegar
2 green onions, thinly sliced
lemon wedges (optional)

In a 5-quart pan bring broth, lemon zest, ginger, and pepper to a boil over high heat; add tofu. Return to a boil, reduce heat, add shrimp, and simmer, uncovered, until shrimp are opaque in center, about 3 minutes.

Place about ⅓ cup rice in each soup bowl. Stir watercress into soup, then vinegar. Ladle soup into rice-filled bowls; top with green onions. Serve immediately with lemon wedges.

EXCHANGES

> 1½ bread; 2 meat per serving; 240 calories; 6.4 grams fat; 64.7 milligrams cholesterol

## LIVELY MEXICAN VEGETABLE SOUP
■

The colors in this soup are full of life, and the flavors bite!

YIELD: 12 (1-cup) servings

PREPARATION TIME: 50 minutes

1 tablespoon oil
1 clove garlic, minced
3 to 5 fresh or bottled chopped jalapeño chilies; stems, seeds, and membranes
    removed
1 large onion, chopped
1 (49½-ounce) can chicken broth, defatted
1 pound (about 3 small) tender chayotes
4 small carrots, thinly sliced
¾ pound banana squash (or other fresh or thawed frozen winter squash) peeled
    and cut into ½-inch cubes
1 (15-ounce) can red or white beans, rinsed and drained, or 1 cup cooked beans
2 tablespoons chopped fresh cilantro, or 1 teaspoon ground coriander
1 teaspoon ground cumin
1 cup corn, thawed if frozen
3 large Italian plum tomatoes (about ¾ pound), diced, or 1 (16-ounce) can
    whole tomatoes with liquid, diced
¾ cup petite peas, thawed if frozen

In 6-quart pot sprayed with nonstick vegetable spray, heat oil over medium heat. Add garlic, chilies, and onion, and cook until onion is tender, 6 to 7 minutes. Add broth, cover, and bring to a boil over medium-high heat.

Cut chayotes with their edible seeds into ½-inch cubes. (Peel the skins off only if they are tough.) Add chayotes, carrots, banana squash, beans, cilantro, and cumin to broth. Cover and simmer until carrots are crisp-tender, 10 to 15 minutes. Add corn and tomatoes; simmer for 1 to 2 minutes. Stir in peas; cook just until hot, about 1 minute.

EXCHANGES

> 1 bread; ½ vegetable; ½ fat per serving; 117 calories; 2.5 grams fat; 0.0 milligram cholesterol

# T.J.'s Vegetarian Chili/Soup

■

A snap to make, essentially fat-free, and delicious. What more could you ask for?

YIELD: 10 main-dish servings

PREPARATION TIME: 50 minutes

1½ cups thinly sliced carrots (about three medium carrots)
1½ cups chopped onions
1 large green pepper, chopped
1½ cups sliced celery
1 (15-ounce) can stewed tomatoes
1 (15-ounce) can tomato purée
1 (6 ounce) can tomato paste
1 cup tomato juice
juice of one lemon
2 (15-ounce) cans red kidney beans, drained (reserve liquid)
1 (15-ounce) can chickpeas (garbanzo beans), rinsed and drained
4 medium cloves garlic, minced
3 tablespoons chili powder
½ teaspoon sugar
1½ teaspoons dried basil
1 teaspoon salt
½ teaspoon pepper
½ teaspoon hot sauce

Spray a large pot with nonstick vegetable spray. Cook carrots, onions, green pepper, and celery until just barely tender, stirring frequently. Add remaining ingredients and mix well. Cover and simmer for about 20 minutes. If the chili gets too thick, add reserved bean liquid. Do not overcook.

Freeze leftovers in single-serving containers or freezer bags to thaw and reheat.

EXCHANGES

> 2 bread; 2 vegetable per serving; 198 calories; 1.6 grams fat; 0.0 milligram cholesterol

## CREAM OF CELERY SOUP
■

Celeriac or celery root tastes like celery, only stronger. Look for heavy, firm bulbs less than 4 inches in diameter. Roots should be firm and clean.

YIELD: 8 servings

PREPARATION TIME: about 45 minutes

½ tablespoon margarine
½ tablespoon extra-light olive oil
1 medium onion, chopped
1½ cups chopped celery
3 cups vegetable stock
½ pound (about 1½ cups) peeled and diced potatoes
1 pound (about 3 cups) peeled and sliced celeriac
¼ cup chopped fresh parsley
½ teaspoon salt (omit if salted stock is used)
¼ teaspoon paprika
⅛ teaspoon pepper
½ cup chopped celery stalk and leaves
1 teaspoon extra-light olive oil
1 cup evaporated nonfat milk
2 tablespoons dry sherry
celery leaves for garnish

Heat margarine and olive oil in 3-quart saucepan. Add onion and celery; cook over medium heat until tender. Stir in vegetable stock, potato, celeriac, parsley, salt, paprika, and pepper. Heat over high heat to boiling; reduce heat, cover, and simmer until vegetables are tender, about 15 minutes.

Sauté chopped celery stalk and leaves in heated olive oil in small pan. After cooling slightly, blend half of the potato mixture in blender at high speed until smooth. Pour into bowl. Blend remaining vegetable mixture. Return puréed mixture to saucepan. Gradually stir in milk, sherry, and sautéed celery. Heat and stir over low heat until heated through. Ladle soup into bowls; garnish with celery leaves.

EXCHANGES

> 1 bread; 1 vegetable; ¾ fat per serving; 138 calories; 3.2 grams fat; 1.2 milligrams cholesterol

# CREAMY LEEK SOUP

∎

The creaminess of this tasty soup comes from nonfat evaporated milk.

YIELD: 6 (1-cup) servings

PREPARATION TIME: 38 minutes

1 onion, chopped
1 leek (white part only), chopped
1 tablespoon margarine
2 cups cubed potato (about 2 medium potatoes)
¼ cup chopped watercress
1 cup chopped celery with leaves (about 2 ribs)
¾ teaspoon salt
2 cups chicken broth, defatted (if salted broth is used, omit salt)
2 (12-ounce) cans nonfat, evaporated milk
1 tablespoon cornstarch
chopped parsley

Cook onion and leek in margarine in nonstick pot until limp. Add potato, watercress, celery, salt, and broth; cover and cook until potato is tender, 15 to 20 minutes. Stir in all but ½ cup of the milk. Heat, but do not boil. Blend cornstarch with remaining milk and add to soup; cook and stir until soup boils. Boil 1 minute. Garnish bowls with parsley.

EXCHANGES

1 milk; 1 bread; ½ fat per serving; 184 calories; 2.7 grams fat; 4.7 milligrams cholesterol

# GAZPACHO
■

Serve chilled with hearty bread and a fresh fruit salad—perfect for a hot day!

YIELD: 5 (⅔-cup) servings

PREPARATION TIME: 12 minutes

1½ cups tomato juice
1 beef bouillon cube
2 tomatoes, chopped
½ cup finely chopped cucumbers
2 tablespoons chopped green peppers
2 tablespoons chopped onions
1 tablespoon wine vinegar
1 teaspoon garlic salt
½ teaspoon Worcestershire sauce
3 drops red pepper sauce
2 tablespoons grated Parmesan cheese

Heat tomato juice to boiling. Stir in bouillon cube until dissolved. Stir in tomato, cucumbers, green peppers, onions, wine vinegar, garlic salt, Worcestershire sauce, and red pepper sauce. Refrigerate in covered container at least 4 hours. Just before serving, pour soup into cups; sprinkle each cup with a little Parmesan cheese.

EXCHANGES

1 vegetable per serving; 36 calories; 0.8 gram fat; 1.5 milligrams cholesterol

## QUICK SINGLE-SERVING FRENCH ONION SOUP (M)
■

This soup makes a quick, satisfying lunch on a nippy day.

YIELD: 1 serving

PREPARATION TIME: 17 minutes

### Special utensil
12-ounce microwave-safe soup bowl

¾ cup sliced white onion
½ tablespoon water
1 cube beef bouillon
1 cup boiling water
dash white pepper
1 teaspoon olive oil
1 slice French bread, toasted
garlic powder
1 tablespoon Parmesan cheese
1½ ounces mozzarella cheese, shredded

Cook onion with water in small nonstick pan, stirring frequently, until tender and golden. Transfer to 12-ounce microwave-safe soup bowl. Dissolve bouillon in boiling water; add broth and pepper to onion. Spread olive oil on toast, then sprinkle with garlic powder and Parmesan cheese. Place toast on soup; top with shredded mozzarella cheese. Microwave on High, uncovered, until cheese is melted, about 1 minute.

---

EXCHANGES

1½ meat; 1 bread; 2 vegetable; 2 fat; 290 calories; 14 grams fat; 29 milligrams cholesterol

# Miso Soup

∙

The customary beginning to many Japanese meals.

YIELD: **4 (1-cup) servings**

PREPARATION TIME: **15 minutes**

3 cups water
½ onion, sliced
3 tablespoons miso (soybean paste available in Oriental markets or
    international sections of the supermarket)
14 ounces medium tofu, diced into ½-inch cubes

In a medium saucepan, bring 2½ cups water to a boil. Add onion and
cook for 2 minutes. Dissolve miso in remaining water. Add miso
mixture and tofu to saucepan. Heat just to a boil; do not overcook.

E X C H A N G E S

> 1 meat; 1 vegetable; ½ fat per serving; 104 calories; 5.4 grams fat; 0.0
> milligram cholesterol

# Salads and Dressings

## Tuna Salad

A staple for the brown-bag lunch crowd.

YIELD: 2 to 3 servings

PREPARATION TIME: 10 minutes

1 (6½-ounce) can white meat water-packed tuna, rinsed and well drained
½ slice fine-textured bread, or 2 tablespoons bread crumbs and 1 tablespoon water
1 small rib celery or 5 water chestnuts, finely chopped
1 tablespoon sweet pickle relish
2 tablespoons reduced-calorie mayonnaise
2 tablespoons nonfat plain yogurt
¼ teaspoon white pepper
¼ teaspoon garlic powder
½ teaspoon sugar
1 green onion (including top), finely chopped (optional)

In medium bowl place tuna and break up with fork. Trim crust from bread; discard. Finely chop bread; add to bowl along with celery and relish. In small bowl blend mayonnaise, yogurt, pepper, garlic powder, and sugar until smooth. Add to tuna and mix well. Cover and refrigerate for up to 3 days.

EXCHANGES

| with 2 servings: | 3 meat; 2 vegetable per serving; 218 calories; 5.2 grams fat; 21.7 milligrams cholesterol |
|---|---|
| with 3 servings: | 2 meat; 1½ vegetable per serving; 146 calories; 3.5 grams fat; 14.4 milligrams cholesterol |

## Chicken Salad Reña
■

A big hit at wedding showers, baby showers, and luncheons, this low-fat version of a well-known salad is perfect for a weight-conscious crowd. And you can double this easy recipe for larger groups.

YIELD: 6 servings

PREPARATION TIME: 30 minutes

¼ cup slivered almonds
3 cups cubed, cooked, skinless chicken breast
1 cup halved seedless red or green grapes
½ cup chopped celery
3 tablespoons chopped onion
½ teaspoon celery salt
2½ tablespoons reduced-calorie mayonnaise
½ cup low-fat or nonfat lemon yogurt
1 tablespoon dry white wine
½ teaspoon prepared mustard

In small nonstick skillet heat almonds over low heat until golden brown, stirring occasionally. In medium bowl, mix almonds, chicken, grapes, celery, onion, and celery salt. In small bowl, blend mayonnaise, yogurt, wine, and mustard until smooth. Pour dressing onto chicken mixture and toss gently until well coated. Refrigerate at least 1 hour before serving.

EXCHANGES

2 meat; 1 vegetable; 1 fat per serving; 178 calories; 7.2 grams fat; 51 milligrams cholesterol

## THREE-BEAN AND CORN SALAD
■

Great as a light lunch or as part of a picnic or barbeque.

YIELD:  14 (½-cup) servings

PREPARATION TIME: 45 minutes

2 (15-ounce) cans red kidney beans, rinsed and drained (or 2 cups dry beans, cooked)
1 (15-ounce) can garbanzo beans or white kidney beans, rinsed and drained (or 1 cup dry beans, cooked)
1 cup cooked fresh or frozen thawed kernel corn
2¼ cups cooked cut fresh green beans or 1 (16-ounce) package frozen cut green beans, thawed and drained
3 medium tomatoes, chopped
½ medium white onion, chopped
2 small fresh or preserved jalapeño peppers, stems, seeds, and membranes removed, minced (optional)
½ cup firmly packed chopped fresh cilantro
½ cup lime juice
¼ cup lemon juice
¼ cup extra-light olive oil
1 teaspoon sugar
pepper to taste

Combine all ingredients in large salad bowl. Cover and refrigerate for 1 to 24 hours.

---

E X C H A N G E S

1½ bread; 1 fat per serving; 152 calories; 4.7 grams fat; 0.0 milligram cholesterol

# CRISP BULGUR WITH CILANTRO
■

Middle East meets Far East in this salad.

YIELD: 8 servings

PREPARATION TIME: 25 minutes

¾ cup bulgur wheat or cracked wheat
1 bunch watercress
1 cup onion, chopped
1 cup shredded Napa or head cabbage
1 cup chopped tomato
¼ cup finely chopped cilantro
1 teaspoon salt
½ teaspoon pepper
a dash each of allspice and Chinese five-spice powder
5 tablespoons fresh squeezed lemon juice
3 tablespoons extra-light olive oil or canola oil
1 tablespoon chicken broth or water

Mix bulgur wheat with just enough water to wet it thoroughly; set aside. Finely chop watercress with knife or in food processor. Place watercress, onion, and cabbage in large salad bowl. Add bulgur wheat to the middle of the bowl and top with tomato; let stand for a few minutes. Add the remaining ingredients and toss well. Cover and refrigerate for several hours before serving.

---

E X C H A N G E S

1 bread; 1 fat per serving; 114 calories; 5.4 grams fat; 0.0 milligram cholesterol

# CUCUMBER NAMASU

∎

This sliced cucumber salad, served as a first course in Japanese restaurants, is quite easy to make.

YIELD: 4 servings

PREPARATION TIME: 15 minutes

1 large cucumber
1 tablespoon finely chopped onion
2 tablespoons finely chopped celery
salt
2 tablespoons sugar
2 tablespoons vinegar
2 tablespoons lime or lemon juice
1 teaspoon fresh ginger, grated
¼ teaspoon MSG (optional)

Peel cucumber, leaving alternate strips of skin on for color if desired. Slice cucumber in half lengthwise, then crosswise into thin slices. Place cucumber in bowl with onion and celery; sprinkle lightly with salt. Set aside for 10 minutes, then squeeze out the excess water.

Dissolve sugar in vinegar and lime or lemon juice in small dish. Add to cucumber mixture along with ginger and MSG; toss. Refrigerate several hours before serving.

---

EXCHANGES

1½ vegetable per serving; 33 calories; 0.1 gram fat; 0.0 milligram cholesterol

# CHILLED WILD RICE WITH SHRIMP
■

A change-of-pace, high-energy salad that's just made for a sizzling day.

YIELD: 4 servings

PREPARATION TIME: 1½ hours

1 cup uncooked wild rice or 2 cups cooked wild rice
6 ounces shelled cooked or drained canned small shrimp
¾ cup orange or mandarin orange segments
2 tablespoons finely chopped green onion
1 tablespoon chopped fresh lemon thyme or ¾ teaspoon dried thyme
½ teaspoon salt
¼ cup Versatile Vinaigrette, page 236
lettuce leaves
2 tablespoons pine nuts, lightly toasted

To prepare uncooked wild rice: Cover wild rice with water and let stand at room temperature overnight. Drain and rinse with fresh water. Or pour boiling water over wild rice and let set for 30 minutes; drain well. Pour rice and 3½ cups water into heavy 3-quart saucepan. Bring to a boil. Cover, reduce heat, and simmer for 45 to 60 minutes or until most of the grains are puffed and some are curly. Fluff with a fork. Rinse rice with cold water; drain well. Use 2 cups; refrigerate the remainder for another meal.

To the wild rice add the shrimp, orange segments, green onion, thyme, salt, and vinaigrette; toss gently. Refrigerate until salad is thoroughly chilled. Arrange lettuce leaves on 4 salad plates; top with rice salad. Sprinkle with pine nuts; serve immediately.

---

EXCHANGES

1½ meat; 2 bread; ½ fat per serving; 276 calories; 6.8 grams fat; 64 milligrams cholesterol

# New Potato Salad (M)

■

A new, lighter version of an old picnic standby.

YIELD: 8 (½ cup) servings

PREPARATION TIME: 30 to 45
minutes, depending on
cooking method used

2 pounds new red potatoes (24 to 32 potatoes)
½ cup sliced celery
¼ cup chopped onions
½ cup chopped yellow bell pepper
2 green onions, finely chopped
1½ tablespoons rice vinegar
½ teaspoon garlic salt
¼ teaspoon fresh ground pepper
½ cup plain nonfat yogurt
½ cup reduced-calorie mayonnaise
½ teaspoon sugar
fresh chopped parsley

In 4- or 5-quart pot, cover unpeeled potatoes with water. Bring to a
boil over high heat. Reduce heat to low, cover, and simmer for 15
minutes or until fork-tender; drain. Cool potatoes until easy to handle. Halve small potatoes; quarter larger ones.

In a large bowl, combine potatoes, celery, onions, bell pepper,
green onions, rice vinegar, garlic salt, and pepper. In small bowl
blend yogurt, mayonnaise, and sugar. Add dressing to potatoes and
mix well. Chill for a few hours or more. Garnish with fresh parsley.

To microwave: Halve small potatoes; quarter larger ones. Place
them in 2-quart microwave-safe casserole with ⅓ cup water; cover.
Microwave on high for 10½ to 15 minutes (longer for ovens with less
than 650 watts of power) or until potatoes are tender, stirring mixture
twice. Let stand, covered, for 2 to 3 minutes. Drain and cool potatoes
enough to handle, and continue as above.

EXCHANGES

1 bread; 1 vegetable; 1 fat per serving; 148 calories; 4.5 grams fat; 4.7
milligrams cholesterol

## Lettuce with Warm Sweet-Sour Sauce
■

The tangy, cooked dressing gives this salad a rich flavor.

YIELD: 6 servings

PREPARATION TIME: 15 minutes

2 ounces Canadian bacon, thinly sliced
1 tablespoon chopped white onion
1 tablespoon virgin olive oil
3 tablespoons red wine vinegar
3 tablespoons ketchup
1 tablespoon Worcestershire sauce
3 tablespoons sugar
3 small heads Boston or leaf lettuce, shredded
½ cup sliced mushrooms

Broil bacon until well done. Chop and set aside. Sauté onion in hot olive oil until tender. Add vinegar, ketchup, Worcestershire sauce, and sugar, and mix well. Toss lettuce with mushrooms and Canadian bacon. Pour hot dressing over salad and toss lightly; serve immediately.

---

EXCHANGES

1 vegetable; ½ fat; ½ fruit per serving; 80 calories; 3.1 grams fat; 4.7 milligrams cholesterol

# ALMOND SNOW PEA SALAD

▪

A refreshing salad with an Oriental flair.

YIELD: 2 servings

PREPARATION TIME: 18 minutes

## *Special utensils*
blancher with basket and cover, or wire basket and kettle, for blanch-
   ing snow peas

2 cups snow peas or sugar snap peas
½ cup sliced water chestnuts
1 clove garlic, minced
1 green onion, finely chopped
2 tablespoons bottled Oriental dressing (if available, use Chinese chicken salad
   dressing)
1 tablespoon rice vinegar
2 cup-shaped iceberg lettuce leaves
½ ounce slivered almonds
½ cup seasoned croutons

Remove stems and strings from peas. Blanch for 2 minutes, then cool
immediately in ice water. Drain and dry peas on towel. In mixing
bowl, combine peas, water chestnuts, garlic, onions, and dressing;
toss lightly. Add rice vinegar and toss again. Place in lettuce cups.
Sprinkle with almonds and croutons; serve.

---

EXCHANGES

1½ bread; 2 vegetable; 2 fat per serving; 251 calories; 11.1 grams fat; 0.0
milligram cholesterol

# Rainbow Pasta Salad
■

Perfect for a light lunch, afternoon picnic, or potluck dinner.

YIELD: 10 (1 cup) servings

PREPARATION TIME: 20 minutes

8 ounces tricolor fusilli (rainbow twirl) pasta
2 tablespoons virgin olive oil
2½ ounces grated fresh Parmesan cheese
5 ounces shredded cooked chicken breast without skin
3 to 4 plum tomatoes, sliced
2 carrots, peeled and sliced diagonally
½ white onion, sliced
1 green onion, chopped
½ cup rice vinegar
3 tablespoons minced parsley
2 tablespoons chopped fresh basil or 2 teaspoons dried basil
1 large clove garlic, minced
1 teaspoon Italian seasoning
1 teaspoon salt
1 teaspoon sugar

Prepare pasta al dente. Rinse with cold water; drain. Pour into large salad bowl; add oil and toss to coat thoroughly. Add remaining ingredients; toss carefully. Refrigerate several hours before serving.

---

E X C H A N G E S

½ meat; 1 bread; 1 vegetable; 1 fat per serving; 181 calories; 5.5 grams fat; 17.2 milligrams cholesterol

## CURLY ENDIVE WITH WARM GOAT CHEESE
■

A nice accompaniment to Veal Piccata on Fresh Pasta (see page 264).

YIELD: 4 servings

PREPARATION TIME: 20 minutes

4 pieces (halves) sun-dried tomato
3 cups lightly packed torn tender chicory or endive (use inner leaves)
4 cups lightly packed crisp leaf lettuce (bibb, Boston, and/or green leaf) torn
    into pieces
2 ounces goat cheese, diced
2 tablespoons nonfat milk
pinch sugar
small shallot, minced
½ cup seasoned croutons
fresh ground pepper to taste

Blanch tomato in boiling water for 2 minutes; drain. Cut tomato into strips; set aside. Toss chicory with leaf lettuce in salad bowl. Melt goat cheese in small saucepan with milk and sugar over low flame, stirring constantly. When smooth, add cheese mixture to salad greens and toss gently. Add tomato (cooled), shallot, and croutons; carefully toss once or twice. Divide salad into serving bowls; serve immediately. Season with pepper at the table.

---

EXCHANGES

½ meat; 3 vegetables per serving; 104 calories; 3.5 grams fat; 12.8 milligrams cholesterol

# JAPANESE SALAD
■

A real favorite among the calorie-conscious, this salad can become a main dish by adding some shredded, cooked chicken breast.

YIELD: **14** (½-cup) servings

PREPARATION TIME: **20 minutes**

3 tablespoons sliced almonds
3 tablespoons sesame seeds
8 green onions, finely sliced
1 head cabbage, finely chopped
2 (3-ounce) packages Ramen noodles (instant Japanese noodle soup), dry,
    without seasoning packets
3 tablespoons sugar
¾ teaspoon pepper
¾ teaspoon salt
3 tablespoons vegetable oil
⅔ cup rice vinegar

Toast almonds and sesame seeds in nonstick pan until lightly browned. Combine onions, cabbage, almonds, and sesame seeds in large bowl. Break up Ramen noodles into small pieces; add to cabbage mixture.

Combine sugar, pepper, salt, vegetable oil, and rice vinegar in small jar and stir vigorously. Add to cabbage mixture and toss well. Refrigerate several hours in covered container before serving.

EXCHANGES

¾ bread; 1 vegetable; 1 fat per serving; 128 calories; 5.2 grams fat; 0.0 milligram cholesterol

## Versatile Vinaigrette

■

Versatile because a variation of this dressing can be used with almost any salad.

YIELD: Makes about 1 cup

PREPARATION TIME: 12 minutes

¼ cup virgin olive, canola, avocado, walnut, or peanut oil
½ cup red wine, rice, balsamic, apple cider, tarragon, or fruit-flavored vinegar
3 tablespoons lemon, lime, or orange juice, or white wine (use sweet wine or orange juice with the more bitter vinegars)
1 tablespoon sugar or honey
1 tablespoon Dijon-style mustard
1 large clove garlic, crushed
salt and freshly ground black pepper, to taste

Blend all ingredients in blender until smooth. Store, covered, in refrigerator. Use within two to three weeks. Shake before using.

---

E X C H A N G E S

¾ fat per tablespoon; 37 calories; 3.5 grams fat; 0.0 milligram cholesterol

# TAHINI

▪

A dressing that complements the nutrients and flavors in garbanzo bean dishes, such as hummus and falafel. This flavorful dressing can also be used as a dip for bread or on bean salads.

YIELD: about 1¼ cups

PREPARATION TIME: 10 minutes

5 cloves garlic, minced
1 teaspoon salt
½ cup sesame seed paste
½ cup fresh lemon juice
¼ cup cold water

Crush garlic and salt into a paste. Beat this mixture with sesame seed paste in small bowl with a fork. Add lemon juice and water, one at a time, beating continuously until blended.

---

E X C H A N G E S

½ bread; 1 fat per 2 tablespoons; 82 calories; 6.6 grams fat; 0.0 milligram cholesterol

# Entrées

## Lemon Chicken

A delicious dish great with rice and steamed broccoli.

YIELD: 4 servings

PREPARATION TIME: 28 minutes

4 skinned chicken breast halves, boned, flattened to ½-inch thickness
1 teaspoon peanut oil
2 teaspoons mild soy sauce
1 teaspoon sherry
½ teaspoon water
dash freshly ground pepper
⅓ cup cornstarch
1 tablespoon extra-light olive oil or canola oil
lemon slices for garnish

*Lemon Sauce*
¾ cup water
¼ cup lemon juice
1½ tablespoons packed light brown sugar
1½ tablespoons cornstarch
1½ tablespoons honey
1 teaspoon instant chicken bouillon
½ teaspoon grated pared fresh ginger root

Wash chicken and pat dry; set aside. Combine peanut oil, soy sauce, sherry, water, and pepper in small bowl. Rub mixture over chicken, allowing excess to drain off. Dredge in cornstarch to coat lightly. Place in single layer on plate or wax paper; refrigerate for 30 minutes.

Heat olive oil or canola oil in 12-inch nonstick skillet over medium heat. Add chicken and sauté until golden brown on both sides and cooked through, 6 to 8 minutes.

Combine all sauce ingredients in medium saucepan, stirring until blended. Cook over medium heat until sauce boils and thickens, stirring constantly, 3 to 4 minutes. Pour sauce over cooked chicken. Garnish with lemon slices; serve.

---

EXCHANGES

3 meat; 1 bread; ⅔ fruit per serving; 282 calories; 7.6 gram fat; 72.4 milligrams cholesterol

## SAVOY CHICKEN ROLL WITH PINEAPPLE DRESSING
∎

A beautiful and unique main-dish salad. Serve with flavorful bread or muffins.

YIELD: 4 servings

PREPARATION TIME: 65 minutes, including baking time

1 head savoy cabbage
1 head radicchio
4 half chicken breasts, skinned and boned
salt and pepper to taste
2 tablespoons reduced-calorie mayonnaise
1 (8-ounce) can crushed pineapple in its own juice, drained (reserve liquid)
2 green onions, finely chopped
¼ cup reduced-calorie mayonnaise
¼ cup plain low-fat or nonfat yogurt
¼ teaspoon curry powder
dash paprika
8 red leaf lettuce leaves
2 tablespoons pine nuts
8 fresh pineapple wedges

Separate four of the large outer leaves from both cabbage and radicchio. Microwave or steam leaves until limp, 2 to 3 minutes; drain and set aside. Flatten chicken breasts with mallet to ¼-inch thickness. Season with salt and pepper. Slit cabbage leaves, if necessary, to flatten. Place one piece of chicken on each cabbage leaf, leaving ¼ inch of the cabbage edge on all sides. (Fold over or cut away excess cabbage.) Place radicchio leaf on chicken, cutting or folding to even edges. Spread ½ tablespoon mayonnaise over each radicchio leaf; top with crushed pineapple and green onion.

Starting with shorter edge, roll up cabbage; fasten with toothpick. Coat casserole with nonstick vegetable spray or oil. Place rolls in casserole; bake, covered, at 400 degrees until done, about 30 minutes.

In small saucepan combine mayonnaise, yogurt, two tablespoons of the reserved pineapple juice, curry powder, and paprika. Stir and heat over low flame until warm; do not boil. Shred and mix enough cabbage and radicchio to make 4 cups. When rolls have cooled slightly, slice them crosswise. Line plates with lettuce leaves and shredded cabbage mixture. Place sliced rolls on cabbage. Drizzle with warm dressing; top with pine nuts. Garnish with pineapple wedges; serve.

---

EXCHANGES

3½ meat; 2 vegetable; 1 fruit; 1 fat per serving; 359 calories; 11.5 grams fat; 80 milligrams cholesterol

---

## Sweet 'n' Spicy Cornish Game Hens (M)

■

The combination of microwave and barbeque cooking makes this a quick and easy dish.

YIELD: **4 servings**

PREPARATION TIME: **22 minutes**

2 Cornish game hens, about 1½ pounds each
1½ tablespoons honey
1½ tablespoons Dijon mustard
1½ tablespoons soy sauce
snipped chives for garnish (optional)

Preheat grill or oven-broiler. Split each hen in two with cleaver or poultry shears. Wash and dry hens thoroughly. Place hen halves in microwave-safe casserole; cover with waxed paper. Microwave on High for 2½ minutes (or longer for ovens with less than 650 watts of power). Turn halves over, with the inner sections facing outside and the outer sections in the center. Microwave for 2½ more minutes.

Combine honey, mustard, and soy sauce; brush both sides of poultry with sauce. Grill or broil until meat is white and juices run clear, about 15 minutes, turning once. Top with chives; serve over wild or seasoned white rice.

EXCHANGES

3½ meat; 1 fat; ½ fruit per serving; 270 calories; 13.9 grams fat; 87.3 milligrams cholesterol

# JUDY'S MISO CHICKEN

■

Tender and juicy, this chicken is a family favorite!

YIELD: 6 servings

PREPARATION TIME: 10 minutes plus marinating/broiling time

½ cup soy sauce
½ cup sugar
½ cup light miso (soybean paste available in the Oriental section of the supermarket)
½ cup beer
1½ pounds boneless, skinless chicken thighs

Blend first four ingredients until smooth. Place chicken in a single layer in the bottom of a glass dish or marinade container. Pour miso-beer mixture over chicken pieces. Cover and marinate for at least 8 hours, or overnight, turning once.

With both sides well coated with the marinade, broil or barbeque the chicken on one side until brown. Turn and cook until meat is firm and juices run clear.

EXCHANGES

3 meat per serving; 196 calories; 8.4 grams fat; 72.4 milligrams cholesterol

# CHICKEN WITH CHINESE PEAS

∎

A super-simple Chinese dish. Serve with white rice, brown rice, or a combination of the two.

YIELD: 2 servings

PREPARATION TIME: 30 minutes

½ pound Chinese peas (about 2½ cups)
1 tablespoon peanut oil
1 large clove garlic, finely chopped
⅓ cup chicken broth
2 tablespoons rice vinegar
1 tablespoon oyster sauce
2 tablespoons soy sauce
6 ounces cooked chicken breast, skinned and shredded or chopped
2 ounces bean sprouts (about 1 cup)
1 tablespoon cornstarch
2 tablespoons cold water
½ cup canned or frozen baby corn, cooked
orange slices for garnish

Remove stems and strings from washed Chinese peas; set aside. Heat peanut oil in nonstick wok or pan over medium heat; add garlic and cook briefly. Add peas and stir-fry for 30 seconds. Add chicken broth, rice vinegar, oyster sauce, and soy sauce; stir-fry for 1 minute. Add chicken and bean sprouts, and stir-fry for an additional 30 to 60 seconds. Blend cornstarch into water; add to wok. Add baby corn and stir-fry until sauce is thickened and bubbly. Serve garnished with orange slices.

EXCHANGES

3 meat; 1 bread; 2 vegetable; ½ fat; 333 calories; 10.8 grams fat; 72.4 milligrams cholesterol

## Marinated Skewered Shark
■

Serve with Almond Snow Pea Salad, p. 232, and Seasoned Wild Rice, p. 278, or white rice for a special outdoor meal.

YIELD: 6 servings

PREPARATION TIME: 55 minutes

### Special utensils
12 thin metal skewers

1½ pounds shark steak (or other firm fish, such as halibut or swordfish), 1 inch thick
½ cup low-sodium soy sauce
1 tablespoon olive oil
2 tablespoons honey
2 tablespoons white wine vinegar
1 clove garlic, minced
½ tablespoon minced fresh ginger
¼ teaspoon pepper
1 medium-sized onion, cut into quarters and separated into pieces
3 oranges, each halved and then quartered
2 dozen cherry tomatoes

Cut fish into 1-inch cubes. In medium-size bowl combine soy sauce, olive oil, honey, vinegar, garlic, ginger, and pepper. Add fish, and toss gently to coat. Cover and refrigerate for 1 to 8 hours.

About 30 to 45 minutes before cooking, mix onion and orange pieces into marinade. Depending on cooking method, light the barbeque or preheat the broiler.

Remove fish, onion, and orange pieces from marinade, reserving marinade. Thread fish, cherry tomatoes, onion, and oranges alternatively onto skewers.

To barbeque: Coals are ready when you can comfortably hold your hand at grill level for 4 to 5 seconds. Place skewers on lightly greased grill set 4 inches above the coals. Cook, turning occasionally and basting frequently with reserved marinade until fish turns opaque and flakes easily, 8 to 10 minutes.

To broil: Prepare as above, using all-metal skewers. Place skewers on lightly greased broiler pan 4 to 6 inches from heat source. Cook as above, basting frequently.

EXCHANGES

3 meat; 1 vegetable; ⅔ fruit per serving; 218 calories; 6.5 grams fat; 57.8 milligrams cholesterol

# SIMMERED HALIBUT

∎

A beautiful presentation; serve with white rice.

YIELD: 4 (3-oz.) servings

PREPARATION TIME: 25 minutes

1 lb. fillets halibut or other firm fish
2 tablespoons flour
1 tablespoon olive oil
½ teaspoon sugar
1 teaspoon fresh minced ginger
1 clove garlic, minced
½ tablespoon soy sauce
¼ cup white wine
water
black pepper to taste
1 green onion, finely chopped
3 tablespoons chopped parsley
2 plum tomatoes, chopped

Wash fillets, shake off excess water, and coat lightly with flour. Heat olive oil in 10-inch nonstick skillet; brown fish over high heat on both sides. Meanwhile, combine sugar, ginger, garlic, soy sauce, white wine, and enough water to make 1 cup. Remove fish from heat, add wine mixture, and return to heat. Simmer, partly covered for 10 minutes per 1-inch thickness. Add black pepper, green onion, parsley, and plum tomatoes. Simmer uncovered until fish flakes with a fork, about 4 minutes.

EXCHANGES

3 meat; 1 vegetable per serving; 185 calories; 6.2 grams fat; 36.3 milligrams cholesterol

# COD DIJONNAIS (M)

∎

A fast, flavorful way to prepare fish.

YIELD: 4 servings

PREPARATION TIME: 20 minutes

1 tablespoon margarine
1 tablespoon white wine
2 tablespoons chopped shallots (about 2 shallots), or 1 tablespoon chopped
    white onion and 1 large clove garlic, minced
1 pound cod or other lean fish fillets, ½ to 1 inch thick
1½ tablespoons fresh lemon juice
1 tablespoon flour
about ⅓ cup nonfat milk
2 teaspoons Dijon mustard
¼ teaspoon salt
2 tablespoons chopped fresh parsley or dill
fresh lemon slices (optional)

In 2-quart microwave-safe dish place margarine, white wine, and shallots. Microwave on High until shallots are tender, 30 to 45 seconds. Place fish in dish with thicker parts to the outside. Pour lemon juice over fish. Cover tightly with lid or vented plastic wrap. Microwave on Medium until the fish flakes when pressed with a finger (it doesn't leave a dent), 7 to 11 minutes (time depends on microwave oven power and thickness of fillets), turning fillets once. Drain, reserving liquid. Let fish stand, covered, for 5 minutes.

Stir flour into reserved liquid. Add milk, if necessary, to yield ⅔ cup. Thin Dijon mustard with a few drops of milk. Stir thinned mustard and salt into liquid. Microwave, uncovered, on High for 1 minute; stir. Microwave on High until sauce thickens and begins to boil lightly, 1 to 1½ minutes. Transfer fillets to serving dish. Pour sauce over fish, top with parsley or dill, and garnish with lemon slices before serving.

EXCHANGES

3 meat per serving; 141 calories; 3.9 grams fat; 49.2 milligrams cholesterol

## SALMON PATTIES

■

Can be served hot, or as a cold sandwich filling.

YIELD: 4 servings

PREPARATION TIME: 35 minutes

### Special utensil
cheesecloth

9 ounces firm tofu
1 (7-ounce) can salmon, drained and flaked
2 egg whites
2 tablespoons seasoned bread crumbs
3 green onions, finely chopped
1 teaspoon prepared horseradish
1 teaspoon prepared mustard
¼ teaspoon black pepper

Squeeze water from tofu in cheesecloth. Break up tofu into small pieces and blend with salmon, using fork or food processor. Add other ingredients and mix well. Form into 4 patties; brown in non-stick pan over medium heat, about 5 minutes per side.

EXCHANGES

3 meat; 1 vegetable per serving; 191 calories; 8.8 grams fat; 27.4 milligrams cholesterol

## TROUT ALMONDINE

■

A traditionally elegant dish.

YIELD: 4 servings

PREPARATION TIME: 20 minutes

¼ cup flour
½ teaspoon seasoned salt
½ teaspoon paprika

1 pound trout fillets or other fresh fillets
2 tablespoons diet margarine, melted
2 tablespoons sliced almonds
2 tablespoons lemon juice
5 to 6 drops hot pepper sauce
1 tablespoon chopped parsley

Combine flour, seasoned salt, and paprika. Dredge fillets in flour mixture and place in single layer, skin side down, in baking dish sprayed with nonstick vegetable spray. Drizzle ½ tablespoon melted margarine over portions. Broil about 4 inches from heat until fish flakes easily with fork, 9 to 12 minutes. Sauté almonds in remaining margarine until golden, stirring continuously. Remove from heat; stir in lemon juice, hot pepper sauce, and parsley. Pour over fillets and serve.

EXCHANGES

3 meat; ½ bread per serving; 190 calories; 8.4 grams fat; 94.2 milligrams cholesterol

## REALLY EASY SALMON STEAKS
■

Serve with a garden salad and garlic toast for a "fast food" meal.

YIELD: 3 servings

PREPARATION TIME: 12 minutes

1 clove garlic, crushed
1 teaspoon olive oil
1 pound salmon steaks, 1 inch thick (3 steaks)
garlic salt to taste
seasoning salt to taste
pepper to taste

Brown garlic in olive oil in 10-inch nonstick pan; remove garlic. Sprinkle pan and salmon with garlic salt, a little seasoning salt, and pepper; add salmon. Cook, uncovered, over bare medium heat, 5 minutes. Turn and cook until fish is lightly browned and flakes easily with fork, about 5 more minutes.

EXCHANGES

> 4 meat per serving; 230 calories; 11.1 grams fat; 83.2 milligrams cholesterol

# QUICK CRAB CAKES
■

An easy seafood dish even steak eaters will love.

YIELD: 3 servings

PREPARATION TIME: 25 minutes

1 slice whole-wheat bread, toasted
2 egg whites
½ pound shelled cooked or drained canned crab, flaked
2 tablespoons drained chopped capers
1 tablespoon reduced-calorie mayonnaise
2 teaspoons lemon juice
1 tablespoon minced shallot
⅛ teaspoon cayenne
1 tablespoon extra-light olive oil
cocktail sauce or lemon wedges

Remove crust from bread; crumble. Combine bread crumbs and egg whites and beat with fork. Add crab, capers, mayonnaise, lemon juice, shallot, and cayenne, and mix thoroughly.

Heat olive oil in 12-inch nonstick skillet over medium heat. Spoon crab mixture into 5 or 6 mounds in skillet; flatten to make 1-inch-thick cakes. Sauté until cakes are lightly browned on both sides, about 10 minutes, turning once. Serve with cocktail sauce or lemon wedges.

EXCHANGES

> 2½ meat; ⅓ bread; 162 calories; 6.4 grams fat; 69.0 milligrams cholesterol

## LINGUINE WITH GARDEN TOMATOES
■

This dish takes advantage of your summer garden's bounty of luscious, fresh tomatoes.

YIELD: 3 servings

PREPARATION TIME: 27 minutes

1 tablespoon virgin olive oil
1 large clove garlic, minced
3 ripe medium-size tomatoes, chopped
3 tablespoons white wine
1 scant teaspoon Italian seasoning
6 ounces skinned, cooked boneless chicken or turkey, sliced
salt to taste
4 ounces dry linguine (other types of pasta may be used)
Parmesan cheese (optional)

Heat water for cooking pasta. In 12-inch nonstick skillet, heat 1 teaspoon of the olive oil over medium-high heat. Add garlic and sauté briefly, about 30 seconds. Add tomatoes, white wine, and Italian seasoning, and cook, stirring occasionally, until most of the liquid is evaporated, about 10 to 12 minutes. Add chicken and salt, and heat through.

Meanwhile, cook pasta al dente about 7 minutes, or according to package instructions. Drain pasta and rinse with hot water. Return to pot; toss with remaining olive oil. Serve pasta topped with tomato sauce, and Parmesan cheese if desired.

---

E X C H A N G E S

(without Parmesan cheese); 2 meat; 2 bread; 1 vegetable; ½ fat; 297 calories; 7.2 grams fat; 48.2 milligrams cholesterol

# SCALLOP PESTO CAPELLINI

■

Bay scallops in a light pesto sauce atop fresh angel hair pasta. Time the preparation so the scallop pesto is ready when the pasta is cooked al dente—so neither will be overcooked. The pesto can be made ahead of time and refrigerated until ready to use.

YIELD: 3 to 4 servings

PREPARATION TIME: 15 minutes

9 ounces fresh angel hair pasta
1 cup chopped, lightly packed basil (1 to 2 bunches)
2 tablespoons virgin olive oil
1 to 1½ tablespoons white wine
1 tablespoon Parmesan cheese
2 tablespoons pine nuts or chopped walnuts
1 clove garlic
½ teaspoon salt, divided
1 pound fresh bay scallops
½ tablespoon white wine
½ tablespoon virgin olive oil
cherry tomatoes for garnish (optional)
lemon wedges

Cook pasta al dente per package instructions; drain. To make pesto, combine basil, olive oil, 1 tablespoon white wine, Parmesan cheese, nuts, garlic, and ¼ teaspoon salt in food processor or blender and whirl until smooth, scraping sides several times. If sauce is too thick, add up to another ½ tablespoon white wine, a little at a time, until sauce is thick but not stiff. Rinse scallops and pat dry. Cook scallops in 10-inch nonstick skillet over medium heat until juices are released, about 1 minute. Add ½ tablespoon white wine. When bubbly, add pesto. Cook until scallops turn opaque and become firm, and excess liquid evaporates, 2 to 4 minutes. Place pasta on warm serving platter; add ½ tablespoon olive oil and remaining salt, and toss to coat thoroughly. Top with scallop pesto; garnish with tomatoes and lemon wedges.

---

EXCHANGES

| | |
|---|---|
| **for 4 servings:** | 3 meat; 2½ bread; ½ fat; 364 calories; 12.0 grams fat; 49.0 milligrams cholesterol |

# ORIENTAL NOODLES
■

This quick and colorful dish is a meal in itself. The MSG, added for extra flavor, can be omitted by those who are sensitive to it or the sodium in it.

YIELD: **4 servings**

PREPARATION TIME: **25 minutes**

3 cloves garlic, minced
½ small onion, chopped
1 tablespoon light olive oil
2 carrots, peeled and cut into strips
1¾ cups skinned, cooked shredded chicken breast (about 9 ounces)
2 tablespoons soy sauce
5 ounces Chinese peas (about 1⅔ cups), stems and strings removed
2 ounces mushrooms, sliced (about ¾ cup)
½ cup chicken broth or bouillon
2 (3-ounce) packages Ramen noodles, any flavor, cooked and drained (save
     seasoning packet for another time, or discard)
½ cup bean sprouts
½ teaspoon MSG
pepper to taste
1 green onion, finely chopped
fresh cilantro sprigs (optional)

Heat garlic and onion in hot olive oil in large nonstick skillet or wok over medium heat. Add carrots and chicken; stir-fry for 4 to 5 minutes. Add soy sauce, Chinese peas, mushrooms, and chicken broth or bouillon; stir-fry for about 2 minutes. Gently fold in noodles; heat briefly. Stir in bean sprouts, MSG, and pepper; cook for 3 to 4 minutes. Top with green onion and cilantro; serve.

---

E X C H A N G E S

> 2½ meat; 1½ bread; 2 vegetables per serving; 299 calories; 6.5 grams fat;
> 54.2 milligrams cholesterol

# EGGPLANT FRITTATA

∎

Great for a brunch or light supper. The cholesterol count is held down by substituting egg whites for some of the yolks.

YIELD: **6 servings**

PREPARATION TIME: **55 minutes**

## *Special utensil*
10- by 15-inch baking pan

1½ pounds small, slender eggplants, stems trimmed
1 large onion, thinly sliced crosswise and separated into rings
1 tablespoon olive oil
2 cloves chopped garlic
4 eggs
4 egg whites
¼ cup fresh grated Parmesan cheese
¼ cup fresh basil leaves, coarsely chopped
⅛ teaspoon ground oregano
⅛ teaspoon pepper
red leaf lettuce leaves for garnish

Line 10- by 15-inch pan with foil; spray with nonstick vegetable spray. Cut eggplants lengthwise into 1-inch strips; lay pieces, skin side down, in pan in a single layer. Mix onion slices with olive oil and garlic in small bowl, then spread evenly over eggplant. Bake in 475-degree oven until eggplant and onion are lightly browned and softened, 15 to 25 minutes. Cool slightly.

Transfer onion with garlic to 10-inch nonstick skillet sprayed generously with nonstick vegetable spray. Top with eggplant pieces side-by-side in a single layer, skin side up. Heat over low setting.

In medium mixing bowl, beat eggs and egg whites slightly. And Parmesan cheese, basil, oregano, and pepper, and beat. Pour egg mixture over eggplant. Cook over medium-low heat without stirring until eggs begin to set around pan rim but aren't cooked through, 8 to 10 minutes.

Transfer skillet to broiler; broil about 8 inches from heat source until the eggs are set, 2 to 3 minutes. Run a spatula around inside rim of pan to loosen eggs. Invert onto round platter. Arrange lettuce leaves on serving dishes. Cut wedges; place on lettuce. Serve warm or at room temperature.

EXCHANGES

> 1 meat; 2 vegetable; 1 fat per serving; 133 calories; 7.1 grams fat; 184.8 milligrams cholesterol

## Egg Burritos
■

Great for a casual brunch or hearty breakfast on the road. Serve with fresh fruit.

YIELD: 2 servings

PREPARATION TIME: 20 minutes

3 ounces ground turkey
2 tablespoons minced onion
2 flour tortillas (8-inch diameter)
1 large egg
3 egg whites or 7 tablespoons egg substitute
2 tablespoons nonfat milk
½ finely chopped serrano chile, seeds and membranes discarded
2 tablespoons salsa, drained
salt and pepper to taste

In 8-inch nonstick skillet cook turkey with onion, breaking it up with spatula as it cooks. (When done, turkey will be firm and cream-colored, with no trace of pink.) Set aside and keep warm.

Lightly moisten tortillas, wrap in foil, and warm in hot 325-degree oven for 10 to 12 minutes. Or cover tortillas with damp paper towel and microwave on High until hot, about 30 seconds, just before filling.

In small bowl beat egg, egg whites or egg substitute, milk, and chile. Spray nonstick omelette pan or 8-inch skillet with nonstick vegetable spray. Heat pan, then pour in egg mixture. As eggs begin to set, lift with spatula to allow uncooked portion to flow underneath.

When almost done, sprinkle ground turkey, onion, and salsa over eggs. Cook until eggs are completely set. Remove from heat. Divide eggs in half. Season with salt and pepper, if desired. Place one serving on one side of each burrito. Fold empty side over eggs, then fold sides over to cover eggs.

If burritos are to be eaten "on the road," enclose each burrito, folded side down, in foil. Wrap burritos in warm towel and place in a small insulated container.

---

E X C H A N G E S

> 2 meat; 1½ bread; 1 fat per serving; 271 calories; 10.2 grams fat; 233.3 milligrams cholesterol

## NILA'S CHICKEN ENCHILADA CASSEROLE
■

A great casual meal kids are guaranteed to love.

YIELD: 6 servings

PREPARATION TIME: 90 minutes

3 pounds chicken, either broiler-fryer or chicken pieces, skinned
3 stalks celery, coarsely chopped
1 large carrot, peeled and coarsely chopped
½ onion
1 clove garlic
½ teaspoon salt
⅛ teaspoon pepper
water
12 corn tortillas
1 (19-ounce) can enchilada sauce (mild to hot)
2 (4-ounce) cans fire-roasted whole green chiles (mild to hot), seeds and
    membranes removed, rinsed and diced
8 ounces low-fat (2 to 3 grams fat per ounce) Cheddar or Swiss cheese,
    shredded or sliced

Place chicken, celery, carrot, onion, garlic, salt, and pepper in large pot. Add water to cover; bring to boil over high heat. Reduce heat, cover, and simmer until chicken is fork-tender, about 35 minutes.

Remove chicken to large bowl; cool enough to handle and shred. Return bones to broth and simmer, uncovered, to make about 10 cups of chicken broth. (Strain broth, cover, and refrigerate for later use, skimming the fat before using.)

Heat tortillas in nonstick skillet over medium heat or on cookie sheet in moderate oven until lightly crisped. (They should hold their shape but not break when bent.) Overlap 6 tortillas to make one layer in a 9- by 13- by 2-inch pan. Top with half of the chicken, sauce, chiles, and cheese. Repeat for second layer. (If you intend to save some for another meal, leave the cheese off of that portion. Add cheese just before reheating.) Bake at 400 degrees until sauce is bubbly and cheese is melted, 10 to 15 minutes, and serve.

---

EXCHANGES

4 meat; 2 bread; 1 vegetable per serving; 409 calories; 12.4 grams fat; 79.4 milligrams cholesterol

## BLUE BUFFALO CALZONE

■

Your family members and guests will enjoy pitching in to fix dinner when this dish is on the menu.

YIELD: 6 servings

PREPARATION TIME: 30 minutes, plus thawing and baking time

6 ounces grated Gorgonzola (Italian blue) cheese
1 tablespoon flour
12 ounces frozen chopped spinach, thawed and squeezed thoroughly dry
1 (4-ounce) can sliced mushrooms
1½ cups seeded chopped plum tomatoes, drained of excess juice
3 green onions, chopped
2 cloves garlic, minced
1 pound pizza or bread dough, thawed
6 ounces shredded buffalo mozzarella cheese

Mix Gorgonzola cheese with flour in bowl. Combine with spinach, mushrooms, tomatoes, onions, and garlic; set aside. Divide dough into 6 sections. Roll each section into circle ¼-inch thick. Spread some of the Gorgonzola cheese mixture evenly over half of each circle. Top with buffalo mozzarella cheese. Fold uncovered half of each circle over the filled half. Press edges together firmly and completely. Place calzones on greased cookie sheet several inches apart. Bake at 425 degrees until golden brown, 20 to 25 minutes.

EXCHANGES

> 2 meat; 2½ bread; 1 vegetable; 2 fat per serving; 414 calories; 18.4 grams fat; 47.3 milligrams cholesterol

# ITALIAN-STYLE TURKEY BURGERS
∎

Low-fat burgers with an Old World flair.

YIELD: 4 burgers

PREPARATION TIME: 12 minutes

1 pound lean ground turkey
¼ cup Italian-style seasoned bread crumbs
½ cup onion, finely chopped
1 egg white
¼ cup oatmeal
1 teaspoon Worcestershire sauce
½ teaspoon poultry or Italian seasoning
½ teaspoon garlic salt
½ teaspoon garlic powder

Combine all ingredients. Form into 4 patties ½-inch thick. Broil, 4 inches from heat, for 4 to 5 minutes. Turn and broil until meat has turned gray from pink, 3 to 4 minutes.

EXCHANGES

> 3 meat; ⅔ bread; ½ fat per serving; 243 calories, 11.5 grams fat; 74.3 milligrams cholesterol

# Falafel Pockets
■

An easy vegetarian dish that any guest will enjoy.

YIELD: 8 servings

PREPARATION TIME: 20 minutes

⅔ cup egg whites or fat-free egg substitute
¾ cup nonfat milk
1 (8-ounce) package falafel mix
2 small or 1 large clove garlic, minced
8 Flatbread Rounds, page 292, or 8 pita bread pockets
3 medium tomatoes, sliced
2 cups shredded iceberg lettuce
6 ounces (1½ cups) shredded Cheddar cheese
1 cup tahini, page 236 (optional); tahini can also be purchased in Middle
    Eastern markets or health food stores

In medium bowl, beat egg whites or egg substitute, milk, falafel mix, and garlic until evenly moistened. Form into 16 patties, each about ¾-inch thick. Place on cookie sheet and bake at 350 degrees until browned, 12 to 15 minutes. To serve, place 2 patties in middle of each flatbread. Top with tomato slices, lettuce, Cheddar cheese, and tahini. Fold up and eat taco-style. (Or slice each pita bread so that one side is bigger than the other. Place the smaller piece inside the larger one at the bottom. Fill with patties and toppings.)

---

E X C H A N G E S (without tahini)

1½ bread; 1 meat; 1 vegetable; 1 fat per serving; 229 calories; 7.6 grams fat; 22.7 milligrams cholesterol

## Mushroom Steak

■

Lean beef simmered in a mushroom-wine sauce.

YIELD: 2 servings

PREPARATION TIME: 22 minutes,
plus marinating time

9 ounces lean steak, ½-inch thick (such as round steak)
¼ cup white wine
1 tablespoon Worcestershire sauce
2 teaspoons light olive oil
2 shallots, thinly sliced
½ cup thinly sliced mushrooms
¼ teaspoon salt
fresh pepper

Trim fat from steak; cut into two servings. Place steaks in flat-bottomed container. Add wine and Worcestershire sauce; marinate for at least 30 minutes. (Refrigerate if marinated longer.)

Heat olive oil in 10-inch nonstick skillet. Remove steaks from marinade, shaking off excess liquid. Add steaks and shallots to pan; brown steaks on both sides over medium-high heat. Turn down heat; add marinade, mushrooms, and salt. Simmer lightly, covered, until done, about 10 minutes for medium. Grind fresh pepper on top before serving.

---

EXCHANGES

3½ meat; 1 vegetable per serving; 258 calories; 12.5 grams fat; 81.4 milligrams cholesterol

# Beef Tomato
■

A great dish for lean cuts of beef or veal—the marinade tenderizes the meat, and the quick cooking method keeps it moist and juicy. Serve over white rice or with warm flour tortillas.

YIELD: 2 to 3 servings

PREPARATION TIME: 30 minutes,
plus marinating time

¾ pound lean beef (such as top round or flank steak)
1 teaspoon blended whiskey
1 tablespoon regular or low-sodium soy sauce
1 tablespoon cornstarch
2 teaspoons sugar
1 tablespoon light olive oil
1 medium-size white onion, sliced
3 stalks celery, chopped
4 medium-size ripe tomatoes, sliced lengthwise
1 teaspoon cornstarch
2 teaspoons water
1 green onion, thinly sliced (including top)

Trim fat from beef and discard. Rinse beef and pat dry. Slice into thin strips across the grain, with knife blade almost parallel to cutting surface. In medium-sized bowl, thoroughly blend whiskey, soy sauce, cornstarch and sugar. Add beef strips and toss to coat. Marinate for at least 30 to 60 minutes.

Heat olive oil in a 10- or 12-inch nonstick skillet over medium heat. Remove beef from marinade with tongs or slotted spoon and add to skillet, reserving marinade. Stir-fry beef until almost done, about 4 minutes. Remove from pan. Add onion and celery and stir-fry until lightly browned, about 3 minutes. Add tomatoes and cook for 2 to 3 minutes (do not let tomatoes get mushy). Return beef and reserved marinade to pan and cook for 1 minute.

Stir cornstarch into water to blend; pour into skillet. Heat and stir until gravy thickens and begins to boil. Top with green onion and serve.

EXCHANGES

| | |
|---|---|
| **for 3 servings:** | 3 meat; 3 vegetable; ½ fat per serving; 282 calories; 11.8 grams fat; 69.8 milligrams cholesterol |

# PORK TOFU
∎

Marinated lean pork and cubed tofu in ginger sauce with colorful vegetables.

YIELD: 3 to 4 servings

PREPARATION TIME: 25 minutes,
plus marinating time

1 tablespoon grated fresh ginger
4 teaspoons soy sauce
½ cup defatted chicken broth
1 teaspoon sugar
½ pound lean pork, sliced thinly into 1½-inch strips
1 (14-ounce) block tofu, drained and cut into 1-inch cubes
1 tablespoon peanut oil
½ large white onion, sliced
½ large red bell pepper, cut into strips
1½ tablespoons cornstarch
½ cup green onion, cut into 1-inch lengths
4 sticks fresh pineapple for garnish (optional)

Combine ginger, soy sauce, chicken broth (reserve 2 tablespoons), and sugar in medium bowl or plastic container. Mix in pork and tofu; marinate for at least 1 hour and up to 24 hours. Drain and separate pork and tofu, reserving marinade. Heat peanut oil in 12-inch non-stick skillet. Add pork, onion, and bell pepper, and sauté over medium-high heat until pork is lightly browned. Add marinade and bring to boil; reduce heat. Simmer until vegetables are crisp-tender. Blend cornstarch into reserved chicken broth until smooth. Add to skillet along with tofu and green onion, stirring carefully until sauce is thickened and bubbly, 3 to 5 minutes. Serve with rice; garnish with fresh pineapple sticks.

E X C H A N G E S

| | |
|---|---|
| **for 4 servings:** | 3 meat; ½ bread; 1 vegetable; 2 fat; ½ fruit; 356 calories; 19.1 grams fat; 40.4 milligrams |

# Seasoned Pork Chops with Wine Sauce
■

A delicious way to serve lean pork.

YIELD: 4 servings

PREPARATION TIME: 1 hour

1 teaspoon dried sage leaves, crumbled
1 teaspoon dried rosemary leaves, crushed
1 teaspoon finely chopped garlic
fresh ground pepper
4 center-cut loin pork chops, very lean, about 1 inch thick (about 12 ounces)
½ tablespoon margarine
1 tablespoon olive oil
¾ cup dry white wine
1 tablespoon finely chopped fresh parsley

Combine sage, rosemary, garlic, and pepper to taste. Trim fat from pork chops; press seasoning mixture firmly into both sides of each pork chop. Heat margarine and olive oil in 10-inch nonstick skillet over medium heat. Add chops and brown for 2 to 3 minutes on each side. Remove chops and set aside.

Pour out any excess fat from pan, add ½ cup white wine, and bring to boil. Return chops to pan, cover, and simmer over very low heat. Cook chops until fork-tender, about 25 to 30 minutes, basting occasionally. Remove chops to heated serving platter.

Add remaining wine to skillet. Boil vigorously over high heat, scraping brown bits from bottom and sides of pan until combination has reduced to a syrupy sauce. Stir in chopped parsley. Pour sauce over pork chops and serve.

EXCHANGES

2½ meat; 1½ fat per serving; 210 calories; 14.7 grams fat; 60.6 milligrams cholesterol

## BROILED LAMB CHOPS WITH MINT DRESSING
■

The nutritional quality of lamb chops is similar to that of beef.

YIELD: 4 servings

PREPARATION TIME: 25 minutes

½ tablespoon olive oil
1 large clove garlic, minced
1 cup sliced mushrooms
2 tablespoons chopped fresh parsley
2 tablespoons chopped fresh mint leaves
¼ teaspoon salt
pepper to taste
1 cup cooked bulgur wheat
3 tablespoons apple juice
4 lamb loin chops, 1 inch thick, well trimmed
mint sprigs for garnish

In 10-inch nonstick skillet heat olive oil; add garlic, mushrooms, parsley, mint leaves, salt, and pepper, and cook over medium heat until vegetables are tender. Add bulgur wheat and apple juice; cook and stir until hot. Starting with fatty side, cut each chop almost to the bone, to form a pocket. Fill each pocket with one quarter of the stuffing; use toothpicks to keep stuffing in place. Broil chops until done, about 15 minutes, turning once. Discard toothpicks; garnish with mint.

---

EXCHANGES

3 meat; 1 bread; 1 fat per serving; 276 calories; 12.0 grams fat; 83.4 milligrams cholesterol

# VEAL PAPRIKA WITH MUSHROOMS

■

Great over noodles or white rice.

YIELD: 6 servings

PREPARATION TIME: 2 hours

2 tablespoons extra-light olive oil
1½ pounds boneless lean veal
1½ onions, chopped
¼ pound fresh mushrooms, sliced
1½ to 2 tablespoons spicy paprika (or use mild paprika and add ⅛ teaspoon
    cayenne pepper)
1 (14½-ounce) can chicken broth, defatted
4 teaspoons cornstrarch
1 tablespoon chopped fresh parsley for garnish

Trim all fat from veal; cube. Heat olive oil in 3-quart saucepan; brown veal over medium-high heat. Remove veal; add onions, mushrooms, and paprika. Sauté for 2 to 3 minutes. Return veal to pan and coat with onion mixture, using wooden spoon. Add all chicken broth except 2 tablespoons. Bring stew to boil. Reduce heat and simmer gently, uncovered, until veal is tender, about 1½ hours. Blend cornstarch into reserved chicken broth; add to stew and bring to boil over medium heat, stirring constantly. Serve topped with fresh parsley.

---

E X C H A N G E S

3½ meat; 1 vegetable; 1 fat; 273 calories; 15.2 grams fat; 86.7 milligrams cholesterol

## VEAL PICCATA ON FRESH PASTA
■

Serve with Caesar salad for a special meal.

YIELD: 3 to 4 servings

PREPARATION TIME: 20 minutes

7 ounces fresh linguine
⅓ cup flour
1 teaspoon salt
¼ teaspoon paprika
2 teaspoons margarine
2 teaspoons virgin olive oil
¾ pound veal cutlets for scaloppine (4 pieces)
2 tablespoons dry white wine
2 tablespoons lemon juice
1 tablespoon capers
2 teaspoons virgin olive oil
1 clove garlic, minced
1½ ounces fresh grated Parmesan cheese
2 to 3 tablespoons minced fresh parsley
lemon slices for garnish

Cook linguine according to package instructions; drain. Combine flour, salt, and paprika on plate. Heat margarine and olive oil in nonstick skillet over medium heat.

Coat cutlets in flour mixture; add to pan, and sauté until meat is browned outside and white inside, 1 to 2 minutes per side. Remove to warm plate. Add white wine to pan and cook, stirring to remove brown bits from bottom of pan. Add lemon juice; heat briefly. Add capers, then cover and turn down heat to lowest setting. Return linguine to pot, and coat with olive oil over low heat. Add garlic, Parmesan cheese, and parsley, and mix completely.

Place pasta on warm platter. Arrange veal cutlets on top of pasta. Pour wine mixture over all. Garnish with lemon slices.

---

EXCHANGES

| | |
|---|---|
| **for 3 servings:** | 3½ meat; 3 bread; 3 fat; 665 calories, 27.5 grams fat; 95.5 milligrams cholesterol |
| **for 4 servings:** | 3 meat; 2 bread; 2½ fat; 499 calories; 20.6 grams fat; 71.6 milligrams cholesterol |

# Side Dishes

## BROCCOLI AU GRATIN (M)

Just about everyone loves broccoli—for its taste and visual appeal as well as its abundance of nutrients. But even old favorites can periodically use some sprucing up. This recipe offers a quick and easy way to add a little pizazz to basic broccoli.

YIELD: 4 servings

PREPARATION TIME: 18 minutes

1 (1-pound) bunch fresh broccoli
1 small clove garlic, minced or pressed
2 tablespoons water
3 tablespoons seasoned bread crumbs
1½ tablespoons chicken bouillon or broth
1 tablespoon chopped fresh tarragon, basil, or parsley or 1 teaspoon dried
½ lemon, thinly sliced

Trim 1 inch from end of broccoli; discard. Slice broccoli into 8 to 12 long spears. Starting at stalk end, cut 2-inch slit lengthwise in thicker spears for more even cooking. Position broccoli in 2-quart microwave-safe dish with flower ends in center and stalk ends facing out. Top with garlic, then water. Cover tightly and microwave on high until stalks can be pierced with fork, 5 to 7½ minutes (the longer time for low-wattage ovens, the shorter time for high-wattage ovens), rotating dish one-quarter turn halfway through cooking time. Let stand, covered, for 3 minutes; drain.

Combine bread crumbs and chicken bouillon or broth; sprinkle this mixture on broccoli; top with chopped herbs. Garnish with lemon slices; serve.

EXCHANGES

> 2 vegetable per serving; 54 calories; 0.7 gram fat; 0.2 milligram cholesterol

# ITALIAN-STYLE COUSCOUS
■

Couscous is steamed semolina best known as the principal ingredient in the North African dish of the same name. Serve either hot as a side dish or as a chilled salad.

YIELD: 6 (¾-cup) servings

PREPARATION TIME: 35 minutes

olive oil-flavored vegetable spray or olive oil
2 to 3 Italian plum tomatoes, finely chopped (about 1 cup)
1 medium onion, chopped
1 tablespoon minced fresh or 1 teaspoon crumbled dry rosemary
3 tablespoons chopped fresh or 1 tablespoon crumbled dry basil
½ tablespoon chopped fresh or ½ teaspoon crumbled dry oregano
1 large clove garlic, minced, or ½ teaspoon garlic powder
1 (14½-ounce) can chicken broth, defatted
2 tablespoons lime juice
1 cup couscous
¼ cup fresh grated Parmesan cheese

Spray 10-inch nonstick skillet with vegetable spray, or coat thinly with olive oil. Over medium-high heat, stir in tomatoes, onion, rosemary, basil, oregano, and garlic powder. Cover and cook until tomatoes get juicy, 2 to 3 minutes. Uncover and simmer, stirring frequently, until juices evaporate, about 5 minutes. Add broth and lime juice and bring to a boil. Stir in couscous, cover, and remove from heat. Let stand until liquid is absorbed, about 8 minutes. Fluff with a fork, then stir in Parmesan cheese.

EXCHANGES

> 1¼ bread; 1 vegetable per serving; 127 calories; 1.7 grams fat; 2.4 milligrams cholesterol

# Peppered Chayote with Cajun Stuffing (M)

■

Pronounced kay-YO-tay and also known as mirliton, this member of the cucumber family is celery-green, pear-shaped, and 3 to 6 inches in length.

YIELD: 4 servings

PREPARATION TIME: 45 minutes, if baking; 25 minutes using a microwave

2 very firm medium-size chayotes (if unavailable, use 2 zucchini and reduce cooking time)
2 teaspoons extra-light olive oil
2 cloves garlic, minced
1 rib celery, finely chopped
½ medium onion, chopped
½ cup each diced red and yellow bell peppers
¼ cup defatted chicken broth
½ teaspoon dried basil leaves or ½ tablespoon fresh chopped basil
½ teaspoon dried oregano leaves or ½ tablespoon fresh chopped oregano
¼ teaspoon paprika
6 to 9 drops red pepper (Tabasco) sauce
1 cup cooked rice
¼ teaspoon salt
parsley for garnish (optional)

Cut chayotes in half lengthwise; remove seed and discard. Bake halves in hot 375-degree oven until fork-tender, 30 to 40 minutes.

Heat olive in nonstick 10-inch skillet over medium-high heat. Add garlic, celery, onion, and peppers. Stir-fry until crisp-tender, 5 to 7 minutes. Stir in chicken broth, basil and oregano leaves, paprika, and red pepper sauce. Bring to boil; reduce heat and simmer until most of the liquid has evaporated. Mix in rice and salt; heat through. Scoop one quarter of the vegetable mixture onto each chayote half. Garnish with parsley; serve.

To microwave: Delete olive oil; reduce chicken broth to 3 tablespoons and red pepper sauce to 4 to 7 drops.

Pierce chayotes with fork in several places. Microwave on high for 5½ to 8½ minutes or until tender (the longer time for low-wattage ovens, the shorter time for high-wattage ovens). Let stand for 5 minutes. Cut in half lengthwise; remove seed.

Combine olive oil, garlic, celery, onion, peppers, broth, basil and oregano leaves, paprika, and red pepper sauce in microwave-safe 1½-

quart casserole; cover with glass lid or vented plastic wrap. Micro-wave on high until vegetables are crisp-tender, 5 to 8 minutes, stirring after 3 minutes. Stir in rice and salt, cover, and microwave on high to heat through, about 30 seconds, stirring once. Scoop one quarter of the vegetable mixture onto each chayote half. Garnish with parsley and serve.

---

E X C H A N G E

> ¾ bread; 2 vegetable; ½ fat per serving; 118 calories; 2.9 grams fat; 0.0 milligram cholesterol

## Asparagus with Mild Peanut Sauce
■

Try this recipe with broccoli when asparagus is out of season. Serve with roasted chicken and rice.

YIELD: **4 servings**

PREPARATION TIME: **25 minutes**

1 pound fresh asparagus
½ tablespoon peanut oil
1 cup sliced mushrooms
2 teaspoons cornstarch
2 tablespoons low-sodium soy sauce
1 tablespoon chunky peanut butter
¼ cup defatted chicken broth
dash sugar
pepper to taste
2 teaspoons minced cilantro
1 tablespoon chopped peanuts

Snap ends from asparagus; discard. Slice asparagus diagonally. Heat peanut oil in nonstick skillet or wok and stir-fry asparagus until it turns bright green, 3 to 5 minutes. Move asparagus to one side; add mushrooms and sauté for 2 minutes.

In small bowl, blend cornstarch into soy sauce until smooth. Add peanut butter and beat with fork or wire whisk until blended. Mix in chicken broth and sugar. Add to asparagus and season with pepper. Cook until sauce is thickened and bubbly, 1 to 2 minutes. Sprinkle with cilantro and peanuts before serving.

EXCHANGES

> 2 vegetable; 1 fat per serving; 94 calories; 5.3 grams fat; 0.0 milligram cholesterol

## GRILLED VEGETABLE WRAPS

∎

Tender summer squash, eggplant, and seasonings combine in this terrific cooked salad.

YIELD: **4 servings**

PREPARATION TIME: **20 minutes**

1 medium-sized zucchini
1 medium-sized yellow squash
1 cup eggplant chunks, 1-inch diameter
1 medium-size red onion, cut into 8 wedges
1 small glove garlic, minced
1 tablespoon virgin olive oil
1 tablespoon white wine vinegar
1 teaspoon dried oregano leaves
½ teaspoon sugar
½ teaspoon salt
heavy-duty aluminum foil

Cut zucchini and yellow squash into ¾-inch slices, then combine all ingredients in large bowl. Tear four 12-inch-square sheets of foil. Divide the vegetables among the foil sheets; bring two opposite sides together and fold over several times. Fold ends together and press tightly to seal all around. Grill or broil pouches, 4 inches from heat, until vegetables are crisp-tender, 10 to 12 minutes, turning once. When serving, open pockets carefully, watching for escaping steam.

EXCHANGES

> 1 vegetable; ¾ fat per serving; 59 calories; 3.6 grams fat; 0.0 milligram cholesterol

# TOFU-VEGETABLE MEDLEY

■

Tofu is mild in flavor, packed with protein, scant on calories, and cholesterol-free. If you don't have some of the vegetables needed for this dish, substitute with whatever is in your fridge.

YIELD: 4 servings

PREPARATION TIME: 35 minutes

2 tablespoons soy sauce
1 tablespoon oyster sauce
2 tablespoons rice vinegar
1 (8-ounce) can pineapple chunks (in its own juice), drained; reserve liquid
10 ounces firm or extra-firm tofu, drained well and cut into ½-inch cubes
1 tablespoon sesame oil
2 large cloves garlic, minced
1 tablespoon grated fresh ginger
½ cup diagonally sliced carrots
¼ pound broccoli florets (about 2 cups)
½ red bell pepper, sliced
¼ pound snow peas, strings and stems removed (about 1¼ cups)
¼ pound mushrooms, sliced (about 1 cup)
½ cup sliced water chestnuts
1 tablespoon cornstarch
2 tablespoons roasted peanuts
2 teaspoons grated lemon zest

Combine soy sauce, oyster sauce, rice vinegar, and reserved pineapple juice in small bowl. Add tofu and marinate in refrigerator for at least 1 hour, or overnight.

Heat sesame oil in nonstick 12-inch skillet or wok over medium heat. Add garlic and ginger, and sauté for 30 seconds. Add carrots; stir-fry for 2 minutes. Add broccoli and bell pepper and stir-fry for 1 to 2 minutes Add snow peas, mushrooms, water chestnuts, and pineapple chunks; stir-fry until vegetables are just crisp-tender, about 2 minutes.

Remove tofu from marinade; carefully add tofu to skillet. Blend cornstarch into marinade; add to skillet and stir-fry until sauce is thickened and begins to boil. Top with roasted peanuts and lemon zest. Serve alone or on top of rice or noodles.

## LEMON GREEN BEANS
∎

Apple and onion make this dish naturally sweet—great with sliced turkey or chicken.

YIELD: 10 (½-cup) servings

PREPARATION TIME: 25 minutes

2 (9-ounce) boxes frozen French-style green beans (about 3 cups cooked)
1 tablespoon margarine
2 teaspoons sugar
¼ teaspoon paprika
4 whole cloves
½ lemon, unpeeled, thinly sliced
1 large unpeeled red apple, cored and cubed
1 cup small white pearl onions
1 tablespoon cornstarch

Cook green beans in water according to package directions. Drain beans, reserving ½ cup of the cooking water. Heat ¼ cup of the reserved water with margarine, sugar, paprika, and cloves. Add lemon slices. Cover and simmer until lemon is translucent, about 8 minutes. Stir in apple and onions and cook until tender. Dissolve cornstarch in ¼ cup remaining reserved water. Blend into lemon sauce; cook until thickened, stirring constantly. Carefully stir in beans and cook until heated through. Remove cloves before serving.

## Green Beans Continental (M)

∎

This delicious recipe can be easily prepared on stovetop or in the microwave.

YIELD: 6 (½-cup) servings

PREPARATION TIME: 30 minutes

1 pound green beans, stemmed and cut into 1-inch pieces
1 carrot, halved and cut into ⅜-inch-thick strips
1 tablespoon margarine
½ pound mushrooms cut into ¼-inch slices
1 medium onion cut into ¼-inch slices
1 clove garlic, minced
1 teaspoon salt
⅛ teaspoon white pepper

Steam green beans and carrot strips for 10 minutes in covered 3-quart saucepan. Meanwhile, heat margarine in nonstick 10-inch skillet. Stir in mushrooms and onion; cook over low heat for 3 minutes. Stir in beans, carrots, garlic, salt, and pepper. Cover and cook until tender, about 5 minutes.

*To microwave:* Reduce garlic to 1 small clove and salt to ⅔ teaspoon. Place green beans and carrot strips with ¼ cup water in 2-quart casserole; cover. Microwave on High for 6 to 10 minutes (the longer time for low-wattage ovens, the shorter time for high-wattage ovens), stirring once halfway through cooking time. Let stand, covered.

In 1½-quart casserole place margarine and onion. Microwave on High for 1 minute or until margarine melts. Add mushrooms, stir, and microwave on High for 1½ to 2½ minutes. Drain beans and carrots; add mushroom-onion mixture, garlic, and pepper. Cover and microwave on High until tender, 1½ to 3 minutes. Stir in salt.

EXCHANGES

1½ vegetable; ½ fat per serving; 61 calories; 2.2 grams fat; 0.0 milligram cholesterol

## Mild Greens Pesto Style (M)
■

For best results, choose crisp, bright-colored greens with no yellow spots. Avoid woody stems or wide veins in the leaves.

YIELD: 4 servings

PREPARATION TIME: 18 minutes

2 pounds fresh Swiss chard, spinach, or other mild-flavored greens
2 teaspoons olive oil
2 cloves minced garlic
½ cup lightly packed chopped fresh basil
2 tablespoons pine nuts, lightly toasted
2 tablespoons grated fresh Parmesan cheese
½ teaspoon salt
¼ teaspoon pepper

Remove stems from leaves; discard. Wash leaves well; cut into ½-inch strips while still wet. In 3-quart casserole combine olive oil, garlic, and greens; cover tightly and microwave on High until tender but firm (not soggy), 2 to 4 minutes, stirring once. Let stand, covered, for 2 minutes. Stir in basil, pine nuts, Parmesan cheese, salt, and pepper. Microwave on High for 10 to 20 seconds; serve.

E X C H A N G E S

2 vegetable; 1 fat per serving; 96 calories; 5.2 grams fat; 1.8 milligrams cholesterol

*Precise cooking time depends on type of greens used and microwave oven power. If more fully cooked greens are desired, increase cooking time to 5½ to 8½ minutes.

## Risotto with Radicchio and Peas (M)

■

The microwave oven was just made for this dish, which takes much longer on the stovetop. The rice should be cooked al dente, or until tender on the outside but still firm in shape and texture.

YIELD: **6 servings**

PREPARATION TIME: **40 minutes**

### Special utensils
microwave-safe 10-inch round dish or 11- by 8½- by 2-inch dish

1 tablespoon olive oil
½ cup minced onion
1 cup Arborio rice (round, short-grain Italian rice); if unavailable, use converted rice
3 cups defatted chicken broth (at room temperature)
1½ packed cups shredded radicchio (approximately 1 small)
1 cup tender frozen peas, thawed
½ teaspoon salt (omit if salted broth is used)
¼ cup grated fresh Parmesan cheese

Heat olive oil and onion in microwave-safe 10-inch round or 11- by 8½- by 2-inch dish, uncovered, on High for 2 to 3 minutes or until the onion is tender. Add rice and stir to coat. Cook for 2 to 3 minutes (the longer time for low-wattage ovens; the shorter time for high-wattage ovens).

Stir in chicken broth and cook, uncovered, on High for 9½ to 13 minutes. Add radicchio; stir. Microwave, uncovered, on High until rice swells and almost all the liquid is gone, about 9 to 11 minutes (the longer time for low-wattage ovens, the shorter time for high-wattage ovens). Stir in peas and salt. Cover and let stand for 5 minutes. Stir in Parmesan cheese; serve.

EXCHANGES

1½ bread; 1½ vegetable; 1 fat; 197 calories; 4.2 grams fat; 2.4 milligrams cholesterol

## Root Vegetable Sauté

■

Simple root vegetables have all but been forgotten in this age of arrugula and radicchio. They reclaim their rightful place in the diet, however, in this easy, tasty, and inexpensive dish.

YIELD: **6 servings**

PREPARATION TIME: **15 minutes**

1 tablespoon margarine
1 medium sweet potato, peeled and cut into 1-inch cubes
1 medium white potato, cut into ½-inch cubes
1 medium parsnip, peeled and sliced
1 carrot, peeled and sliced
1 medium turnip, peeled and sliced
½ teaspoon salt
⅛ teaspoon pepper
¼ teaspoon ground nutmeg
1 tablespoon finely chopped green onion (including tops) or chives

In 12-inch skillet sprayed with nonstock vegetable spray, melt margarine over medium-low heat. Add sweet potato, white potato, parsnip, carrot, turnip, salt, pepper, and nutmeg. Sauté until vegetables are tender and browned, stirring occasionally, 10 to 12 minutes. Sprinkle with green onion; serve.

---

E X C H A N G E S

¾ bread; ½ fat per serving; 72 calories; 2.1 grams fat; 0.0 milligram cholesterol

# BOK CHOY WITH WATERCRESS

■

Also known as Chinese mustard cabbage, bok choy has long, white, stringless stalks and dark green leaves. Its satisfying crunch and delicate flavor make it a popular vegetable in Oriental cuisine.

YIELD: 6 (½-cup) servings

PREPARATION TIME: 27 minutes

1¼ pounds bok choy
⅔ cup chicken broth, defatted
2 tablespoons soy sauce
1 tablespoon cornstarch
1 teaspoon sugar
1 tablespoon peanut oil
1 teaspoon grated fresh ginger
1 clove garlic, minced
¼ pound shitake mushrooms, sliced
2 green onions, chopped
1 medium carrot, sliced diagonally
1 bunch watercress, chopped

Separate leaves and stalks of bok choy. Cut stalks into ¼- to ½-inch slices. Combine ⅓ cup chicken broth, soy sauce, cornstarch, and sugar until smooth; set aside. Heat peanut oil in 12-inch nonstock skillet or wok. Add ginger, garlic, mushrooms, and green onions and sauté for 2 minutes. Remove from wok and set aside. Add bok choy stalks, carrot, and ⅓ cup chicken broth to wok and simmer until tender-crisp, about 4 minutes. Add soy sauce mixture and stir over medium heat until mixture boils and thickens. Add mushroom mixture, bok choy leaves, and watercress; stir-fry until leaves and watercress wilt.

EXCHANGES

2 vegetables; ½ fat per serving; 69 calories; 2.7 grams fat; 0.0 milligram cholesterol

# Polenta Marinara
∎

Polenta—coursely ground, boiled cornmeal high in complex carbohy-drates and low in fat—doesn't sound like much. But put it with a tasty marinara sauce and it will really surprise you!

YIELD: 8 servings

PREPARATION TIME: 1 hour

*Special utensil*
5-quart saucepan

1 tablespoon oilive oil
1 large onion, chopped
3 cloves garlic, minced
8 large Italian plum tomatoes (about 2 pounds), or 1 (28-ounce) can whole
    tomatoes (including juice), quartered
1 (6-ounce) can tomato paste
½ pound mushrooms, sliced
½ cup finely chopped green pepper
½ cup dry red wine
1 cube chicken bouillon
½ cup water
⅓ cup chopped fresh basil
1 teaspoon Italian seasoning
1 teaspoon sugar
1½ cups polenta or yellow cornmeal
7 cups water
½ cup freshly grated Parmesan cheese

Heat olive oil in 5-quart saucepan over medium heat. Add onion and garlic and sauté until onion is soft, about 10 minutes, stirring fre-quently. Stir in tomatoes, tomato paste, mushrooms, green pepper, red wine, chicken bouillon, water, basil, Italian seasoning, and sugar. Bring sauce to boil over high heat; cook and stir until sauce is very thick, 30 to 40 minutes.

Bring water to boil in 4- or 5-quart pan. Gradually add polenta or yellow cornmeal, stirring until blended. Reduce heat to low and stir frequently until polenta or yellow cornmeal is smooth and has a consistency similar to that of mayonnaise, about 8 to 10 minutes.

Into serving bowl immediately pour Polenta or yellow cornmeal, smoothing it out into layer 1- to 1½ inches thick. Top with marinara sauce and Parmesan cheese.

EXCHANGES

1½ bread; 1 vegetable; 1 fat per serving; 183 calories; 4.6 grams fat; 3.7 milligrams cholesterol

## SEASONED WILD RICE
▪

A special accompaniment to poultry or broiled fish.

YIELD:  8 (½-cup) servings

PREPARATION TIME: 1½ hours

1 cup wild rice
3½ cups chicken broth, defatted (2 [14½-ounce] cans)
¼ teaspoon dried or 1 teaspoon each crushed fresh sage, thyme, and marjoram
2 green onions, finely chopped (including tops)
2 teaspoons margarine

Cover wild rice with water and let stand at room temperature overnight. Drain and rinse with fresh water. Or pour boiling water over wild rice and let set for 30 minutes; drain well. Transfer rice, chicken broth, and spices to heavy 3-quart saucepan. Bring to boil. Cover, reduce heat, and simmer for 45 to 60 minutes or until most of the liquid has been absorbed. Fluff rice with fork; stir in green onions and margarine. Cook uncovered to evaporate any excess moisture, if needed.

EXCHANGES

1 bread; ½ fat per serving; 100 calories; 1.8 grams fat; 1.1 milligrams cholesterol

## Stir-Fried Rice
∎

A welcome accompaniment to a simple entrée such as broiled chicken or steamed fish.

YIELD: 6 to 8 servings

PREPARATION TIME: 15 minutes

1 egg
2 egg whites or ¼ cup nonfat egg substitute
1 tablespoon peanut oil
½ cup diced lean ham (or leftover meat of any kind)
½ cup frozen baby peas
½ cup sliced fresh mushrooms or bamboo shoots
1 medium carrot cut into 1½-inch slivers
1 tablespoon soy sauce
1 tablespoon oyster sauce (available in the Oriental section of large markets)
3 cups cooked rice
¼ cup thinly sliced green onions

Beat egg with egg whites lightly; set aside. Heat peanut oil over medium-high heat in nonstick 12-inch skillet or wok. Add ham, peas, mushrooms or bamboo shoots, and carrot; stir-fry until carrot slivers are crisp-tender, about 3 minutes. Add soy sauce and oyster sauce; cook 1 minute. Add egg mixture and rice; heat until egg is thoroughly cooked, stirring occasionally. Sprinkle with green onions and serve.

E X C H A N G E S

for 8 (¾-cup) servings:
1 bread; ¼ meat; 1 vegetable; ½ fat per serving; 142 calories; 3.0 grams fat; 38.4 milligrams cholesterol

## SPECIAL SWEET POTATOES WITH BAKED APPLES (M)

∎

A special addition to Thanksgiving turkey dinner!

YIELD: 6 to 8 servings

PREPARATION TIME: 40 minutes

### Special utensil
9-inch microwave pie plate

4 sweet potatoes (about 2 pounds)
¼ cup water
2 large tart apples, peeled and sliced
1 tablespoon orange juice
1 tablespoon brown sugar
½ teaspoon cinnamon
1 teaspoon lemon juice
powdered butter substitute equal to 3 tablespoons butter
¼ cup nonfat evaporated milk
¼ cup orange juice
¼ teaspoon ground nutmeg

Pierce potato skins with knife. Place them around perimeter of microwave-safe 9-inch pie plate, leaving center empty. Pour water over potatoes. Cover tightly and microwave on High until fork-tender, 10 to 15 minutes (the longer time for low-wattage ovens, the shorter time for high-wattage ovens), rearranging once. Let stand, covered, for 5 to 10 minutes.

Combine apple slices, orange juice, brown sugar, cinnamon, and lemon juice in medium bowl. Cover with wax paper and microwave on High until apples are tender, 3 to 4 minutes, stirring once. Keep covered and set aside.

Peel and dice potatoes; place in blender or food processor. Add butter substitute, nonfat evaporated milk, orange juice, and nutmeg; whirl until smooth, scraping sides of bowl several times. Spoon mixture into 9-inch pie plate and spread to even out. Top with apple mixture. Cover with wax paper and microwave on High until heated through, 3 to 5 minutes, rotating plate one-quarter turn halfway through if necessary. Slice and serve.

## VEGETABLE MEDLEY WITH HONEYED POTATOES (M)

■

This attractive side dish tastes a little like German potato salad.

YIELD: 6 servings

PREPARATION TIME: 30 minutes in microwave; 45 minutes on stovetop

4 medium-size potatoes (about 1 pound), peeled and cut into ¾-inch cubes
½ cup sliced red onions
1 tablespoon olive oil
½ tablespoon honey
2 tablespoons red wine vinegar
3 cloves garlic, minced
¼ teaspoon salt
1 each small green and red bell peppers, stems, seeds, and membranes removed
    and thinly sliced lengthwise
2 medium-size carrots, thinly sliced diagonally

Place potatoes and onions in medium saucepan. Cover with water and bring to boil over high heat. Reduce heat to low, cover, and simmer until tender, 20 to 25 minutes. Drain water; stir in olive oil, honey, vinegar, garlic, and salt. Steam bell peppers and carrots until crisp-tender, about 15 minutes; drain. Stir carrots and bell peppers into potato-onion mixture. Serve immediately.

To microwave: Decrease garlic to 2 cloves. Place potatoes and onions in 2-quart casserole with ¼ cup water; cover tightly. Microwave on High until tender, about 9 to 13 minutes (the longer time for low-wattage ovens, the shorter time for high-wattage ovens), stirring twice. Drain potatoes, then stir in olive oil, honey, vinegar, garlic, and salt, in that order. Cover and set aside.

Place bell peppers and carrots in 1-quart casserole with 2 tablespoons water. Cover tightly and microwave on High until crisp-tender, 2½ to 4 minutes, stirring once. Let stand for 2 minutes; drain. Stir carrots and bell peppers into potato-onion mixture. Serve immediately.

E X C H A N G E S

½ bread; 2 vegetable; ½ fat per serving; 107 calories; 2.5 grams fat; 0.0 milligram cholesterol

## Tender New Potatoes in Mild Basil Cheese Sauce (M)

If you've had it with plain baked potatoes, try this deceptively easy dish, prepared in no time using the range and microwave.

YIELD: 8 servings

PREPARATION TIME: 30 minutes

2 pounds small new red potatoes (24 to 32 potatoes)
⅓ cup water
1 small onion, thinly sliced crosswise and separated into rings
¼ teaspoon salt
2 ounces reduced-calorie pasteurized process cheese product (low-fat Laughing Cow cheese wedges—green label)
2 teaspoons cornstarch
½ teaspoon garlic salt
⅛ teaspoon ground white pepper
½ cup nonfat milk
¼ cup defatted chicken broth, cooled (omit salt if salted broth is used)
2 tablespoons snipped fresh basil or 2 teaspoons dried basil

Halve any large potatoes. With vegetable peeler, remove a strip around center of each remaining whole potato. In 1½- or 2-quart microwave-safe casserole, combine potatoes, water, onion, and salt; cover with glass lid or vented plastic wrap. Microwave on High until potatoes are tender, 13½ to 20 to 22 minutes (the longer time for low-wattage ovens, the shorter time for high-wattage ovens), stirring twice during cooking. Let stand for 2 to 3 minutes.

Thinly slice cheese, using knife dusted with flour. In medium saucepan combine cornstarch, garlic salt, white pepper, milk, and chicken broth. Cook over medium heat, stirring constantly, until smooth. Add cheese and continue stirring over low heat until cheese is melted and sauce is thickened and begins to boil.

Drain potato mixture. Add cheese sauce and gently toss until potatoes are well coated. Spoon onto serving platter; sprinkle with basil.

---

E X C H A N G E S

1¼ bread; ¼ meat per serving; 118 calories; 1.3 grams fat; 0.9 milligram cholesterol

## OVEN-CRISPED POTATOES
■

A low-fat alternative to hash browns or scalloped potatoes.

YIELD: 6 servings

PREPARATION TIME: 40 minutes

1½ pounds russet potatoes, cut in eighths or sixteenths
1 tablespoon soft margarine
1 teaspoon garlic salt
¼ cup chopped fresh basil
1 tablespoon minced shallot

Brush margarine evenly on potatoes to coat. Sprinkle with garlic salt. Roast potatoes in 450-degree oven until brown and crispy, about 20 to 30 minutes, turning once or twice. Stir in fresh basil and shallot. Transfer to serving dish; serve.

---

E X C H A N G E S

1 bread per serving; 86 calories; 2 grams fat; 0.0 milligram cholesterol

# Whole-Grain Stuffed Cabbage (M)

∎

Tender cabbage stuffed with savory whole grains is an attractive dish to serve with roast chicken, pork, or beef.

YIELD: 6 servings

PREPARATION TIME: 45 minutes
plus cooking/standing time
of about 40 minutes

⅓ cup brown rice
1½ cups chicken broth or stock
1 (2-pound) head of savoy or other cabbage
¼ cup bulgur wheat, soaked and drained
¼ cup seasoned bread crumbs
½ cup finely chopped onions
1 tablespoon chopped fresh or 1 teaspoon dried parsley
¼ cup chopped pine nuts
2 egg whites, beaten slightly
¼ teaspoon salt
2 tablespoons tomato paste
½ teaspoon dried thyme
¼ teaspoon pepper

Boil brown rice in 1 cup chicken broth or stock until it puffs up, about 10 minutes; drain and set aside. Meanwhile, trim cabbage stem to form flat bottom; remove discolored outer leaves. Steam cabbage until leaves become limp. (To microwave, place cabbage in 3-quart casserole with lid and add 2 tablespoons water. Cover and cook on high for 5 to 8 minutes.) Rinse with water to cool.

Carefully pull back 2 to 3 layers of outer cabbage leaves and lay flat. Cut the remaining head away from the stem, being careful not to cut off the outer leaves. Remove 2 leaves from the head and set aside. Finely chop the head to make 2 cups. In medium bowl, combine chopped cabbage, brown rice, bulgur wheat, bread crumbs, onions, parsley, pine nuts, egg whites, and salt. Place mixture in center of outer cabbage leaves, molding the mixture into a ball. Place the 2 reserved leaves over top of ball. Bring outer leaves back into original position, and fasten outer leaves together with about 4 toothpicks inserted at the top.

Place cabbage, top side down, in 3-quart casserole. Add remaining chicken broth or stock. Cover and microwave on High for 10 minutes. Carefully turn cabbage over, using oven mitts or potholders. Cover and microwave on medium until cabbage is cooked but not brown, about 15 to 45 minutes (the longer time for low-wattage ovens, the shorter time for high-wattage ovens). Transfer cabbage to serving platter—reserving liquid in casserole—and let stand, covered with foil, for 5 to 10 minutes. Stir tomato paste, thyme, and pepper into the juice in the casserole. Microwave on High until slightly thickened, 2 to 4 minutes. Cut cabbage into wedges and spoon sauce over each wedge.

EXCHANGES

1½ bread; 1 vegetable; ½ fat per serving; 162 calories; 2.9 grams fat; 0.2 milligram cholesterol

# Breads and Spreads

### GENEVA'S ZUCCHINI BREAD
•

Great for breakfast or with a luncheon salad.

YIELD: 32 slices

PREPARATION TIME: 30 minutes,
plus baking time

*Special utensils*
two pans 9 by 5 by 3 inches*

1 egg
4 egg whites
1 cup sugar
6 tablespoons vegetable oil
1 tablespoon vanilla
2 cups plus 2 tablespoons unpeeled, grated zucchini
1½ cups sifted all-purpose flour
½ cup nonfat dry milk
2 cups oat bran
1 tablespoon cinnamon
2 teaspoons baking soda
1 teaspoon salt
¼ teaspoon baking powder
1 cup chopped raisins

  *Three pans 8 by 4 by 2 inches can also be used. Reduce baking time to about 45 minutes.

Grease bottoms only of 2 pans 9 by 5 by 3 inches. Preheat oven to 350 degrees. Beat egg and egg whites in large bowl until fluffy. Blend in sugar, vegetable oil, and vanilla. Stir in zucchini. Blend in flour, dry milk, oat bran, cinnamon, baking soda, salt, and baking powder. Stir in chopped raisins. Pour into pans. Bake until wooden tooth pick inserted in center comes out clean, 50 to 60 minutes. Let cool for 10 minutes. Loosen sides of loaves from pans; remove loaves. Cool completely before slicing.

E X C H A N G E S

> 1 bread; ½ vegetable; ½ fat per slice; 113 calories; 3.3 grams fat; 8.9 milligrams cholesterol

# PUMPKIN BREAD
■

Wrap up the second loaf for a special homemade gift.

YIELD: 32 slices

PREPARATION TIME: 25 minutes, plus baking time

## *Special utensils*
two pans 9 by 5 by 3 inches

⅓ cup extra-light olive oil
2 cups packed brown sugar
1 teaspoon vanilla
2 eggs
4 egg whites
1 (1-pound) can pumpkin
1 cup nonfat milk
3⅓ cups sifted all-purpose flour
1 cup nonfat dry milk
2 teaspoons baking soda
½ teaspoon baking powder
1½ teaspoons salt
1 teaspoon each cinnamon, pumpkin pie spice, ground cloves
⅔ cup raisins

Combine olive oil and brown sugar in large bowl. Add vanilla, eggs, egg whites, and pumpkin; mix. Stir in milk. Blend in flour, dry milk, baking soda, baking powder, salt, cinnamon, pumpkin pie spice and cloves. Stir in raisins. Pour into two greased pans 9 by 5 by 3 inches. Bake at 350 degrees for about 70 minutes, until toothpick inserted in center comes out clean. Cool slightly before removing from pans.

EXCHANGES

> 1 bread; 1 fruit per slice; 148 calories; 2.8 grams fat; 17.6 milligrams cholesterol

# LENTIL BREAD
■

High in soluble fiber, lentils are made for more than just soup! To give this bread a golden hue, use small, red-orange decorticated lentils known as "Persians."

YIELD: 16 slices

PREPARATION TIME: 45 minutes, plus baking time

### Special utensil
one pan 9 by 5 by 3 inches

¾ cup Persian lentils (found in Indian or Middle Eastern markets or
    international food section of well-stocked supermarket)
3 tablespoons sesame seeds
2 tablespoons extra-light olive oil
¾ cup honey
2 egg whites
1½ cups all-purpose flour
1 teaspoon baking soda
½ teaspoon salt
½ teaspoon curry powder
¾ teaspoon baking powder
¾ cup chopped, dried dates

Sift lentils to remove any debris; rinse and drain. Bring lentils to boil in 3 cups water over high heat. Cover and simmer until lentils are tender, about 15 minutes. Drain and cool. In small pan over medium heat, lightly brown sesame seeds, shaking pan frequently. Set aside.

In a large bowl, combine olive oil, honey, and egg whites; stir in lentils. In separate bowl mix flour, baking soda, salt, curry powder, baking powder, dates, and all but 2 teaspoons of the sesame seeds. Add dry ingredients to liquid and blend well.

Pour batter into greased and floured pan 9 by 5 by 3 inches and sprinkle top with remaining sesame seeds. Bake at 350 degrees until bread is browned and just begins to pull from sides of pan, for about 1 hour. Cool for 10 minutes before removing from pan.

---

EXCHANGES

2 bread; ½ fat per slice; 169 calories; 2.8 grams fat; 0.0 milligram cholesterol

## SWEET BREAKFAST BREAD

∎

Dimpling the dough before baking produces a luscious marbled effect in the sliced bread.

YIELD: 8 servings

PREPARATION TIME: 15 minutes,
plus rising/baking time

*Special utensil*
7 by 11 inches pan

1 (1-pound) loaf white or wheat bread dough, thawed
¼ cup sugar
1 teaspoon cinnamon
½ cup currants or dark seedless raisins
2 tablespoons melted margarine

Spray bottom of pan 7 by 11 inches with nonstick vegetable spray. Place dough in pan, pressing and stretching dough to fill pan evenly and completely. (If dough is too elastic, let rest a few minutes and try again.) Cover pan lightly with plastic wrap or towel and let dough rise in warm place until doubled, 45 to 60 minutes.

Combine sugar, cinnamon, and currants or raisins. Brush raised dough with margarine; sprinkle with currant or raisin mixture. With fingers, gently press dough down all over, forming deep dimples in surface and fitting dough into pan corners. (Some of the raisin mixture will fall into the dimples, forming the "marbled" effect.) Bake at 400 degrees until bread is golden brown, about 10 minutes. Cover lightly with foil and bake until done, 8 to 12 minutes more. Cut and serve warm or cool, or wrap uncut bread in foil to store and reheat when ready to serve.

---

EXCHANGES

1¾ bread; 1 fat; 1 fruit; 229 calories; 4.7 grams fat; 1.7 milligrams cholesterol

# Sun-Kissed Muffins
∎

Top with a little plain yogurt for a delicious, lowfat breakfast.

YIELD: 12 (1-ounce) muffins

PREPARATION TIME: 48 minutes

*Special utensil*
1 muffin pan

1 cup all-purpose flour
½ cup whole-wheat flour
2 teaspoons baking powder
¼ teaspoon baking soda
¼ teaspoon salt
2 egg whites, lightly beaten
½ cup honey
½ teaspoon finely shredded lemon peel
5 tablespoons lemon juice
2 tablespoons extra-light olive oil

Preheat oven to 400 degrees. Spray muffin cups with nonstick vegetable spray or line with paper baking cups; set aside. Mix flours, baking powder, baking soda, and salt in large bowl. Make a well in the center. In small bowl, combine egg whites, honey, lemon peel, lemon juice, and olive oil. Add all at once to flour mixture; stir just until moistened. (Batter will be lumpy.) Pour batter into muffin cups. Bake until toothpick inserted in center comes out clean; 17 to 18 minutes. Remove from pans. Serve warm or cool.

EXCHANGES

> 1 bread; ½ fat; ½ fruit per muffin; 119 calories; 2.5 grams fat; 0.0 milligram cholesterol

# ITALIAN SNACKING BREAD (FOCACCIA)*
■

Sure to please as a snack, side dish, or cut into smaller pieces as an appetizer.

YIELD: 12 to 16 servings

PREPARATION TIME: 20 minutes,
plus rising/baking time

### Special utensil
baking pan 10 by 15 by 1 inches

2 (1-pound) loaves frozen white or wheat bread dough, thawed (1½ to 2½ hours) and kneaded together
6 pieces (halves) dried tomato
1½ tablespoons virgin olive oil
¼ cup capers
1 tablespoon chopped fresh or 1 teaspoon crumbled dried rosemary
coarse salt to taste
2 tablespoons chopped Italian parsley

Spray bottom of baking pan 10 by 15 by 1 inches with nonstick vegetable spray. Place dough in pan and press and stretch it to fill pan evenly and completely. (If dough is too elastic, let rest a few minutes and try again.) Cover pan lightly with plastic wrap or towel and let

*This recipe can be reduced by cutting all ingredients in half, using a smaller pan, and baking for total of 15 to 20 minutes. Follow directions as above.

dough rise in warm place free of drafts until doubled, 45 to 60 minutes.

Blanch tomatoes in boiling water for 2 minutes. Drain and cut into strips. Brush olive oil over dough. With fingers, gently press dough down, forming dimples in surface and fitting dough into pan corners. Place tomato pieces, capers, and rosemary into dimples, pushing down lightly. Sprinkle surface with salt.

Bake at 400 degrees until dough is lightly browned on edges and bottom, 15 to 20 minutes. Sprinkle with parsley; bake until golden brown, another 5 to 10 minutes. (Cover lightly with foil at this point if topping is already brown.) Cool slightly; serve.

EXCHANGES

> 2 bread per serving; 152 calories; 2.8 grams fat; 1.7 milligrams cholesterol

# FLATBREAD ROUNDS
■

Grilled with garlic and herbs, made into minipizzas, filled with sandwich fixings, or simply enjoyed by themselves, these flatbread rounds taste great!

YIELD: 8 flatbreads

PREPARATION TIME: 40 minutes

1 (1-pound) loaf whole-wheat or white dough, thawed
1½ tablespoons virgin olive oil

On bread board dusted with flour, divide dough into 8 equal pieces, and shape each into ball. Roll out each ball into a 3- to 4-inch round. Lightly brush top with olive oil; place on cookie sheet, oil side down, leaving several inches between rounds. Again lightly brush top with olive oil; flatten round with hands to ⅛-inch thickness and about 4 to 5 inches wide. Let stand, uncovered, at room temperature until slightly puffy, 15 to 25 minutes.

Bake at 425 degrees until both sides are golden brown but still pliable, 5 to 12 minutes, checking frequently and removing individual breads as they are done. (Or grill directly over moderate heat, 2 to 3 minutes on each side.) Serve warm.

For garlic rounds, sprinkle with garlic salt or powder, a little freshly ground pepper, and Parmesan cheese. Bake as above.

---

EXCHANGES

1¾ bread; 1 fat per round; 175 calories; 4.4 grams fat; 1.7 milligrams cholesterol

## BLUEBERRY PANCAKES

∎

Make a batch and freeze the leftovers in individual servings, to pop in the microwave for an instant, old-fashioned breakfast. Top cakes with a little syrup, fresh fruit, or a dollop of fruited yogurt.

YIELD: about 12 pancakes

PREPARATION TIME: 30 minutes

¾ cup sifted whole-wheat flour
½ cup all-purpose flour
3 teaspoons baking powder
½ teaspoon salt
½ cup nonfat milk
½ cup evaporated nonfat milk
3 egg whites, slightly beaten
1 tablespoon raspberry or strawberry jam or preserves
1 cup blueberries

In large bowl, combine flours, baking powder, and salt. Add milk, evaporated milk, egg whites, and jam or preserves; stir just until flour is moistened. Fold in blueberries. Spray nonstick 12-inch skillet or griddle with nonstick vegetable spray. Heat griddle over medium heat until drop of water sizzles. Pour batter into skillet by scant quarter cupfuls. Cook until tops bubble, edges are dry, and bottoms are browned. Turn and cook until golden brown. Place on warm platter.

---

EXCHANGES

1 bread per pancake; 71 calories; 0.3 gram fat; 0.6 milligram cholesterol

# FRENCH TOAST SUPREME

■

A creamy center makes this French toast a surprising delight.

YIELD: 2 servings

PREPARATION TIME: 20 minutes

2 (1½ inches thick) slices day-old white bread (4 ounces total)
¼ cup Yogurt Cheese, page 294
1 tablespoon blackberry or raspberry jam
1 egg white, slightly beaten
1 tablespoon evaporated nonfat milk
1 tablespoon orange juice
dash cinnamon
2 teaspoons powdered sugar

Cut bread slices diagonally in half. Using sharp, pointed knife, cut pocket into each piece, stopping just short of crust. Mix jam with yogurt cheese; spread about 1 tablespoon into each pocket and gently seal bread closed.

In medium-size bowl, combine egg white, milk, orange juice, and cinnamon. Dip bread slices in egg mixture, turning to coal all sides. Brown slices over medium heat in nonstick skillet sprayed with nonstick vegetable spray. Sprinkle with powdered sugar; serve immediately.

EXCHANGES

2 bread; ½ milk; ½ fruit; 233 calories; 1.9 grams fat; 2.8 milligrams cholesterol

# Yogurt Cheese

■

Great as a very low-calorie substitute for cream cheese in recipes or on bagels, muffins, and crackers. Use fruited yogurt to make a sweet cheese and plain yogurt for a tart cheese. Add jam, preserves, or savory herbs for a flavored cheese spread.

YIELD: 8 fluid ounces

PREPARATION TIME: 3 minutes,
plus draining time

## *Special utensil*
cheesecloth

16 ounces nonfat or lowfat yogurt, plain or fruited, as desired

Place yogurt in double-layered cheesecloth and then in strainer. Suspend strainer over large bowl and refrigerate. Turn cheesecloth occasionally during straining process to facilitate drainage of liquid. For a product the consistency of cream cheese, let yogurt drain over night or until about 1 cup of yogurt cheese remains in cheesecloth. Discard the liquid.

---

EXCHANGES

**for plain nonfat yogurt:** ¼ milk per 2-tablespoon serving; 24 calories; 0.0 gram fat; 0.8 milligram cholesterol

# Desserts

## PEANUT BUTTER COOKIES

•

These little gems are packed with lots of goodies, such as oat bran, whole-wheat flour, and peanut butter, and with fewer than 2 grams of fat each, they contain less than half the fat of traditional peanut butter cookies!

YIELD: 40 cookies

PREPARATION TIME: 35 minutes, plus baking time

½ cup packed brown sugar
½ cup peanut butter, smooth or crunchy
½ cup light corn syrup
¼ cup mashed ripe banana
1 egg
½ teaspoon vanilla
⅔ cup oat bran
1¼ cups sifted whole-wheat flour
¾ teaspoon baking soda
¼ teaspoon salt
½ teaspoon baking powder

Combine brown sugar, peanut butter, corn syrup, banana, egg, and vanilla in large mixing bowl. In separate bowl mix oat bran, flour, baking soda, salt, and baking powder. Stir dry ingredients into wet, a little at a time, until blended, scraping bottom and sides of bowl with rubber scraper several times. Dough will be stiff. Spray cookie sheets with nonstick vegetable spray. Drop dollops of dough 1½ inches in diameter onto baking sheets; flatten with fork dipped in flour. Bake in

375-degree oven until lightly browned on bottom, 9 to 10 minutes. Let cool a few minutes before removing from pan. Store in airtight container. A slice of fresh bread placed inside the container will help keep the cookies fresh.

EXCHANGES

½ bread; ¼ fruit per cookie; 61 calories; 1.8 grams fat; 6.8 milligrams cholesterol

## LIGHT-STYLE CHOCOLATE CRUNCH COOKIES
■

Ruth Wakefield, a dietitian, served her chocolate crunch cookies to countless guests at the Toll House Inn in Whitman, Massachusetts, during the 1930s. These cookies are reminiscent of her famous treat, but with much less fat and fewer calories.

YIELD: about 48 cookies (½ ounce each)

PREPARATION TIME: 30 minutes, plus baking time

2 cups all-purpose flour
¾ cup whole-wheat flour
½ teaspoon baking soda
2 teaspoons baking powder
½ teaspoon salt
3 tablespoons extra-light olive oil or canola oil
½ cup light corn syrup
¾ cup packed brown sugar
7 tablespoons plain nonfat yogurt
3 tablespoons mashed ripe banana
1½ teaspoons vanilla
4 ounces semisweet chocolate minichips

Combine all-purpose and whole-wheat flours, baking soda, baking powder, and salt; set aside. Blend olive oil or canola oil, corn syrup, brown sugar, yogurt, banana, and vanilla in large bowl until smooth, using hand strokes or electric mixer. Gradually add flour mixture and mix well. Stir in chocolate pieces. Drop dough by rounded teaspoonfuls onto baking sheets sprayed with nonstick vegetable spray. Bake at 375 degrees until bottoms brown, 10 to 12 minutes. Cool slightly before removing from pan.

EXCHANGES

¾ bread; ¼ fat per cookie; 69 calories; 1.8 grams fat; 0.0 milligram cholesterol

# APRICOT-RAISIN BARS

■

Eat as you would commercial granola bars for a wholesome snack that's low in fat.

YIELD: 24 bars

PREPARATION TIME: 45 minutes

## Special utensil
baking pan 9 by 9 by 2 inches

1 (8-ounce) package chopped, dried apricots
2 cups water
¼ cup raisins
1 cup uncooked oat bran cereal or quick-cooking oats
1 cup whole-wheat flour
⅓ cup apricot nectar
3 tablespoons margarine, melted
¼ cup firmly packed light brown sugar
½ teaspoon cinnamon
¼ teaspoon ground ginger
¼ teaspoon salt

In 2-quart saucepan, bring apricots and water to boil over medium heat. Reduce heat and simmer until tender, about 10 minutes. Drain well. Mix with raisins and set aside.

Mix oat bran, flour, apricot nectar, margarine, brown sugar, cinnamon, ginger, and salt in medium-size bowl. Press half of this mixture into bottom of greased baking pan 9 by 9 by 2 inches. Spread apricots and raisins on top evenly. Crumble the rest of the mixture over the top. Bake at 375 degrees until golden brown, about 20 minutes. Cool thoroughly in pan before cutting. Bars can be individually wrapped in plastic wrap or foil and frozen for handy anytime snacks.

---

EXCHANGES

½ bread; ¾ fruit per bar; 88 calories; 1.8 grams fat; 0.0 milligram cholesterol

## BLUEBERRY CHEESECAKE

∎

There's a fruity surprise baked inside!

YIELD: 12 servings

PREPARATION TIME: 30 minutes, plus baking/cooling time of about 2 hours

*Special utensil*
*springform pan 9 inches*

CRUST:
20 graham cracker squares
4 tablespoons margarine, melted
2 tablespoons sugar

FILLING:
2 pounds low-fat cottage cheese, well drained
¾ cup sugar
3 eggs
1 tablespoon flour
1 teaspoon vanilla
1 cup fresh blueberries, washed and patted dry (or frozen blueberries, thawed and well drained)

TOPPING:
1 cup plain yogurt, firm (if yogurt is runny, hang it from faucet in triple-layered cheesecloth for 1 to 2 hours to remove excess liquid)
3 tablespoons sugar
1½ teaspoons vanilla

To prepare pie crust, place graham crackers in sturdy plastic bag and roll them into fine crumbs with rolling pin. (Or, pulverize them in blender or food processor using knife blade attachment.) Mix in margarine and sugar to make fine-crumb mixture. Press into the bottom of a 9 inch springform pan. Bake at 350 degrees for 10 minutes; set aside.

To prepare filling, blend cottage cheese, sugar, eggs, flour, and vanilla in blender or food processor until smooth. Pour two-thirds of filling into pie crust; sprinkle blueberries on top to within ½ inch of edge. Pour remaining filling over the blueberries and smooth with a rubber scraper. Bake at 350 degrees for 70 minutes. Turn off oven but *leave cake inside, with door open slightly,* to cool gradually, about 1 hour.

To prepare topping, blend yogurt, sugar and vanilla. Spread over baked cheesecake. Refrigerate before serving.

---

E X C H A N G E S

> 1 milk; 1 fruit; ½ bread; 1½ fat per serving; 249 calories; 7.5 grams fat; 72 milligrams cholesterol

## MINI CHEESECAKES
∎

A surprise ingredient—"yogurt cheese"—is used instead of cream cheese for these light, flavorful, low-cal cakes.

YIELD: 8 servings

> PREPARATION TIME: 20 minutes, plus baking time of 35 minutes

*Special utensils*
cheesecloth
8 souffle cups

32 ounces vanilla low-fat yogurt
⅔ cup sugar
½ cup evaporated whole milk
½ cup plain nonfat yogurt
1 teaspoon vanilla
3-4 drops lemon juice
3 tablespoons egg white or fat-free egg substitute
1 tablespoon graham cracker crumbs

To prepare yogurt cheese, spoon the yogurt into a double-layered cheesecloth, then place the cheesecloth in a strainer. Suspend the strainer over a large bowl and refrigerate it overnight or longer, turning the cheesecloth occasionally. It is ready when about 2 cups of yogurt cheese the firmness of cream cheese remain in the cheesecloth. Discard the liquid whey that has dripped into the bowl.

Preheat oven to 325 degrees. Put cheese in medium-sized bowl and add sugar, evaporated milk, plain yogurt, vanilla, and lemon juice. Mix until smooth. Stir in egg whites, a little at a time, just until smooth (do not overmix).

Pour yogurt mixture into souffle cups. Bake until set, 30 to 35 minutes. Sprinkle the top of each cup with graham cracker crumbs. Cool on a wire rack. Refrigerate until chilled. Before serving, top each cake with fresh banana slices and shaved chocolate, warm fruit sauce, or fresh berries.

EXCHANGES

1 milk; 1⅓ fruit; ½ fat per serving; 182 calories; 2.5 grams fat; 9.5 milligrams cholesterol

## GUILT-FREE CHOCOLATE LOAF

∎

The fat is gone, but a subtle chocolate flavor remains. Serve with slices of low-fat cheese and fresh fruit.

YIELD: 12 (¾ inch) slices

PREPARATION TIME: 80 minutes, including baking time

*Special utensil*
loaf pan 9 by 5 inches

2 cups whole-wheat flour
1 cup all-purpose flour
½ cup cocoa
¼ cup raisins
½ cup firmly packed brown sugar
1½ teaspoons baking soda
½ teaspoon salt

3 egg whites
3 tablespoons light corn syrup
1½ cups nonfat or low-fat buttermilk
powdered sugar (optional)

In a large mixing bowl blend whole-wheat flour, white flour, cocoa, raisins, brown sugar, baking soda, and salt. In a small bowl, beat egg whites, corn syrup, and buttermilk to blend. Add liquid to dry ingredients, mixing just until moistened.

Pour batter into a loaf pan 9 by 5 inches sprayed with nonstick vegetable spray. Bake at 350 degrees until edges begin to pull from pan sides and toothpick inserted in center comes out clean, about 1 hour. Cool in pan for 10 minutes, then remove loaf to a rack to continue cooling. Sift powdered sugar over top before serving, if desired. Store wrapped loaf at room temperature.

### EXCHANGES

> 1½ bread; 1 fruit per serving; 184 calories; 1.1 grams fat; 1.1 milligrams cholesterol

## APRICOT COMPOTE (M)
■

A delicious alternative to fruit pie. Peaches or nectarines can be used instead of apricots.

YIELD: 6 servings

PREPARATION TIME: 10 minutes,
plus standing/baking time

### Special utensils
6 compote cups

1½ pounds ripe apricots, pitted and coarsely chopped (4½ cups fruit)
1 tablespoon lemon juice
⅓ cup granulated sugar
⅓ cup firmly packed brown sugar
3 tablespoons quick-cooking tapioca
1½ to 2 cups firm vanilla frozen yogurt or quality ice milk

Combine apricots and lemon juice in large bowl. In small bowl, mix sugars and tapioca, then stir gently into fruit. Set aside for 15 to 60 minutes to let tapioca soften, stirring carefully several times.

Pour mixture into 9-inch pie pan sprayed with nonstick vegetable spray. Bake on bottom rack of 400-degree oven until bubbly, 45 to 55 minutes. Cool slightly on rack.

Line 6 compote cups with ½-inch thickness of frozen yogurt or ice milk. Spoon warm fruit mixture into cups; serve immediately. If fruit has cooled, carefully transfer to microwave-safe bowl if necessary, cover, and warm in microwave before adding to yogurt- or ice-milk-lined cups.

To microwave: Prepare apricot mixture as above. Spoon it into 1½-quart casserole and cover loosely with waxed paper. Microwave on High until apricots are tender and mixture is bubbly, 6 to 10 minutes (the longer time for low-wattage ovens, the shorter time for high-wattage ovens), turning once. Let stand for 2 minutes and continue as above.

---

EXCHANGES

¾ milk; 3 fruit per serving; 233 calories; 1.1 grams fat; 0.0 milligram cholesterol

## BANANA-STRAWBERRY SORBET

■

Keep some frozen strawberries on hand to serve this dessert on a moment's notice.

YIELD: 6 (1 cup) servings

PREPARATION TIME: 20 minutes, plus freezing time

*Special utensils*
baking pan 13 by 9 inches, chilled beater, and bowl

1¼ pounds ripe bananas (about 3 medium)
⅓ cup lemon juice
2 cups hulled fresh or unsweetened frozen strawberries
¼ cup granulated sugar
⅓ cup cold evaporated nonfat milk
6 whole strawberries

Peel and slice bananas and purée with lemon juice to make 2 cups. Purée strawberries with sugar to make almost 2 cups. Blend purées together. Pour into baking pan 13 by 9 inches.

Cover with foil or waxed paper and freeze until firm around the edges but soft in the middle, about 2 hours.

Beat milk with chilled beater in chilled bowl until it makes soft peaks. Gradually beat in strawberry mixture until smooth but still frozen. Return mixture to pan. Cover and freeze until firm, about 2 hours.

Let sorbet stand at room temperature for 15 minutes before serving. Spoon into stemmed compotes and garnish with strawberries.

EXCHANGES

2½ fruit; 151 calories; 0.7 gram fat; 0.5 milligram cholesterol

# Peach Frozen Yogurt
∎

Refreshing and light, this dessert is made easily in your freezer and doesn't require a special container or ice-cream maker. Serve alone, or top with fresh blueberries for a special treat.

YIELD: about 3½ cups

PREPARATION TIME: 15 minutes, plus freezing/standing time

*Special utensils*
blender, chilled bowl and chilled electric beaters, or food processor

5 large ripe peaches, peeled
⅛ teaspoon almond flavoring
⅛ teaspoon vanilla
½ cup sugar
1 teaspoon lemon juice
1 cup plain low-fat yogurt
2 ounces firm tofu

Pit and chop four peaches. Reserve fifth peach for garnish. Place peaches in blender, food processor, or in bowl with chilled electric beaters and add almond flavoring, vanilla, sugar, lemon juice, yogurt, and tofu. Whirl on high speed until smooth. Pour into shallow pan or ice-cube trays. Freeze, stirring occasionally, until partially frozen, 2 to 3 hours. Turn mixture into food processor or chilled mixing bowl and break up. Process or beat until smooth but not melted. Freeze again in individual molds, 1-quart mold, or freezer container until firm, 3 to 4 hours for 1-quart container.

When ready to serve, unmold by running warm water on outside of container. Let yogurt mixture stand for several minutes (or micro-wave for 10 seconds on High), then spoon into dessert glasses. Top with slices of reserved peach; serve.

---

EXCHANGES

| | |
|---|---|
| **for 5 servings:** | 1 milk; 1½ fruit per serving; 177 calories; 1.2 grams fat; 0.8 milligram cholesterol |

# Recipes for Kitchen Phobics

## SAUTÉED CHICKEN
·

chicken pieces, skinned
garlic salt or garlic powder
seasoning salt
pepper
nonstick frying pan
margarine and waxed paper (optional)

Skin chicken pieces, rinse, and pat dry. Season with garlic salt or garlic powder, seasoning salt, and pepper. If you're cooking breasts only, wipe nonstick frying pan with the waxed paper coated with margarine prior to placing chicken in pan (chicken breasts have less fat than other parts, so you'll need the margarine for cooking).

Cooking chicken over medium heat until outside is browned, the inside of the meat is white, and the juices run clear, approximately 15 to 40 minutes, turning once. Cooking time depends on the size and number of pieces.

## MOM'S MEATLOAF
·

1 pound extra-lean ground beef (less than 15 percent fat)
1 pound ground turkey (2 pounds turkey can be used instead of ground beef)
1 egg and 2 egg whites
1 medium onion, diced
about ½ cup Italian bread crumbs
1 teaspoon Italian seasoning

¾ teaspoon each salt and garlic salt
dash of pepper
carrots, halved or quartered lengthwise
potatoes, halved or quartered

Combine all ingredients (except potatoes and carrots) in large bowl and form into loaf. Place loaf on rack in roasting pan. Place potatoes and carrots in pan. Cover and bake at 350 degrees for 1¼ hours. Uncover and bake another 15 minutes.

## LINGUINE WITH CLAM SAUCE
■

canned whole or chopped clams, drained
1 jar low-fat spaghetti sauce (check ingredients; some are high in fat)
linguine

Combine clams with spaghetti sauce in medium saucepan and heat. Cook linguine according to package instructions and drain. Top linguine with clam sauce and serve.

## LITESTYLE TOSTADA
■

1 (6- or 8-inch) warmed flour or toasted corn tortilla
1 to 2 ounces ground turkey, optional
a bit of packaged taco mix, optional
about ½ cup canned pinto beans, drained, mashed, and heated
4 tablespoons (1 ounce) shredded low-fat jack or Cheddar cheese
chopped tomato, onion, shredded lettuce
salsa

Cook turkey with taco mix. Place on tostada and top with the other ingredients.

## VEGETARIAN OMELETTE
■

Use vegetables suggested below or any you have on hand:
1 egg and 2 to 3 egg whites (or ¼ cup fat-free egg substitute)

2 to 3 tablespoons nonfat milk
several large mushrooms, sliced
about 1 tablespoon each onion and green pepper, chopped
2 to 3 tablespoons spinach, coarsely chopped
1 to 2 pieces sun-dried tomato
1 teaspoon margarine or oil
½ ounce low-fat cheese

Beat egg and egg whites (or egg substitute) until smooth. Stir in nonfat milk and set aside.

Cook vegetables in 10-inch nonstick skillet, stirring constantly, until lightly cooked. Transfer to plate.

Heat 1 teaspoon margarine or oil in pan. Pour in egg mixture. When egg begins to turn dry and golden around edges, gently lift edges with spatula to allow uncooked egg to flow underneath.

Add cooked vegetables and cheese to eggs, and cook for several minutes longer. Fold omelette in half with spatula to cover vegetables. Cover, if desired, and cook until egg is set and lightly golden brown.

# Really Easy Recipes

## INSTANT LUNCH
■

Fortify 1 package oriental noodles by stirring in shredded cabbage, grated carrot, and 1 egg into soup along with boiling water. Close and let sit according to package instructions.

## TOMATO SALAD
■

Combine 1 tomato, coarsely chopped and drained, with 1 ounce diced mozarella cheese, fresh-snipped basil, and a sprinkle of pepper.

## SPINACH SALAD (a good source of vitamins, minerals, and fiber)
■

Thoroughly wash spinach by immersing leaves in sink or large bowl of water. Lift from the water and spin or pat dry with clean towel.

Gently toss 2 cups lightly packed spinach with ⅓ cup mandarin orange sections, ½ small chopped apple, 2 chopped walnuts, and seasoned vinegar (such as rice vinegar or wine vinegar).

## CHEESE BREAD
■

Heat or toast 1 (1 ounce) slice of Italian or sourdough bread topped with 4 tablespoons (1 ounce) shredded cheddar and sprinkled with garlic salt.

## FRUIT SPRITZER
■

Mix equal parts fruit juice and sparkling water, diet Seven-Up, or diet lemon-lime soda. Serve over ice.

# APPENDIX A

## Diet Assessment

The food diary and the food frequency charts in this section will help you improve your knowledge and awareness of the fat content in the foods you've been eating.

Pick a day and fill out the food diary, recording everything you eat and drink that day. Then follow the directions on page 314 to detect the fat in your diet, including "visible" and "invisible" sources of fat.

Visible fats, of course, are the obvious ones. They include margarine, butter, oil, sour cream, cream cheese, whipped cream, salad dressing, mayonnaise, tartar sauce, shortening, lard, and coffee creamer or cream, plus the outside fat on meats and the skin on poultry.

Invisible fats are harder to detect. They hide in foods that are naturally high in fat, including whole milk, low-fat milk, cheese, eggs, avocados, olives, nuts, seeds, peanut butter, and fresh, cured, and processed meats.

And don't forget the many foods prepared with fat, including biscuits, muffins, croissants, pies, pastries, doughnuts, cakes, cookies, potato chips, crackers, french fries, refried beans, fried vegetables, cheese sauces, cream sauces, cream soups, gravies, fried chicken, and fried fish.

Once you have detected the fat in your diet, read the directions for calculating the percentage of fat you've consumed. Then fill out the Food Frequency Chart to see how balanced—or unbalanced—your overall diet is.

If you're like most people, you'll be surprised at how much fat (and how many calories) you've been consuming. Use the Fat and Cholesterol Comparison Charts in this section to help reduce the amount of fat, calories, and cholesterol in your diet from now on.

## FOOD DIARY

NAME _____

DATE FOOD CONSUMED _____

| TIME | FOOD ITEM: DESCRIPTION and QUANTITY | grams FAT | CALORIES |
|------|-----------------------------------|-----------|----------|
|      |                                   |           |          |
|      |                                   |           |          |
|      |                                   |           |          |
|      |                                   |           |          |
|      |                                   |           |          |
|      |                                   |           |          |
|      |                                   |           |          |
|      |                                   |           |          |
|      |                                   |           |          |
|      |                                   |           |          |
|      |                                   |           |          |
|      |                                   |           |          |

Step 1: Circle all sources of visible fat. Write in grams of fat and calories for these foods (See the food exchange lists on page 172 and the Fat and Cholesterol Comparison Chart in this section).

Step 2: Underline all sources of invisible fat. Write in grams of fat and calories for these foods.

## FOOD DIARY

NAME _____

DATE FOOD CONSUMED _____

| Time | Food Item: Description And Quantities | Grams Fat | Calories |
|------|----------------------------------------|-----------|----------|
| 8 AM | 2 slices whole-wheat toast with: | | |
| | 1 tablespoon (margarine) | 11 | 102 |
| | ½ cup orange juice | | |
| | 1 cup coffee with: | | |
| | 1 tablespoon (liquid creamer) | 1.5 | 20 |
| 10 AM | 1 medium banana | | |
| 12 NOON | Sandwich with: 2 slices white bread | | |
| | 2 ounces roast beef | 15 | 200 |
| | 2 slices American cheese - 1½ oz. | 13.4 | 159 |
| | 1 tablespoon mayonnaise | 11 | 99 |
| | 1 small bag potato chips (1 ounce) | 10.1 | 147 |
| | 1 cup (2%) lowfat milk | 4.7 | 121 |
| 3 PM | ½ bag microwave popcorn (w/oil, salt & oil) 5 cups | 15 | 275 |
| | 12 ounces soda | | |
| 6 PM | (grilled chicken with skin) ½ breast & 1 leg | 10.9/5.3 | 222/84 |
| | 2 cups garden salad with: | | |
| | 2 tablespoons (Thousand Island dressing) | 11 | 118 |
| | 1 cup white rice | | |
| | 1 corn on the cob with: | | |
| | 1 tablespoon (margarine) | 11 | 102 |
| | ice tea with lemon - 8 ounces | | |
| 9 PM | 4 chocolate chip cookies (2¼ inch diameter) | 11 | 185 |
| | 1 cup hot tea with lemon | | |

Step 3: Write in calories for all remaining foods (fruits, vegetables and other fat free foods). Determine % fat in your diet using the instructions on the next page.

| FOOD DIARY | NAME | | |
|---|---|---|---|
| | DATE FOOD CONSUMED | | |
| Time | Food Item: Description And Quantities | Grams Fat | Calories |
| 8AM | 2 slices whole-wheat toast with: | | 140 |
| | 1 tablespoon margarine | 11 | 102 |
| | ½ cup orange juice | | 56 |
| | 1 cup coffee with: | | 0 |
| | 1 tablespoon liquid creamer | 1.5 | 20 |
| 10AM | 1 medium banana | | 105 |
| 12 NOON | Sandwich with: 2 slices white bread | | 130 |
| | 2 ounces roast beef | 15 | 200 |
| | 2 slices American cheese - 1½ oz. | 13.4 | 159 |
| | 1 tablespoon mayonnaise | 11 | 99 |
| | 1 small bag potato chips (1 ounce) | 10.1 | 147 |
| | 1 cup (2%) lowfat milk | 4.7 | 121 |
| 3 PM | ½ bag microwave popcorn (wth salt foil) 5 cups | 15 | 215 |
| | 12 ounces soda | | 0 |
| 6PM | grilled chicken with skin- ½ breast & 1 leg | 109/5.3 | 222/84 |
| | 2 cups garden salad with: | | 25 |
| | 2 tablespoons Thousand Island dressing | 11 | 118 |
| | 1 cup white rice | | 225 |
| | 1 corn on the cob with: | | 100 |
| | 1 tablespoon margarine | 11 | 102 |
| | ice tea with lemon -8 ounces | | 0 |
| 9PM | 4 chocolate chip cookies (2¼ inch diameter) | 11 | 185 |
| | 1 cup hot tea with lemon | | 0 |

## To Calculate the Percentage of Fat

Take the total number of grams of fat consumed for the day. Say, for example, 131 grams of fat were consumed.

Multiply by 9 (1 gram of fat has 9 calories) to get the total number of calories that came from fat.

$$131 \times 9 = 1179$$

Now, divide the total number of calories from fat, 1179, by the total number of calories for the day, 2615.

$$\frac{1179}{2615} = .45 \times 100 \text{ or 45 percent.}$$

So, in this example, 45 percent of the calories came from fat. Your goal is 30 percent or less.

You can also use this calculation to determine the percentage of fat from calories on various food items to find lower fat alternatives to high-fat products. Here's how:

When choosing yogurt, for example, look at the ingredient list for the number of calories and the grams of fat per serving. Multiply the grams of fat by 9 to get the total number of calories from fat. Then divide that number by the total number of calories per serving:

Brand A has 160 calories per serving and 9 grams of fat.

$$9 \times 9 = 81 \text{ calories from fat}$$

$$\frac{81}{160} = .506 \times 100, \text{ or 50.6 percent calories from fat}$$

Brand B has 250 calories per serving and 4 grams of fat.

$$4 \times 9 = 36 \text{ calories from fat}$$

$$\frac{36}{250} = .144 \times 100, \text{ or 14.4 percent calories from fat}$$

As you can see, there's a big difference between Brand A and Brand B. Which yogurt would you rather have?

# FOOD FREQUENCY

How many servings of the following foods do you eat per week, including snacks?
Please check the appropriate box for each question below.

| FOOD | GOAL | less than 1 | 1-2 | 3-5 | 6 or more |
|---|---|---|---|---|---|
| Fried, deep-fat fried, or breaded foods (fried chicken or fish, hash browns, french fries, etc.). | less than one per week | | | | |
| Fatty meats (bacon, sausage, hamburger, lunchmeat, ribs, prime rib, corned beef and hot dogs). | less than one per week | | | | |
| Lean red meats (round or sirloin steak, London broil, lean ham, pork loin, Canadian bacon, veal). | up to 3 to 4 3-ounce servings per week | | | | |
| Sea food (fish and shellfish -- other than fried). | 3-4 servings per week | | | | |
| Egg yolks (including those in baked and cooked foods). | 3-4 per week | | | | |
| Whole milk, high-fat cheese (such as cheddar, cream and Swiss). | depends on other fat sources | | | | |
| Butter, coffee creamer, whipped cream, sour cream. | less than one per week | | | | |
| High-fat desserts such as pies, pastries, ice cream, cookies, cake and chocolate. | less than one per week or in small amts. | | | | |
| High-fat snacks such as crackers, chips, buttered popcorn, etc. | less than one per week or in small amts. | | | | |
| Nuts, avocado, olive oil, olives, peanut butter. | small amts. | | | | |
| Whole grains, whole-wheat or rye bread, whole-wheat paste, brown rice, bran or whole-wheat cereals. | 6 or more servings per week | | | | |
| Oat bran, oatmeal, legumes (dark beans, peas, and lentils). | depends | | | | |
| Fresh or frozen, raw or lightly cooked vegetables. | 2 or more per day | | | | |
| Whole, fresh or dried fruit. | 2 or more per day | | | | |
| Margarine, salad dressing, vegetable oil (in cooking etc.). | small amts. | | | | |

## FOOD FREQUENCY
How many servings of the following foods do you eat per week, including snacks?

| FOOD | GOAL | EXPLANATION |
|---|---|---|
| Fried, deep-fat fried, or breaded foods (fried chicken or fish, hash browns, french fries, etc.). | less than one per week | *Very high in fat and calories.* |
| Fatty meats (bacon, sausage, hamburger, lunchmeat, ribs, prime rib, corned beef and hot dogs). | less than one per week | *Very high in fat and calories.* |
| Lean red meats (round or sirloin steak, London broil, lean ham, pork loin, Canadian bacon, veal). | up to 3 to 4 3-ounce servings per week | *Moderate amounts of lean red meat will not lead to excessive fat/chol. intake and help promote a well balanced diet.* |
| Sea food (fish and shellfish -- other than fried). | 3-4 servings per week | *Low in fat; source of desirable Omega 3 fats.* |
| Egg yolks (including those in baked and cooked foods). | 3-4 per week | *Yolks should be limited due to cholesterol, but need not be eliminated - they are nutrient rich and relatively low in fat.* |
| Whole milk, high-fat cheese (such as cheddar, cream and Swiss). | depends on other fat sources | *Rich in calcium and other nutrients but high in fat and saturated fat. Non-fat/low-fat choices are preferred.* |
| Butter, coffee creamer, whipped cream, sour cream. | less than one per week | *Very high in fat, saturated fat and calories.* |
| High-fat desserts such as pies, pastries, ice cream, cookies, cake and chocolate. | less than one per week or in small amts. | *High in fat/calories and low in nutrients. Low-fat alternatives are preferred, such as angel food cake, fig newtons, vanilla wafers, sherbet, frozen yogurt& hard candy.* |
| High-fat snacks such as crackers, chips, buttered popcorn, etc. | less than one per week or in small amts. | *High in fat/calories and low in nutrients. Low-fat snacks are lower in calories than things such as pretzels, plain popcorn, fruit, crispbread.* |
| Nuts, avocado, olive oil, olives, peanut butter. | small amts. | *High in fat, but monounsaturates are preferred type.* |
| Whole grains, whole-wheat or rye bread, whole-wheat paste, brown rice, bran or whole-wheat cereals. | 6 or more servings per week | *Eat daily for insoluble fiber, promotes regularity and decreases cancer risk.* |
| Oat bran, oatmeal, legumes (dark beans, peas, and lentils). | depends | *Sources of soluble fiber which helps decrease blood sugar and serum cholesterol in those with elevated levels.* |
| Fresh or frozen, raw or lightly cooked vegetables. | 2 or more per day | *Rich in fiber and nutrients; fat and cholesterol-free low in calories.* |
| Whole, fresh or dried fruit. | 2 or more per day | *Rich in fiber and nutrients; fat and cholesterol-free; naturally sweet.* |
| Margarine, salad dressing, vegetable oil (in cooking etc.). | small amts. | *Very high in fat and calories.* |

■

# FAT AND CHOLESTEROL COMPARISON CHARTS

■

## MEATS

| Product 3½ ounces, cooked)* | Saturated Fatty Acids (grams) | Cholesterol (milligrams) | Total Fat† (grams) | Calories From Fat‡(%) | Total Calories |
|---|---|---|---|---|---|
| *Beef* | | | | | |
| Kidneys, simmered§ | 1.1 | 387 | 3.4 | 21 | 144 |
| Liver, braised§ | 1.9 | 389 | 4.9 | 27 | 161 |
| Round, top round, lean only, broiled | 2.2 | 84 | 6.2 | 29 | 191 |
| Round, eye of round, lean only, roasted | 2.5 | 69 | 6.5 | 32 | 183 |
| Round, tip round, lean only, roasted | 2.8 | 81 | 7.5 | 36 | 190 |
| Round, full cut, lean only, choice, broiled | 2.9 | 82 | 8.0 | 37 | 194 |
| Round, bottom round, lean only, braised | 3.4 | 96 | 9.7 | 39 | 222 |
| Short loin, top loin, lean only, broiled | 3.6 | 76 | 8.9 | 40 | 203 |
| Wedge-bone sirloin, lean only, broiled | 3.6 | 89 | 8.7 | 38 | 208 |
| Short loin, tenderloin, lean only, broiled | 3.6 | 84 | 9.3 | 41 | 204 |

Source: *Eating to Lower Your Blood Cholesterol.* Developed by National Heart, Lung, and Blood Institute.

*Composition of Foods: Beef Products—Raw•Processed•Prepared, Agriculture Handbook 8–13.* Washington, D.C.: U.S. Department of Agriculture, Human Nutrition Information Service (August 1986).

*Composition of Foods: Pork Products—Raw•Processed•Prepared, Agriculture Handbook 8–10.* Washington, D.C.: U.S. Department of Agriculture, Human Nutrition Information Service (August 1983).

*Home and Garden Bulletin. Nutritive Value of Foods,* No. 72. Washington, D.C.: U.S. Department of Agriculture, Human Nutrition Information Service (1986).

*3½ ounces = 100 grams (approximately).

†Total fat = saturated fatty acids plus monounsaturated fatty acids plus polyunsaturated fatty acids.

‡Percent calories from fat = total fat calories divided by total calories, multiplied by 100; total fat calories = total fat (grams) multiplied by 9.

§Liver and most organ meats are low in fat but high in cholesterol. If you are eating to lower your blood cholesterol, consider your total cholesterol intake before selecting an organ meat.

| Product 3½ ounces, cooked)* | Saturated Fatty Acids (grams) | Cholesterol (milligrams) | Total Fat† (grams) | Calories From Fat‡(%) | Total Calories |
|---|---|---|---|---|---|
| Chuck, arm pot roast, lean only, braised | 3.8 | 101 | 10.0 | 39 | 231 |
| Short loin, T-bone steak, lean only, choice, broiled | 4.2 | 80 | 10.4 | 44 | 214 |
| Short loin, porter house steak, lean only, choice, broiled | 4.3 | 80 | 10.8 | 45 | 218 |
| Brisket, whole, lean only, braised | 4.6 | 93 | 12.8 | 48 | 241 |
| Rib eye, small end (ribs 10–12), lean only, choice broiled | 4.9 | 80 | 11.6 | 47 | 225 |
| Rib, whole (ribs 6–12), lean only, roasted | 5.8 | 81 | 13.8 | 52 | 240 |
| Flank, lean only, choice, braised | 5.9 | 71 | 13.8 | 51 | 244 |
| Rib, large end (ribs 6–9), lean only, broiled | 6.1 | 82 | 14.2 | 55 | 233 |
| Chuck, blade roast, lean only, braised | 6.2 | 106 | 15.3 | 51 | 270 |
| Corned beef, cured, brisket, cooked | 6.3 | 98 | 19.0 | 68 | 251 |
| Flank, lean and fat, choice, braised | 6.6 | 72 | 15.5 | 54 | 257 |
| Ground, lean, broiled meium | 7.2 | 87 | 18.5 | 61 | 272 |
| Round, full cut, lean and fat, choice, braised | 7.3 | 84 | 18.2 | 60 | 274 |
| Rib, short ribs, lean only, choice, braised | 7.7 | 93 | 18.1 | 55 | 295 |
| Salami, cured, cooked, smoked, 3–4 slices | 9.0 | 65 | 20.7 | 71 | 262 |
| Short loin, T-bone steak, lean and fat, choice, broiled | 10.2 | 84 | 24.6 | 68 | 324 |
| Chuck, arm pot roast, lean and fat, braised | 10.7 | 99 | 26.0 | 67 | 350 |
| Sausage, cured, cooked, smoked, about 2 | 11.4 | 67 | 26.9 | 78 | 312 |

| Product<br>(3½ ounces,<br>cooked)* | Saturated<br>Fatty Acids<br>(grams) | Cholesterol<br>(milligrams) | Total Fat†<br>(grams) | Calories<br>From<br>Fat‡(%) | Total<br>Calories |
|---|---|---|---|---|---|
| Bologna, cured, 3–4 slices | 12.1 | 58 | 28.5 | 82 | 312 |
| Frankfurter, cured, about 2 | 12.0 | 61 | 28.5 | 82 | 315 |
| *Lamb* | | | | | |
| Leg, lean only, roasted | 3.0 | 89 | 8.2 | 39 | 191 |
| Loin chop, lean only, broiled | 4.1 | 94 | 9.4 | 39 | 215 |
| Rib, lean only, roasted | 5.7 | 88 | 12.3 | 48 | 232 |
| Arm chop, lean only, braised | 6.0 | 122 | 14.6 | 47 | 279 |
| Rib, lean and fat, roasted | 14.2 | 90 | 30.6 | 75 | 368 |
| *Pork* | | | | | |
| Cured, ham steak, boneless, extra lean, unheated | 1.4 | 45 | 4.2 | 31 | 122 |
| Liver, braised§ | 1.4 | 355 | 4.4 | 24 | 165 |
| Kidneys, braised§ | 1.5 | 480 | 4.7 | 28 | 151 |
| Fresh, loin, tenderloin, lean only, roasted | 1.7 | 93 | 4.8 | 26 | 166 |
| Cured, shoulder, arm picnic, lean only, roasted | 2.4 | 48 | 7.0 | 37 | 170 |
| Cured, ham, boneless, regular, roasted | 3.1 | 59 | 9.0 | 46 | 178 |
| Fresh, leg (ham), shank half, lean only, roasted | 3.6 | 92 | 10.5 | 44 | 215 |
| Fresh, leg (ham), rump half, lean only, roasted | 3.7 | 96 | 10.7 | 43 | 221 |
| Fresh, loin, center loin, sirloin, lean only, roasted | 4.5 | 91 | 13.1 | 49 | 240 |
| Fresh, loin, sirloin, lean only, roasted | 4.5 | 90 | 13.2 | 50 | 236 |
| Fresh, loin, center rib, lean only, roasted | 4.8 | 79 | 13.8 | 51 | 245 |
| Fresh, loin, top loin, lean only, roasted | 4.8 | 79 | 13.8 | 51 | 245 |
| Fresh, shoulder, blade, Boston, lean only, roasted | 5.8 | 98 | 16.8 | 59 | 256 |

| Product 3½ ounces, cooked)* | Saturated Fatty Acids (grams) | Cholesterol (milligrams) | Total Fat† (grams) | Calories From Fat‡(%) | Total Calories |
|---|---|---|---|---|---|
| Fresh, loin, blade, lean only, roasted | 6.6 | 89 | 19.3 | 62 | 279 |
| Fresh, loin, sirloin, lean and fat, roasted | 7.4 | 91 | 20.4 | 63 | 291 |
| Cured, shoulder, arm picnic, lean and fat, roasted | 7.7 | 58 | 21.4 | 69 | 280 |
| Fresh, loin, center loin, lean and fat, roasted | 7.9 | 91 | 21.8 | 64 | 305 |
| Cured, shoulder, blade roll, lean and fat, roasted | 8.4 | 67 | 23.5 | 74 | 287 |
| Fresh, Italian sausage, cooked | 9.0 | 78 | 25.7 | 72 | 323 |
| Fresh, bratwurst, cooked | 9.3 | 60 | 25.9 | 77 | 301 |
| Fresh, chitterlings, cooked | 10.1 | 143 | 28.8 | 86 | 303 |
| Cured, liver sausage, liverwurst | 10.6 | 158 | 28.5 | 79 | 326 |
| Cured, smoked link sausage, grilled | 11.3 | 68 | 31.8 | 74 | 389 |
| Fresh, spareribs, lean and fat, braised | 11.8 | 121 | 30.3 | 69 | 397 |
| Cured, salami, dry or hard | 11.9 | N.A. | 33.7 | 75 | 407 |
| Bacon, fried | 17.4 | 85 | 49.2 | 78 | 576 |
| *Veal* | | | | | |
| Rump, lean only, roasted | N.A. | 128 | 2.2 | 13 | 156 |
| Sirloin, lean only, roasted | N.A. | 128 | 3.2 | 19 | 153 |
| Arm steak, lean only, cooked | N.A. | 90 | 5.3 | 24 | 200 |
| Loin chop, lean only, cooked | N.A. | 90 | 6.7 | 29 | 207 |
| Blade, lean only, cooked | N.A. | 90 | 7.8 | 33 | 211 |
| Cutlet, medium fat, braised or broiled | 4.8 | 128 | 11.0 | 37 | 271 |
| Foreshank, medium fat, stewed | N.A. | 90 | 10.4 | 43 | 216 |
| Plate, medium fat, stewed | N.A. | 90 | 21.2 | 63 | 303 |
| Rib, medium fat, roasted | 7.1 | 128 | 16.9 | 70 | 218 |

| Product (3½ ounces, cooked)* | Saturated Fatty Acids (grams) | Cholesterol (milligrams) | Total Fat† (grams) | Calories From Fat‡(%) | Total Calories |
|---|---|---|---|---|---|
| Flank, medium fat, stewed | N.A. | 90 | 32.3 | 75 | 390 |

## POULTRY

| Product (3½ ounces, cooked)* | Saturated Fatty Acids (grams) | Cholesterol (milligrams) | Total Fat† (grams) | Calories From Fat‡(%) | Total Calories |
|---|---|---|---|---|---|
| Turkey, fryer-roasters, light meat without skin, roasted | 0.4 | 86 | 1.9 | 8 | 140 |
| Chicken, roasters, light meat without skin, roasted | 1.1 | 75 | 4.1 | 24 | 153 |
| Turkey, fryer-roasters, light meat with skin, roasted | 1.3 | 95 | 4.6 | 25 | 164 |
| Chicken, broilers or fryers, light meat without skin, roasted | 1.3 | 85 | 4.5 | 24 | 173 |
| Turkey, fryer-roasters, dark meat without skin, roasted | 1.4 | 112 | 4.3 | 24 | 162 |
| Chicken, stewing, light meat without skin, stewed | 2.0 | 70 | 8.0 | 34 | 213 |
| Turkey roll, light and dark | 2.0 | 55 | 7.0 | 42 | 149 |
| Turkey, fryer-roasters, dark meat with skin, roasted | 2.1 | 117 | 7.1 | 35 | 182 |
| Chicken, roasters, dark meat without skin, roasted | 2.4 | 75 | 8.8 | 44 | 178 |

Source: *Eating to Lower Your Blood Cholesterol.* Developed by National Heart, Lung, and Blood Institute.

*Composition of Foods: Poultry Products—Raw•Processed•Prepared, Agriculture Handbook 8-5.* Washington, D.C.: U.S. Department of Agriculture, Science and Education Administration (August 1979).
*3½ ounces = 100 grams (approximately).
†Total fat = saturated fatty acids plus monounsaturated fatty acids plus polyunsaturated fatty acids.
‡Percent calories from fat = total fat calories divided by total calories, multiplied by 100; total fat calories = total fat (grams) multiplied by 9.
§Source: Practorcare/Nutripractor. Nutripractor 600 Software program. Practorcare, Inc. San Diego, CA.

| Product (3½ ounces, cooked)* | Saturated Fatty Acids (grams) | Cholesterol (milligrams) | Total Fat† (grams) | Calories From Fat‡(%) | Total Calories |
|---|---|---|---|---|---|
| Chicken, broilers or fryers, dark meat without skin, roasted | 2.7 | 93 | 9.7 | 43 | 205 |
| Chicken, broilers or fryers, light meat with skin, roasted | 3.0 | 85 | 10.9 | 44 | 222 |
| Chicken, stewing, dark meat without skin, stewed | 4.1 | 95 | 15.3 | 53 | 258 |
| Duck, domesticated, flesh only, roasted | 4.2 | 89 | 11.2 | 50 | 201 |
| Chicken, broilers or fryers, dark meat with skin, roasted | 4.4 | 91 | 15.8 | 56 | 253 |
| Goose, domesticated, flesh only, roasted | 4.6 | 96 | 12.7 | 48 | 238 |
| Turkey bologna, about 3½ slices | 5.1 | 99 | 15.2 | 69 | 199 |
| Chicken frankfurter, about 2 | 5.5 | 101 | 19.5 | 68 | 257 |
| Turkey frankfurter, about 2 | 5.9 | 107 | 17.7 | 70 | 226 |
| Turkey ham, 1 oz.§ | 0.48 | 16 | 1.44 | 36 | 36 |

## FISH AND SHELLFISH

| Product (3½ ounces, cooked)* | Saturated Fatty Acids (grams) | Cholesterol (milligrams) | Omega-3 Fatty Acids (grams) | Total Fat† (grams) | Calories From Fat‡(%) | Total Calories |
|---|---|---|---|---|---|---|
| *Finfish* | | | | | | |
| Haddock, dry heat | 0.2 | 74 | 0.2 | 0.9 | 7 | 112 |
| Cod, Atlantic, dry heat | 0.2 | 55 | 0.2 | 0.9 | 7 | 105 |

Source: *Eating to Lower Your Blood Cholesterol.* Developed by National Heart, Lung, and Blood Institute.

*Composition of Foods: Finfish and Shellfish Products—Raw•Processed•Prepared, Agriculture Handbook 8-15.* Washington, D.C.: U.S. Department of Agriculture (in press).
*3½ ounces = 100 grams (approximately)
†Total fat = saturated fatty acids plus monounsaturated fatty acids plus polyunsaturated fatty acids.
‡Percent calories from fat = total fat calories divided by total calories, multiplied by 100; total fat calories = total fat (grams) multiplied by 9.
§Source: Practorcare/Nutripractor.

| Product (3½ ounces, cooked)* | Saturated Fatty Acids (grams) | Cholesterol (milligrams) | Omega-3 Fatty Acids (grams) | Total Fat† (grams) | Calories From Fat‡(%) | Total Calories |
|---|---|---|---|---|---|---|
| Pollock, walleye, dry heat | 0.2 | 96 | 1.5 | 1.1 | 9 | 113 |
| Perch, mixed species, dry heat | 0.2 | 42 | 0.3 | 1.2 | 9 | 117 |
| Grouper, mixed species, dry heat | 0.3 | 47 | N.A. | 1.3 | 10 | 118 |
| Whiting, mixed species, dry heat | 0.3 | 84 | 0.9 | 1.7 | 13 | 115 |
| Snapper, mixed species, dry heat | 0.4 | 47 | N.A. | 1.7 | 12 | 128 |
| Halibut, Atlantic and Pacific, dry heat | 0.4 | 41 | 0.6 | 2.9 | 19 | 140 |
| Rockfish, Pacific, dry heat | 0.5 | 44 | 0.5 | 2.0 | 15 | 121 |
| Sea bass, mixed species, dry heat | 0.7 | 53 | N.A. | 2.5 | 19 | 124 |
| Trout, rainbow, dry heat | 0.8 | 73 | 0.9 | 4.3 | 26 | 151 |
| Swordfish, dry heat | 1.4 | 50 | 1.1 | 5.1 | 30 | 155 |
| Tuna, bluefin, dry heat | 1.6 | 49 | N.A. | 6.3 | 31 | 184 |
| Tuna salad§ (1 cup) | 3.21 | 27 | N.A. | 19.22 | 44.5 | 389 |
| Salmon, sockeye, dry heat | 1.9 | 87 | 1.3 | 11.0 | 46 | 216 |
| Anchovy, European, canned | 2.2 | N.A. | 2.1 | 9.7 | 42 | 210 |
| Herring, Atlantic, dry heat | 2.6 | 77 | 2.1 | 11.5 | 51 | 203 |
| Eel, dry heat | 3.0 | 161 | 0.7 | 15.0 | 57 | 236 |

| Product (3½ ounces, cooked)* | Saturated Fatty Acids (grams) | Cholesterol (milligrams) | Omega-3 Fatty Acids (grams) | Total Fat† (grams) | Calories From Fat‡(%) | Total Calories |
|---|---|---|---|---|---|---|
| Mackerel, Atlantic, dry heat | 4.2 | 75 | 1.3 | 17.8 | 61 | 262 |
| Pompano, Florida, dry heat | 4.5 | 64 | N.A. | 12.1 | 52 | 211 |
| *Crustaceans* | | | | | | |
| Lobster, northern | 0.1 | 72 | 0.1 | 0.6 | 6 | 98 |
| Crab, blue, moist heat | 0.2 | 100 | 0.5 | 1.8 | 16 | 102 |
| Shrimp, mixed species, moist heat | 0.3 | 195 | 0.3 | 1.1 | 10 | 99 |
| *Mollusks* | | | | | | |
| Whelk, moist heat | 0.1 | 130 | N.A. | 0.8 | 3 | 275 |
| Clam, mixed species, moist heat | 0.2 | 67 | 0.3 | 2.0 | 12 | 148 |
| Mussel, blue, moist heat | 0.9 | 56 | 0.8 | 4.5 | 23 | 172 |
| Oyster, Eastern, moist heat | 1.3 | 109 | 1.0 | 5.0 | 33 | 137 |

## FRUITS AND VEGETABLES*

| Product | Total Calories | Total Fat (grams) | Calories from Fat (%) |
|---|---|---|---|
| Apple, 1 g. (10 oz.) | 167 | 1.02 | 5.0 |
| Pear, 1 g. (10 oz.) | 167 | 1.13 | 6.0 |
| Banana, 1 g. (10 oz.) | 183 | 0.95 | 5.0 |
| Coleslaw, 0.5 cup | 41 | 1.56 | 34.0 |
| Carrot and raisin salad, 0.5 cup | 152 | 10.78 | 64.0 |
| Potato salad, 0.5 cup | 144 | 8.25 | 52.0 |
| Baked Potato, 1 g., 10 oz. | 309 | 0.28 | 0.8 |
| McDonald's French fries, regular serving | 220 | 11.5 | 47.0 |
| Hash browns, ckd. (1 cup) | 345 | 18.19 | 47.0 |

*Source: Practorcare/Nutripractor.

## DAIRY AND EGG PRODUCTS

| Product | Saturated Fat (grams) | Cholesterol (milligrams) | Total Fat* (grams) | Calories From Fat†(%) | Total Calories |
|---|---|---|---|---|---|
| *Milk* (8 oz.) | | | | | |
| Skim milk | 0.3 | 4 | 0.4 | 5 | 86 |
| Buttermilk | 1.3 | 9 | 2.2 | 20 | 99 |
| Low-fat milk, 1% fat | 1.6 | 10 | 2.6 | 23 | 102 |
| Low-fat milk, 2% fat | 2.9 | 18 | 4.7 | 35 | 121 |
| Whole milk, 3.3% fat | 5.1 | 33 | 8.2 | 49 | 150 |
| *Yogurt* (4 oz.) | | | | | |
| Plain yogurt, low fat | 0.1 | 2 | 0.2 | 3 | 63 |
| Plain yogurt | 2.4 | 14 | 3.7 | 47 | 70 |
| *Cheese* | | | | | |
| Cottage cheese, low-fat, 1% fat, 4 oz. | 0.7 | 5 | 1.2 | 13 | 82 |
| Mozzarella, part-skim, 1 oz. | 2.9 | 16 | 4.5 | 56 | 72 |
| Helluva Good low-fat Cheddar cheese, 1 oz.‡ | 3 | 20 | 6 | 60 | 90 |
| Weight Watchers low-fat Cheddar cheese, 1 oz.‡ | 3 | 20 | 5 | 50 | 90 |
| Kraft low-fat Cheddar cheese, 1 oz.‡ | 3 | 20 | 5 | 56 | 80 |
| Kraft Light Singles American pasturized processed, 1 oz.‡ | 3 | 15 | 4 | 51 | 70 |
| Cottage cheese, creamed, 4 oz. | 3.2 | 17 | 5.1 | 39 | 117 |
| Mozzarella, 1 oz. | 3.7 | 22 | 6.1 | 69 | 80 |
| Sour cream, 1 oz. | 3.7 | 12 | 5.9 | 87 | 61 |
| American processed cheese spread, pasteurized, 1 oz. | 3.8 | 16 | 6.0 | 66 | 82 |
| Feta, 1 oz. | 4.2 | 25 | 6.0 | 72 | 75 |
| Neufchâtel, 1 oz. | 4.2 | 22 | 6.6 | 81 | 74 |
| Camembert, 1 oz. | 4.3 | 20 | 6.9 | 73 | 85 |
| American processed cheese food, pasteurized, 1 oz. | 4.4 | 18 | 7.0 | 68 | 93 |
| Provolone, 1 oz. | 4.8 | 20 | 7.6 | 68 | 100 |

Source: *Eating to Lower Your Blood Cholesterol.* Developed by National Heart, Lung, and Blood Institute.

*Composition of Foods: Dairy and Egg Proucts—Raw•Processed•Prepared, Agriculture Handbook 8-1.* Washington, D.C.: U.S. Department of Agriculture, Agricultural Research Service (November 1976).
*Total fat = saturated fatty acids plus monounsaturated fatty acids plus polyunsaturated fatty acids.
†Percent calories from fat = total fat calories divided by total calories, multiplied by 100; total fat calories = total fat (grams) multiplied by 9.
‡Source: Manufacturer information.

| Product | Saturated Fat (grams) | Cholesterol (milligrams) | Total Fat* (grams) | Calories From Fat†(%) | Total Calories |
|---|---|---|---|---|---|
| Limburger, 1 oz. | 4.8 | 26 | 7.7 | 75 | 93 |
| Brie, 1 oz. | 4.9 | 28 | 7.9 | 74 | 95 |
| Romano, 1 oz. | 4.9 | 29 | 7.6 | 63 | 110 |
| Gouda, 1 oz. | 5.0 | 32 | 7.8 | 69 | 101 |
| Swiss, 1 oz. | 5.0 | 26 | 7.8 | 65 | 107 |
| Edam, 1 oz. | 5.0 | 25 | 7.9 | 70 | 101 |
| Brick, 1 oz. | 5.3 | 27 | 8.4 | 72 | 105 |
| Blue, 1 oz. | 5.3 | 21 | 8.2 | 73 | 100 |
| Gruyère, 1 oz. | 5.4 | 31 | 9.2 | 71 | 117 |
| Muenster, 1 oz. | 5.4 | 27 | 8.5 | 74 | 104 |
| Parmesan, 1 oz. | 5.4 | 22 | 8.5 | 59 | 129 |
| Monterey Jack, 1 oz. | 5.5 | 25 | 8.6 | 73 | 106 |
| Roquefort, 1 oz. | 5.5 | 26 | 8.7 | 75 | 105 |
| Ricotta, part-skim, 4 oz. | 5.6 | 25 | 9.0 | 52 | 156 |
| American processed cheese, pasteurized, 1 oz. | 5.6 | 27 | 8.9 | 75 | 106 |
| Colby, 1 oz. | 5.7 | 27 | 9.1 | 73 | 112 |
| Cheddar, 1 oz. | 6.0 | 30 | 9.4 | 74 | 114 |
| Cream cheese, 1 oz. | 6.2 | 31 | 9.9 | 90 | 99 |
| Ricotta, whole milk, 4 oz. | 9.4 | 58 | 14.7 | 67 | 197 |
| *Eggs* | | | | | |
| Egg, chicken, white | 0 | 0 | tr. | 0 | 16 |
| Egg, chicken, whole | 1.7 | 274 | 5.6 | 64 | 79 |
| Egg, chicken, yolk | 1.7 | 272 | 5.6 | 80 | 63 |

## FROZEN DESSERTS

| Product (1 cup) | Saturated Fatty Acids (grams) | Cholesterol (milligrams) | Total Fat* (grams) | Calories From Fat†(%) | Total Calories |
|---|---|---|---|---|---|
| Fruit Popsicle, 1 bar | N.A. | N.A. | 0.0 | 0 | 65 |
| Fruit ice | N.A. | N.A. | tr. | 0 | 247 |
| Fudgsicle | N.A. | N.A. | 0.2 | 2 | 91 |

Source: *Eating to Lower Your Blood Cholesterol.* Developed by National Heart, Lung, and Blood Institute.

*Composition of Foods: Dairy and Egg Products—Raw•Processed•Prepared, Agriculture Handbook 8-1.*Washington, D.C.: U.S. Department of Agriculture, Agricultural Research Service (November 1976).

J. Pennington, and H. Church, *Bowes and Church's Food Values of Portions Commonly Used* 14th ed. Philadelphia: J. B. Lippincott Company (1985).
*Total fat = saturated fatty acids plus monounsaturated fatty acids plus polyunsaturate fatty acids.
†Percent calories from fat = total fat calories divided by total calories, multiplied by 100; total fat calories = total fat (grams) multiplied by 9.
‡Source: Manufacturer information.

| Product (1 cup) | Saturated Fatty Acids (grams) | Cholesterol (milligrams) | Total Fat* (grams) | Calories From Fat†(%) | Total Calories |
|---|---|---|---|---|---|
| Frozen yogurt, fruit-flavored | N.A. | N.A. | 2.0 | 8 | 216 |
| Sherbet, orange | 2.4 | 14 | 3.8 | 13 | 270 |
| Pudding pops, 1 pop | 2.5 | 1 | 2.6 | 25 | 94 |
| Ice milk, vanilla, soft serve | 2.9 | 13 | 4.6 | 19 | 223 |
| Ice milk, vanilla, hard | 3.5 | 18 | 5.6 | 28 | 184 |
| Ice cream, vanilla, regular | 8.9 | 59 | 14.3 | 48 | 269 |
| Ice cream, French vanilla, soft-serve | 13.5 | 153 | 22.5 | 54 | 377 |
| Ice cream, vanilla, rich, 16% fat | 14.7 | 88 | 23.7 | 61 | 349 |
| Nonfat frozen yogurt‡ 8 fluid oz. | 0 | 0 | 0 | 0 | 160 |

## FATS AND OILS

| Product (1 tablespoon) | Saturated Fatty Acids (grams) | Cholesterol (milligrams) | Poly-unsaturated Fatty Acids (grams) | Mono-unsaturated Fatty Acids (grams) | Total Fat (grams)* | Total Calories* |
|---|---|---|---|---|---|---|
| Rapeseed oil (canola oil) | 0.9 | 0 | 4.5 | 7.6 | 13.0 | 117 |
| Safflower oil | 1.2 | 0 | 10.1 | 1.6 | 12.9 | 116 |
| Sunflower oil | 1.4 | 0 | 5.5 | 6.2 | 13.1 | 118 |
| Peanut butter, smooth | 1.5 | 0 | 2.3 | 3.7 | 7.5 | 68 |
| Corn oil | 1.7 | 0 | 8.0 | 3.3 | 13.0 | 117 |
| Olive oil | 1.8 | 0 | 1.1 | 9.9 | 12.8 | 115 |
| Hydrogenated sunflower oil | 1.8 | 0 | 4.9 | 6.3 | 13.0 | 117 |

Source: *Eating to Lower Your Blood Cholesterol.* Developed by National Heart, Lung, and Blood Institute.

*Composition of Foods: Fats and Oils—Raw•Processed•Prepared, Agriculture Handbook 8-4.* Washington, D.C.: U.S. Department of Agriculture, Science and Education Administration (June 1979).

*Composition of Foods: Legumes and Legume Products—Raw•Processed•Prepared, Agriculture Handbook 8-16.* Washington, D.C.: U.S. Department of Agriculture, Human Nutrition Information Service (December 1986).

*Source: Practorcare/Nutripractor.

| Product (1 tablespoon) | Saturated Fatty Acids (grams) | Cholesterol (milligrams) | Poly-unsaturated Fatty Acids (grams) | Mono-unsaturated Fatty Acids (grams) | Total Fat (grams)* | Total Calories* |
|---|---|---|---|---|---|---|
| Margarine, liquid, bottled | 1.8 | 0 | 5.1 | 3.9 | 10.8 | 97 |
| Margarine, soft, tub | 1.8 | 0 | 3.9 | 4.8 | 10.5 | 95 |
| Sesame oil | 1.9 | 0 | 5.7 | 5.4 | 13.0 | 117 |
| Soybean oil | 2.0 | 0 | 7.9 | 3.2 | 13.1 | 118 |
| Margarine, stick | 2.1 | 0 | 3.6 | 5.1 | 10.8 | 97 |
| Peanut oil | 2.3 | 0 | 4.3 | 6.2 | 12.8 | 115 |
| Cottonseed oil | 3.5 | 0 | 7.1 | 2.4 | 13.0 | 117 |
| Lard | 5.0 | 12 | 1.4 | 5.8 | 12.2 | 110 |
| Beef tallow | 6.4 | 14 | 0.5 | 5.3 | 12.2 | 110 |
| Palm oil | 6.7 | 0 | 1.3 | 5.0 | 13.0 | 117 |
| Butter | 7.1 | 31 | 0.4 | 3.3 | 10.8 | 97 |
| Cocoa butter | 8.1 | 0 | 0.4 | 4.5 | 13.0 | 117 |
| Palm kernel oil | 11.1 | 0 | 0.2 | 1.5 | 12.8 | 115 |
| Coconut oil | 11.8 | 0 | 0.2 | 0.8 | 12.8 | 115 |

## NUTS AND SEEDS

| Product (1 ounce) | Saturated Fatty Acids (grams) | Cholesterol (milligrams) | Total Fat* (grams) | Calories From Fat†(%) | Total Calories |
|---|---|---|---|---|---|
| European chestnuts | 0.2 | 0 | 1.1 | 9 | 105 |
| Filberts or hazelnuts | 1.3 | 0 | 17.8 | 89 | 179 |
| Almonds | 1.4 | 0 | 15.0 | 80 | 167 |
| Pecans | 1.5 | 0 | 18.4 | 89 | 187 |
| Sunflower seed kernels, roasted | 1.5 | 0 | 1.4 | 77 | 165 |

Sources: *Eating to Lower Your Blood Cholesterol.* Developed by National Heart, Lung, and Blood Institute.

*Composition of Foods: Legumes and Legume Products—Raw•Processed•Prepared, Agriculture Handbook 8-16.* Washington, D.C.: U.S. Department of Agriculture, Human Nutrition Information Service (December 1986).

*Composition of Foods: Nut and Seed ProductsRaw•Processed•Prepared, Agriculture Handbook 8-12.* Washington, D.C.: U.S. Department of Agriculture, Human Nutrition Information Service (September 1984).

*Total fat = saturated fatty acids plus monounsaturated fatty acids plus polyunsaturated fatty acids.
†Percent calories from fat = (total fat calories divided by total calories) multiplied by 100; total fat calories = total fat (grams) multiplied by 9.

| Product (1 ounce) | Saturated Fatty Acids (grams) | Cholesterol (milligrams) | Total Fat* (grams) | Calories From Fat†(%) | Total Calories |
|---|---|---|---|---|---|
| English walnuts | 1.6 | 0 | 17.6 | 87 | 182 |
| Pistachio nuts | 1.7 | 0 | 13.7 | 75 | 164 |
| Peanuts | 1.9 | 0 | 14.0 | 76 | 164 |
| Hickory nuts | 2.0 | 0 | 18.3 | 88 | 187 |
| Pine nuts, pignolia | 2.2 | 0 | 14.4 | 89 | 146 |
| Pumpkin and squash seed kernels | 2.3 | 0 | 12.0 | 73 | 148 |
| Cashew nuts | 2.6 | 0 | 13.2 | 73 | 163 |
| Macadamia nuts | 3.1 | 0 | 20.9 | 95 | 199 |
| Brazil nuts | 4.6 | 0 | 18.8 | 91 | 186 |
| Coconut meat, unsweetened | 16.3 | 0 | 18.3 | 88 | 187 |

## BREADS, CEREALS, PASTA, RICE, AND DRIED PEAS AND BEANS

| Product | Saturated Fatty Acids (grams) | Cholesterol (milligrams) | Total Fat* (grams) | Calories From Fat†(%) | Total Calories |
|---|---|---|---|---|---|
| *Breads* | | | | | |
| Melba toast, 1 plain | 0.1 | 0 | tr. | 0 | 20 |
| Pita, ½ large shell | 0.1 | 0 | 1.0 | 5 | 165 |
| Corn tortilla | 0.1 | 0 | 1.0 | 14 | 65 |
| Rye bread, 1 slice | 0.2 | 0 | 1.0 | 14 | 65 |
| English muffin | 0.3 | 0 | 1.0 | 6 | 140 |
| Bagel, 1, 3½" diameter | 0.3 | 0 | 2.0 | 9 | 200 |
| White bread, 1 slice | 0.3 | 0 | 1.0 | 14 | 65 |
| Ry-Krisp, 2 triple crackers | 0.3 | 0 | 1.0 | 16 | 56 |
| Whole-wheat bread, 1 slice | 0.4 | 0 | 1.0 | 13 | 70 |
| Saltines, 4 | 0.5 | 4 | 1.0 | 18 | 50 |
| Hamburger bun | 0.5 | tr. | 2.0 | 16 | 115 |

Source: *Eating to Lower Your Blood Cholesterol*. Developed by National Heart, Lung, and Blood Institute.

*Composition of Foods: Breakfast Cereals—Raw•Processed•Prepared, Agriculture Handbook 8-8*. Washington, D.C.: U.S. Department of Agriculture, Human Nutrition Information Service (July 1982).

*Composition of Foods: Legume and Legume Products, Agriculture Handbook 8-16*. Washington, D.C.: U.S. Department of Agriculture, Nutrition Monitoring Division (December 1986).

*Home and Garden Bulletin. Nutritive Value of Foods*, No. 72. Washington, D.C.: U.S. Department of Agriculture. Human Nutrition Information Service (1986).

*Total fat = saturated fatty acids plus monounsaturated fatty acids plus polyunsaturated fatty acids.

†Percent calories from fat = total fat calories divided by total calories, multiplied by 100; total fat calories = total fat (grams) multiplied by 9.

‡Source: Practorcare/Nutripractor.

§Source: Wendy's Old-Fashioned Hamburgers of New York International.

| Product | Saturated Fatty Acids (grams) | Cholesterol (milligrams) | Total Fat* (grams) | Calories From Fat†(%) | Total Calories |
|---|---|---|---|---|---|
| Hot dog bun | 0.5 | tr. | 2.0 | 16 | 115 |
| Pancake, 1, 4″ diameter | 0.5 | 16 | 2.0 | 30 | 60 |
| Bran muffin, 1, 2½″ diameter | 1.4 | 24 | 6.0 | 43 | 125 |
| Corn muffin, 1, 2½″ diameter | 1.5 | 23 | 5.0 | 31 | 145 |
| Plain doughnut, 1, 3¼″ diameter | 2.8 | 20 | 12.0 | 51 | 210 |
| Croissant, 1, 4½″ by 4″ | 3.5 | 13 | 12.0 | 46 | 235 |
| Waffle, 1, 7″ diameter | 4.0 | 102 | 13.0 | 48 | 245 |
| Flour tortilla, 6″‡ | N.A. | N.A. | 1.35 | 17 | 71 |
| Flour tortilla, 8″‡ | N.A. | N.A. | 1.8 | 17 | 95 |
| *Cereals* (1 cup) | | | | | |
| Corn flakes | tr. | N.A. | 0.1 | 0 | 98 |
| Cream of wheat, cooked | tr. | N.A. | 0.5 | 3 | 134 |
| Corn grits, cooked | tr. | N.A. | 0.5 | 3 | 146 |
| Oatmeal, cooked | 0.4 | N.A. | 2.4 | 15 | 145 |
| Granola | 5.8 | N.A. | 33.1 | 50 | 595 |
| 100% Natural Cereal with raisins and dates | 13.7 | N.A. | 20.3 | 37 | 496 |
| *Pasta* (1 cup) | | | | | |
| Spaghetti, cooked | 0.1 | 0 | 1.0 | 6 | 155 |
| Elbow macaroni, cooked | 0.1 | 0 | 1.0 | 6 | 155 |
| Egg noodles, cooked | 0.5 | 50 | 2.0 | 11 | 160 |
| Chow mein noodles, canned | 2.1 | 5 | 11.0 | 45 | 220 |
| *Rice* (1 cup, cooked) | | | | | |
| Rice, white | 0.1 | 0 | 0.5 | 2 | 225 |
| Rice, brown | 0.3 | 0 | 1.0 | 4 | 230 |
| *Dried peas and beans* (1 cup, cooked) | | | | | |
| Split peas | 0.1 | 0 | 0.8 | 3 | 231 |
| Kidney beans | 0.1 | 0 | 1.0 | 4 | 225 |
| Lima beans | 0.2 | 0 | 0.7 | 3 | 217 |
| Black-eyed peas | 0.3 | 0 | 1.2 | 5 | 200 |
| Garbanzo beans | 0.4 | 0 | 4.3 | 14 | 269 |
| Refried beans, ½ c.§ | 2.0 | tr. | 6.0 | 39 | 140 |

## SWEETS AND SNACKS

| Product | Saturated Fatty Acids (grams) | Cholesterol (milligrams) | Total Fat* (grams) | Calories From Fat†(%) | Total Calories |
|---|---|---|---|---|---|
| *Beverages* | | | | | |
| Ginger ale, 12 oz. | 0.0 | 0 | 0.0 | 0 | 125 |
| Cola, regular, 12 oz. | 0.0 | 0 | 0.0 | 0 | 160 |
| Chocolate shake, 10 oz. | 6.5 | 37 | 10.5 | 26 | 360 |
| *Candy* (1 oz). | | | | | |
| Hard candy | 0.0 | 0 | 0.0 | 0 | 110 |
| Gum drops | tr. | 0 | tr. | tr. | 100 |
| Fudge | 2.1 | 1 | 3.0 | 24 | 115 |
| Milk chocolate, plain | 5.4 | 6 | 9.0 | 56 | 145 |
| *Cookies* | | | | | |
| Vanilla wafers, 5 cookies, 1¾" diameter | 0.9 | 12 | 3.3 | 32 | 94 |
| Fig bars, 4 cookies, 1⅝" × 1⅝" × ⅜" | 1.0 | 27 | 4.0 | 17 | 210 |
| Chocolate brownie with icing, 1½" × 1¾" × ⅞" | 1.6 | 14 | 4.0 | 36 | 100 |
| Oatmeal cookies, 4 cookies, 2⅝" diameter | 2.5 | 2 | 10.0 | 37 | 245 |
| Chocolate-chip cookies, 4 cookies, 2¼" diameter | 3.9 | 18 | 11.0 | 54 | 185 |
| Chocolate chip cookies, commercial, 1 oz.‡ | 1.81 | 11.06 | 5.95 | 40 | 133 |
| Chocolate chip cookies, Homemade, 1 oz.‡ | 3.75 | 27.8 | 7.97 | 51 | 141 |
| Graham bears, all types, 1 oz.§ | N.A. | 0 | 4 | 30 | 120 |
| Honey, 1 tbsp.‡ | 0 | 0 | 0 | 0 | 64 |
| Sugar, granulated, 1 tbsp.‡ | 0 | 0 | 0 | 0 | 49 |
| Jelly, 1 tbsp.‡ | 0 | 0 | 0.02 | 0.3 | 55 |
| Fig bars, 1 oz.‡ | 0.43 | 11.05 | 1.59 | 14 | 102 |

Source: *Eating to Lower Your Blood Cholesterol*. Developed by National Heart, Lung, and Blood Institute.

*Home and Garden Bulletin, Nutritive Value of Foods*, No. 72. Washington, D.C.: U.S. Department of Agriculture, Human Nutrition Information Service (1986).
*Total fat = saturated fatty acids plus monounsaturated fatty acids plus polyunsaturated fatty acids.
†Percent calories from fat = total fat calories divided by total calories, multiplied by 100; total fat calories = total fat (grams) multiplied by 9.
‡Source: Practorcare/Nutripractor.
§Source: Manufacturer information.

| Product | Saturated Fatty Acids (grams) | Cholesterol (milligrams) | Total Fat* (grams) | Calories From Fat†(%) | Total Calories |
|---|---|---|---|---|---|
| Animal crackers, 1 oz.‡ | 0.68 | 0 | 2.66 | 20 | 122 |
| Vanilla wafers, 1 oz‡ | 1.13 | 11.06 | 4.57 | 31 | 131 |
| Gingersnaps, 1 oz.‡ | 0.66 | 11.05 | 2.52 | 19 | 119 |
| *Cakes and pies* | | | | | |
| Angel food cake, 1/12 of 10" cake | tr. | 0 | tr. | tr. | 125 |
| Gingerbread, 1/9 of 8" cake | 1.1 | 1 | 4.0 | 21 | 175 |
| White layer cake with white icing, 1/16 of 9" cake | 2.1 | 3 | 9.0 | 32 | 260 |
| Yellow layer cake with chocolate icing, 1/16 of 9" cake | 3.0 | 36 | 8.0 | 31 | 235 |
| Pound cake, 1/17 of loaf | 3.0 | 64 | 5.0 | 41 | 110 |
| Devil's-food cake with chocolate icing, 1/16 of 9" cake | 3.5 | 37 | 8.0 | 31 | 235 |
| Lemon meringue pie, 1/6 of 9" pie | 4.3 | 143 | 14.0 | 36 | 355 |
| Apple pie, 1/6 of 9" pie | 4.6 | 0 | 18.0 | 40 | 405 |
| Cream pie, 1/6 of 9" pie | 15.0 | 8 | 23.0 | 46 | 455 |
| *Snacks* | | | | | |
| Popcorn, air-popped, 1 cup | tr. | 0 | tr. | tr. | 30 |
| Pretzels, stick, 2¼", 10 pretzels | tr. | 0 | tr. | tr. | 10 |
| Popcorn with oil and salted, 1 cup | 0.5 | 0 | 3.0 | 49 | 55 |
| Corn chips, 1 oz. | 1.4 | 25 | 9.0 | 52 | 155 |
| Potato chips, 1 oz. | 2.6 | 0 | 10.1 | 62 | 147 |
| *Pudding* | | | | | |
| Gelatin | 0.0 | 0 | 0.0 | 0 | 70 |
| Tapioca, ½ cup | 2.3 | 15 | 4.0 | 25 | 145 |
| Chocolate pudding, ½ cup | 2.4 | 15 | 4.0 | 24 | 150 |

## MISCELLANEOUS

| Product | Saturated Fatty Acids (grams) | Cholesterol (milligrams) | Total Fat* (grams) | Calories From Fat†(%) | Total Calories |
|---|---|---|---|---|---|
| *Gravies* (½ cup) | | | | | |
| Au jus, canned | 0.1 | 1 | 0.3 | 3 | 80 |
| Turkey, canned | 0.7 | 3 | 2.5 | 37 | 61 |
| Beef, canned | 1.4 | 4 | 2.8 | 41 | 62 |
| Chicken, canned | 1.7 | 3 | 6.8 | 65 | 95 |
| *Sauces* (½ cup) | | | | | |
| Sweet and sour | tr. | 0 | 0.1 | <1 | 147 |
| Barbecue | 0.3 | 0 | 2.3 | 22 | 94 |
| White | 3.2 | 17 | 6.7 | 50 | 121 |
| Cheese | 4.7 | 26 | 8.6 | 50 | 154 |
| Sour cream | 8.5 | 45 | 15.1 | 53 | 255 |
| Hollandaise | 20.9 | 94 | 34.1 | 87 | 353 |
| Bearnaise | 20.9 | 99 | 34.1 | 88 | 351 |
| *Salad dressings* (1 tbsp.) | | | | | |
| Russian, low-calorie | 0.1 | 1 | 0.7 | 27 | 23 |
| French, low-calorie | 0.1 | 1 | 0.9 | 37 | 22 |
| Italian, low-calorie | 0.2 | 1 | 1.5 | 85 | 16 |
| Thousand Island, low-calorie | 0.2 | 2 | 1.6 | 59 | 24 |
| Imitation mayonnaise | 0.5 | 4 | 2.9 | 75 | 35 |
| Thousand Island, regular | 0.9 | N.A. | 5.6 | 86 | 59 |
| Italian, regular | 1.0 | N.A. | 7.1 | 93 | 69 |
| Russian, regular | 1.1 | N.A. | 7.8 | 92 | 76 |
| French, regular | 1.5 | N.A. | 6.4 | 86 | 67 |
| Blue cheese | 1.5 | N.A. | 8.0 | 93 | 77 |
| Mayonnaise | 1.6 | 8 | 11.0 | 100 | 99 |
| *Other* | | | | | |
| Olives, green, 4 medium | 0.2 | 0 | 1.5 | 90 | 15 |
| Nondairy creamer, powdered, 1 tsp. | 0.7 | 0 | 1.0 | 90 | 10 |
| Avocado, Florida | 5.3 | 0 | 27.0 | 72 | 340 |

Source: *Eating to Lower Your Blood Cholesterol.* Developed by National Heart, Lung, and Blood Institute.

*Composition of Foods: Fats and Oils—Raw•Processed•Prepared, Agriculture Handbook 8-4.* Washington, D.C.: U.S. Department of Agriculture, Science and Education Administration (June 1979).

*Composition of Foods: Soups, Sauces and Gravies—Raw•Processed•Prepared, Agriculture Handbook 8-6.* Washington, D.C.: U.S. Department of Agriculture, Science and Education Administration (February 1980).

*Home and Garden Bulletin. Nutritive Value of Foods,* No. 72. Washington, D.C.: U.S. Department of Agriculture, Human Nutrition Information Service (1986).

*Total fat = saturated fatty acids plus monounsaturated fatty acids plus polyunsaturated fatty acids.

†Percent calories from fat = total fat calories divided by total calories, multiplied by 100; total fat calories = fat (grams) multiplied by 9.

| Product | Saturated Fatty Acids (grams) | Cholesterol (milligrams) | Total Fat* (grams) | Calories From Fat†(%) | Total Calories |
|---|---|---|---|---|---|
| Pizza, cheese, ⅛ of 15″ diameter | 4.1 | 56 | 9.0 | 28 | 290 |
| Quiche lorraine, ⅛ of 8″ diameter | 23.2 | 285 | 48.0 | 72 | 600 |
| White wine, 3.5 oz.‡ | 0 | 0 | 0 | 0 | 71 |
| Salsa, 1.8 oz.‡ | 0 | 0 | 0 | 0 | 10 |

# APPENDIX B

# Stretching Exercises

Warm-ups, cool-downs, and stretching are essential to any safe, comfortable workout. While warming up prepares your muscles for vigorous activity by increasing the blood flow and improving flexibility, cooling down and stretching help you avoid stiffness and soreness by preventing the muscles from tightening up. These exercises, in effect, allow you to "ease in" and "ease out" of your workout. And they help focus your mind on what you're doing.

To warm your muscles, walk, cycle, or stair-step at a slower pace than usual for five minutes or so, then speed it up. Do the same thing to cool down, then do the following stretching exercises (which can also be used for warming up):

**1. Overall stretch.** Lie on the floor with your back flat, and arms and hands on the floor above your head. Keeping your arms and legs as flat against the mat or carpet as possible, stretch your body in opposite directions by reaching up with your arms and down with your legs. Good for overall flexibility.

**2. Hips.** Lie flat on the floor on your back. Pull one knee up toward your chest, keeping the opposite leg flat on the floor. Slowly return the bent leg to the start position. Repeat with the other leg. Good for walking, tennis, golf, or any activity requiring hip flexibility.

**3. Spine rotation.** Sit on the floor with your legs stretched out flat in front of you. (If you can't straighten your legs, then bend them cross-legged.) With your arms folded across your chest, slowly turn your entire upper torso to the right, then to the left, keeping your legs and hips in place. Good for any activity requiring turning, twisting, or reaching.

**4. Shoulders.** Lie flat on the floor on your back, with your arms straight down at your sides, palms down. Bend your knees, and slide your feet up close to your buttocks. Keep your lower back flat and elbows straight as you raise your arms in the air, then slowly lower them until the backs of your hands touch the mat above your head. Good for tennis, golf, or any activity that uses the shoulders.

**5. Hamstrings.** Sit on the floor with one leg stretched out in front of you. Bend the other leg and cross it above the stretched leg's knee. Planting your hands on the mat next to your hips for support, bend forward from the hips, keeping your arms straight. Make sure you bend from the hips and not the upper back. Focusing attention on an object directly in front of you may help you do this properly. Good for most activities that require walking or running.

**6. Upper calves.** Stand facing a wall about eighteen inches away from it, with your feet apart and your hands on the wall for balance. With your legs straight and your toes pointed ahead, lean toward the wall as you would in a push-up. Keep your body straight during the stretch. Good for any activity requiring walking or running.

**7. Spine and hip rotation.** Stand with your hands on your hips. Do the same twisting motion that you did for the spine rotation, but include the hips as you rotate. Keep your knees in place and your feet pointing straight ahead, aproximately your shoulders' width apart. Good for walking, golf, tennis, or any activity requiring reaching or hip rotation.

**8. Achilles tendons.** Do the same exercise as for upper calves (stretch number 6), but bend your knees. Good for any activity requiring walking or running.

# APPENDIX C

## Your Walking Program

To begin the *Rockport Fitness Walking Test:*

■ Take your pulse by putting your second and third fingers together and placing them on your radial artery, just inside your wristbone, or on your neck's carotid artery, on either side of the Adam's apple. Take your pulse for ten seconds and multiply by 6 to obtain your heart rate in beats per minute.

■ Find or mark a mile-length track, choosing a route that's as flat and smooth as possible. If you don't use the local high-school track, then mark a route, instead, with your car's odometer, staying away from streets with lots of stoplights, crowded sidewalks, and traffic.

■ Warm up and stretch for five minutes before you start. You can use the stretches that appear in Appendix B.

■ Walk your one-mile route at a brisk but steady pace and record the time it took you.

■ Take your pulse immediately after finishing, before your heart rate starts to slow down.

■ Record your pulse and your time, which should range between 10 and 25 minutes, to the nearest second, on the vital-statistics chart in Appendix G.

Once you have your results, find the relative fitness chart in this section that corresponds to your age and sex. Plot your time against your heart rate to determine your relative fitness level: low, high, average, above average, or high. Do the same to find your exercise program color.

**Example of Relative Fitness Chart for 50-to-59-Year-Old Woman**

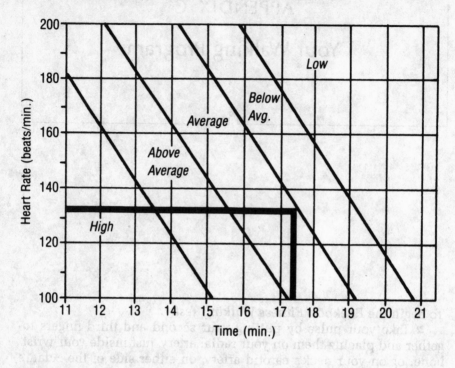

Here's an example of how to do it: Mary, a 55-year-old, walked one mile in 17 minutes, 15 seconds. Her heart rate at the end of the walk was 132 beats per minute. On the relative fitness chart for a 50–59-year-old-woman Mary locates 17 minutes, 15 seconds on the horizontal line (time) and draws a vertical line from that point. She finds 132 on the vertical line (heart rate), and draws a vertical line from that point. The point at which the two lines meet shows that Mary's relative fitness level is average.

To find her exercise program color, Mary locates the exercise program chart for a 50–59-year-old woman. Once again she plots her time against her heart rate. The point at which they meet is in the Green color group (see sample chart). Mary knows she should start with the Green section of the walking program in the Thirty-Day Eating and Exercise Starter Plan in Chapter 3.

**Example of Exercise Program Chart for 50–59-Year-Old Woman**

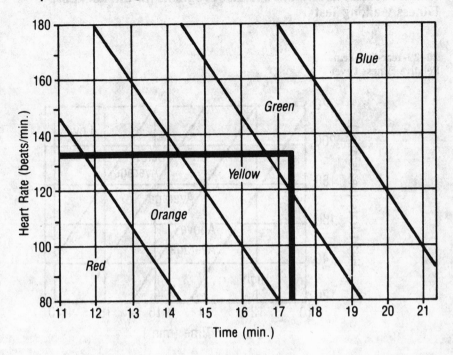

Now that you know your fitness level and your color, turn to Chapter 3 and get started with your thirty-day program. Once you have finished that, continue with week five in the Twenty-Week Walking Program in Chapter 4. Chapter 7 also offers a wealth of tips for motivating yourself to stay with exercise.

To check your progress, retest yourself at week ten and week twenty, and record the results again on the vital-statistics chart. Use the walking log in this section to keep track of your daily and weekly progress.

Note: All the charts in Appendix C are from James M. Rippe and Ann Ward, *Dr. James M. Rippe's Complete Book of Fitness Walking* (New York: Prentice Hall Press, 1989).

## Relative Fitness Levels and Exercise Programs for the Rockport Fitness Walking Test

**20–29-Year-Old Females**
**Relative Fitness Level**

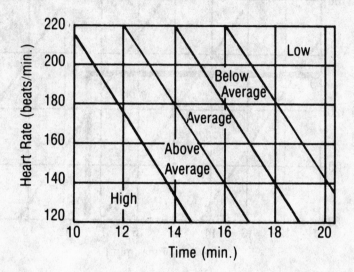

**20–29-Year-Old Females**
**Exercise Program**

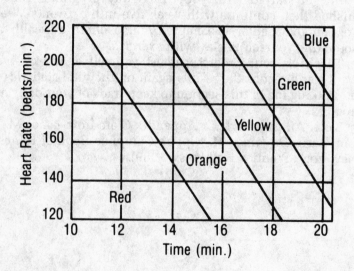

**20–29-Year-Old-Males
Relative Fitness Level**

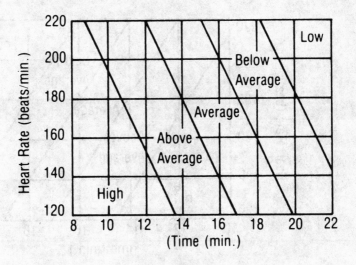

**20–29-Year-Old Males
Exercise Program**

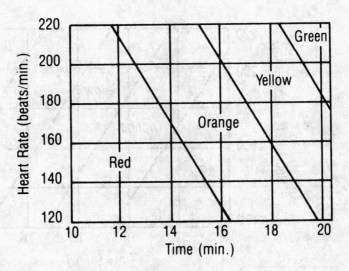

**30–39-Year-Old Females
Relative Fitness Level**

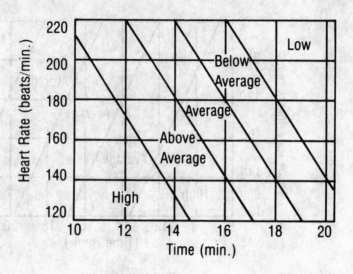

**30–39-Year-Old Females
Exercise Program**

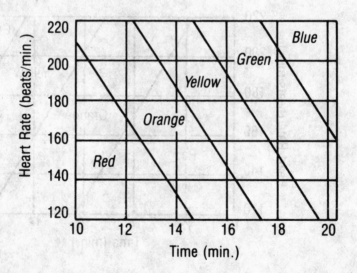

**30–39-Year-Old Males
Relative Fitness Level**

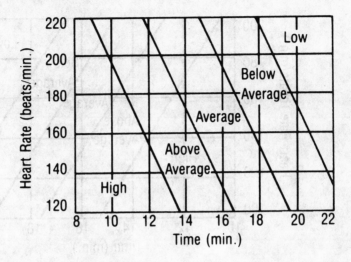

**30–39-Year-Old Males
Exercise Program**

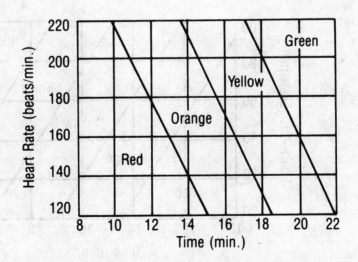

**40–49-Year-Old Females**
**Relative Fitness Level**

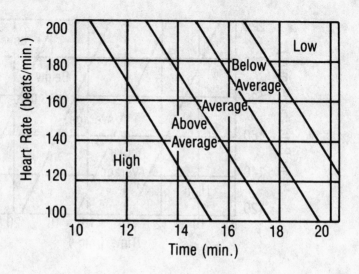

**40–49-Year-Old Females**
**Exercise Program**

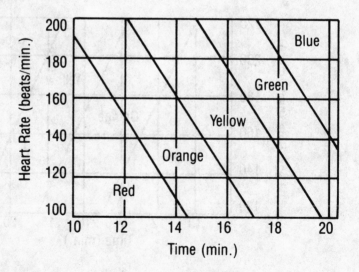

**40–49-Year-Old Males
Relative Fitness Level**

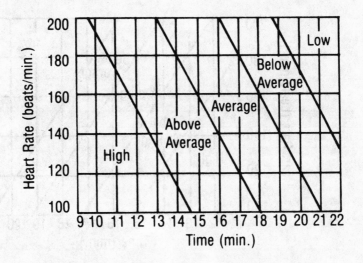

**40–49-Year-Old Males
Exercise Program**

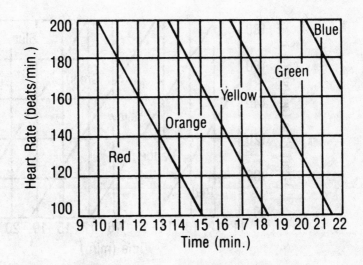

**50–59-Year-Old Females
Relative Fitness Level**

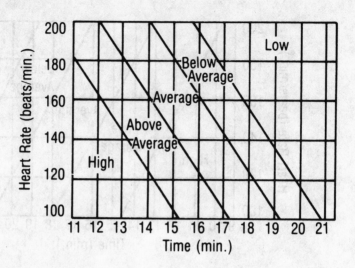

**50–59-Year-Old Females
Exercise Program**

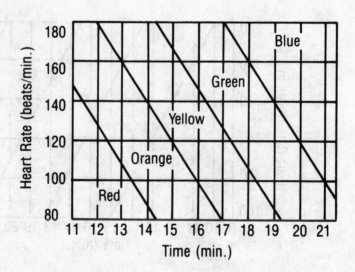

**50–59-Year-Old Males
Relative Fitness Level**

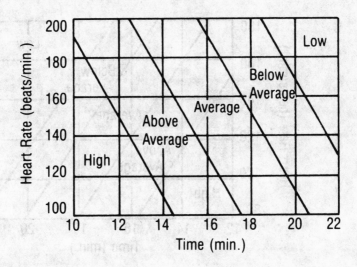

**50–59-Year-Old Males
Exercise Program**

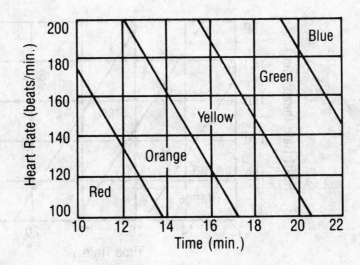

**60 + Year-Old Females
Relative Fitness Level**

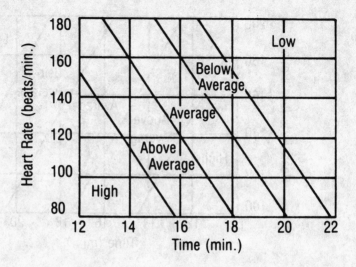

**60 + Year-Old Females
Exercise Program**

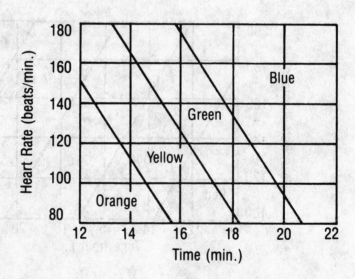

**60 + Year-Old Males
Relative Fitness Level**

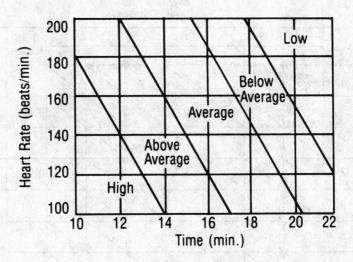

**60 + Year-Old Males
Exercise Program**

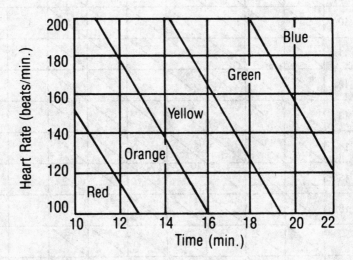

# WALKING LOG

| | EXERCISE LOG Mileage/Duration | | | | | | | | |
|---|---|---|---|---|---|---|---|---|---|
| Week | Days | | | | | | | Total Mileage | Comments |
| | 1 | 2 | 3 | 4 | 5 | 6 | 7 | | |
| 1 | Mileage Duration | | | | | | | | |
| 2 | | | | | | | | | |
| 3 | | | | | | | | | |
| 4 | | | | | | | | | |
| 5 | | | | | | | | | |
| 6 | | | | | | | | | |
| 7 | | | | | | | | | |
| 8 | | | | | | | | | |
| 9 | | | | | | | | | |
| 10 | | | | | | | | | |
| 11 | | | | | | | | | |
| 12 | | | | | | | | | |
| 13 | | | | | | | | | |
| 14 | | | | | | | | | |
| 15 | | | | | | | | | |
| 16 | | | | | | | | | |
| 17 | | | | | | | | | |
| 18 | | | | | | | | | |
| 19 | | | | | | | | | |
| 20 | | | | | | | | | |

# APPENDIX D

# Your Lifecycle Program

In this program:
  ■ Warm up and stretch for five minutes before you start. You can use the stretches that appear in Appendix B.
  ■ Then follow the directions on the Lifecycle console, which will guide you through the *Lifecycle FIT Test*.
  ■ Be sure to record that score on the vital-statistics chart in Appendix G.

Now find the chart for your sex in this section and plot your score (also known as VO2 max) against your *age* to determine your relative fitness level: very poor, poor, below average, average, above average, good, excellent, or elite.

**Relative Fitness Classification for Men**

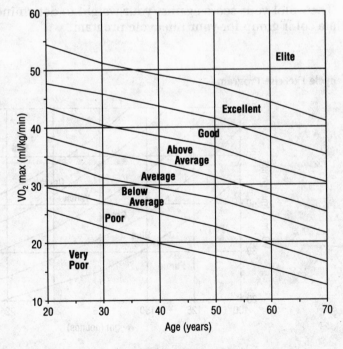

**Relative Fitness Classification for Women**

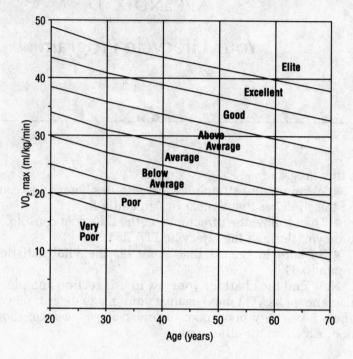

Then plot your score against your *weight* to determine the appropriate color group for your Lifecycle program.

**Lifecycle Exercise Program**

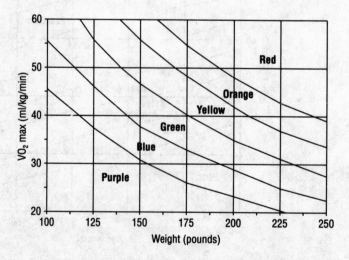

For example, if you are a 40-year-old man weighing 175 pounds whose FIT test score was 35, your relative fitness level would be above average (age vs. score). Your color for the Lifecycle program would be Green (score vs. weight).

Now that you know your fitness level and your color, turn to the Lifecycle program in the Thirty-Day Eating and Exercise Starter Plan in Chapter 3. Once you have finished all thirty days, you can continue with week five of the Twenty-Week Lifecycle Program in Chapter 4. You'll find a wealth of tips for motivating yourself to stay with exercise in Chapter 7.

Retest yourself at week ten and week twenty, and record the results again on the vital-statistics chart in Appendix G. To keep track of your daily and weekly progress, use the Lifecycle log in this section.

# LIFECYCLE TRAINING LOG

| Week | Days | | | | | | | Total Mileage | Comments |
|------|---|---|---|---|---|---|---|---|---|
| | 1 | 2 | 3 | 4 | 5 | 6 | 7 | | |
| 1 | Level/Duration | | | | | | | | |
| 2 | | | | | | | | | |
| 3 | | | | | | | | | |
| 4 | | | | | | | | | |
| 5 | | | | | | | | | |
| 6 | | | | | | | | | |
| 7 | | | | | | | | | |
| 8 | | | | | | | | | |
| 9 | | | | | | | | | |
| 10 | | | | | | | | | |
| 11 | | | | | | | | | |
| 12 | | | | | | | | | |
| 13 | | | | | | | | | |
| 14 | | | | | | | | | |
| 15 | | | | | | | | | |
| 16 | | | | | | | | | |
| 17 | | | | | | | | | |
| 18 | | | | | | | | | |
| 19 | | | | | | | | | |
| 20 | | | | | | | | | |

EXERCISE LOG
Level/Duration

# APPENDIX E

## Your Lifestep Program

In this program:

■ Warm up and stretch for five minutes before you start. You can use the stretches that appear in Appendix B.

■ Follow the instructions on the Lifestep console for the *Lifestep Electronic FIT Test.*

■ Now record your score on the vital-statistics chart in Appendix G.

Look at the relative fitness table below that corresponds to your sex and find your FIT test score, also known as VO2 max, and your age. This will indicate your relative fitness level: very poor, poor, below average, average, above average, good, excellent, or elite. Now look at the program color chart to determine the color of your Lifestep program: Purple, Blue, Green, Yellow, Orange, or Red.

| FIT Test Scoring Table | | | | | |
| --- | --- | --- | --- | --- | --- |
| (Estimated VO$_2$ Max) | | | | | |
| MEN | AGE | | | | |
| RATING | 20-29 | 30-39 | 40-49 | 50-59 | 60-69 |
| Elite | 55+ | 52+ | 50+ | 48+ | 45+ |
| Excellent | 50-54 | 47-51 | 45-49 | 43-47 | 40-44 |
| Good | 45-49 | 42-46 | 40-44 | 38-42 | 35-38 |
| Above Average | 40-44 | 37-41 | 35-39 | 33-37 | 30-34 |
| Average | 36-39 | 33-36 | 31-34 | 29-32 | 26-29 |
| Below Average | 31-35 | 28-32 | 26-30 | 24-28 | 21-25 |
| Poor | 26-30 | 23-27 | 20-25 | 18-23 | 16-20 |
| Very Poor | <26 | <23 | <20 | <18 | <16 |

| WOMEN | AGE | | | | |
|---|---|---|---|---|---|
| RATING | 20-29 | 30-39 | 40-49 | 50-59 | 60-69 |
| Elite | 49+ | 46+ | 44+ | 42+ | 40+ |
| Excellent | 44-48 | 41-45 | 39-43 | 37-41 | 35-39 |
| Good | 39-43 | 36-40 | 34-38 | 32-36 | 30-34 |
| Above Average | 34-38 | 31-35 | 29-33 | 27-31 | 25-29 |
| Average | 30-33 | 27-30 | 25-28 | 23-26 | 21-24 |
| Below Average | 25-29 | 22-26 | 20-24 | 18-22 | 16-20 |
| Poor | 20-24 | 17-21 | 15-19 | 13-17 | 11-15 |
| Very Poor | <20 | <17 | <15 | <13 | <11 |

## LIFESTEP PROGRAM COLOR CHART

| FIT Test Score $(VO_{2max})$ (ml/kg/min) | Program |
|---|---|
| <20 | Purple/Blue |
| 20–30 | Green |
| 31–40 | Yellow |
| 41–50 | Orange |
| >50 | Red |

For example, 40-year-old John had a score of 40 on his FIT test. According to the tables, that puts him in the "good" fitness category and in the Yellow Lifestep program.

(Note: We have included a Purple level for those of you who have been inactive for some time. Use the Purple program as long as you need to get used to the machine. But feel free to move into Blue program as soon as you're ready for more of a challenge.)

Now that you know your fitness level and your color, turn to Chapter 3 and get started with your thirty-day program. Once you have finished that, continue with week five in the Twenty-Week Lifestep program in Chapter 4.

To check your progress, retest yourself at week ten and week twenty, and record the results again on the vital-statistics chart in Appendix G. Use the Lifestep log in this section to keep track of your daily and weekly progress.

## LIFESTEP TRAINING LOG

| Week | Days | | | | | | | Total Mileage | Comments |
|---|---|---|---|---|---|---|---|---|---|
| | 1 | 2 | 3 | 4 | 5 | 6 | 7 | | |
| 1 | Mileage / Duration | | | | | | | | |
| 2 | | | | | | | | | |
| 3 | | | | | | | | | |
| 4 | | | | | | | | | |
| 5 | | | | | | | | | |
| 6 | | | | | | | | | |
| 7 | | | | | | | | | |
| 8 | | | | | | | | | |
| 9 | | | | | | | | | |
| 10 | | | | | | | | | |
| 11 | | | | | | | | | |
| 12 | | | | | | | | | |
| 13 | | | | | | | | | |
| 14 | | | | | | | | | |
| 15 | | | | | | | | | |
| 16 | | | | | | | | | |
| 17 | | | | | | | | | |
| 18 | | | | | | | | | |
| 19 | | | | | | | | | |
| 20 | | | | | | | | | |

**EXERCISE LOG**
**Mileage/Duration**

# APPENDIX F

# Your Strength Training Program

To all interested in strength training, take the following sit-up and push-up test to get a measure of your overall muscular endurance. That goes for everyone; those using the Lifecircuit program, the Generic/Home Strength Training Program. Doing so will place you in the appropriate color group for the Thirty-Day Eating and Exercise Starter Plan.

To do the sit-up test:

■ Find an exercise mat, a watch or clock with a sweep second hand, and a partner or a heavy piece of furniture to hold your feet in place.

■ On the mat, lie on your back with your knees bent, feet stabilized, and arms folded across your chest.

■ To do the sit-up properly, curl forward off the ground until your elbows reach your thighs (but not in a sitting position). Finish the sit-up by slowly returning your shoulders to the floor.

■ When your partner gives you the starting signal, do as many sit-ups as possible in one minute, counting only the number of correctly performed sit-ups. Record the number on the vital-statistics chart in Appendix G.

To do the push-up test:

■ While still on the mat, lie face down with your palms flat on the floor, arms placed shoulder-width apart. Lift your body off the floor, with your back straight and rigid and supported by the balls of the feet (standard push-up), or with your back supported by your knees (modified push-up). Do as many as you can correctly.

Now that you have the results, find the appropriate relative strength chart in this section that corresponds to your age. Plot your sit-up score on the horizontal line against your push-up score on the vertical line. For example, twenty-seven-year-old Sue completed twenty-four sit-ups and thirteen push-ups in one minutes. That places her in the Green group.

358

Now that you know the color group that is appropriate to your fitness level, follow the instructions below for the type of strength training you have chosen.

## The Lifecircuit Program

We chose to feature Lifecircuit strength training equipment, made by Life Fitness, Inc., of Irvine, California, because it offers computerized training and one-touch weight adjustment, which, we believe, yields the most thorough, safe, and efficient workout now possible.

A recent study by my laboratory at the University of Massachusetts showed that men who performed one set of twelve repetitions on the Lifecircuit showed similar improvements in strength, self-esteem, and mood as those who performed three sets of twelve, ten, or eight repetitions on a well-known brand of conventional strength training equipment. And when it came to increasing lean muscle tissue, one set of twelve repetitions on Lifecircuit outperformed three sets on the conventional equipment.

Our conclusion: On Lifecircuit you get the maximum benefit from the minimum amount of workout time.

Other Lifecircuit features include:

■ *The "set-up test."* Instead of estimating your proper training weight and setting iron plates and bars manually, as you would on traditional weight machines, you perform this simple test by lifting the most weight you can comfortably.

As you lift, sensors measure the force you've applied and set the appropriate weight for you automatically. The machine also measures *range* of motion performed on the first repetition of each set, and limits your motion to that range for the remainder of that set. It also means that you're lifting the maximum you can lift safely, and there's no guesswork. And it enables inexperienced lifters and people with orthopedic limitations to train safely without risking injury.

■ *Pyramid-style training.* You lift 75 percent of your maximum on the first repetition, 80 percent on the second, 90 percent on the third, 100 on the next six repetitions, 90 percent on the tenth, 80 percent on the eleventh, and 70 percent on the twelfth repetition. This type of training allows for maximal muscle stimulation while maintaining proper form.

■ *Additional negative resistance.* Lifecircuit adds 25 to 40 percent additional negative resistance on the downstroke of each repetition. We believe that this extra "eccentric" work is the key to why Lifecircuit is so effective at building lean body mass.

■ *The "regular" option.* However, if you prefer a more traditional workout, you can choose this program mode, which does not call for

**Relative Strength Chart for 20–29-Year-Olds**

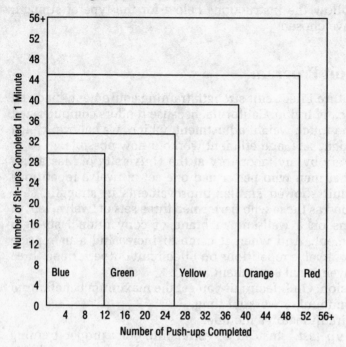

**Relative Strength Chart for 30–39-Year-Olds**

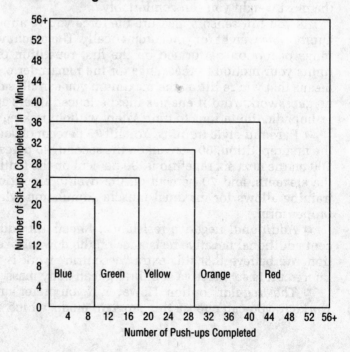

**Relative Strength Chart for 40–49-Year-Olds**

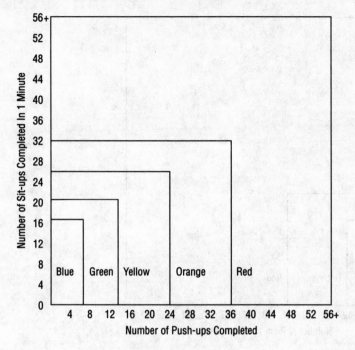

**Relative Strength Chart for 50–59-Year-Olds**

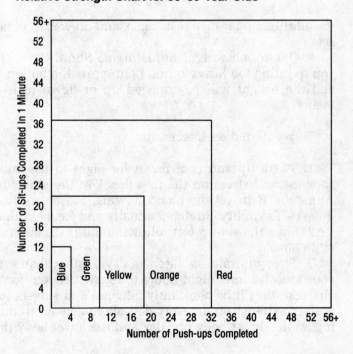

**Relative Strength Chart for 60–69-Year-Olds**

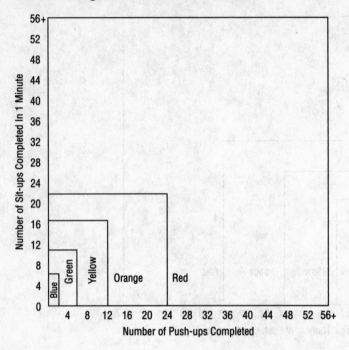

the additional negative resistance, and do your standard one-to-three sets.

■ *One-touch weight adjustment.* Should you find the weight you're lifting too heavy or too light, press the button on the console, and the weight will be adjusted up or down in five-pound increments.

To get started on Lifecircuit:

1. Warm up and cool down for eight to ten minutes to reduce soreness and stress on the muscles. Use the stretching exercises in Appendix B to get the blood flowing, loosen up the muscles, and increase flexibility. Stretch gradually and easily with no bouncing.

2. Take the set-up test following the instructions on the Lifecircuit console.

3. Strength-train on alternate days, rather than every day, to give your muscles forty-eight hours to recover. If you don't let your muscles rest, they'll be constantly fatigued and subject to injury. (If you prefer to strength-train every day, alternate your training, concentrating on the upper body one day and the lower body the next.) Follow

the instructions pictured on each machine to ensure proper technique.

4. Consult the Lifecircuit program section of the Thirty-Day Eating and Exercise Starter Plan in Chapter 3, which will tell you the number of repetitions and sets to do for your color group. As we said, only one set is necessary if you choose the Lifecircuit mode that calls for additional negative resistance. However, the program in Chapter 3 specifies additional sets for those choosing the regular mode.

5. Use the Lifecircuit strength training log in this section to keep track of your progress. Once you have completed all thirty days, go on to the Twenty-Week Lifecircuit Strength Training Program chart in Chapter 4, starting with week five of that chart.

## The Generic Program

We realize that some readers may not have access to Lifecircuit equipment. For that reason, we offer the following strength training tips for working out with all other major brands of strength-training equipment.

How many repetitions should you do? That depends on what you want to accomplish. To improve muscular strength and endurance, work up to fifteen to twenty repetitions at the same weight per set. To increase size or bulk of muscles, do fewer repetitions—six to eight— at a higher weight. The strength-training programs in this book offer a balance of both approaches.

The number of sets you do will be determined by your level of fitness, your fitness goals, and the type of equipment you're using. Generally you should expect to do one to three sets at each station, depending on your fitness level.

| MACHINE | MUSCLES |
|---|---|
| Leg extension | Quadriceps (front of thighs) |
| Leg curl | Hamstrings (back of thighs) |
| Rower or arm cross | Back, chest |
| Chest or bench press | Chest, arms (upper body) |
| Back or hip extension | Hip, lower back |
| Abdominal curl | Stomach |
| Arm curl | Biceps (front of upper arm) |
| Tricep extension | Tricep (back of upper arm) |
| Hip abductor/adductor | Inner/outer thighs |

Now to get started:

1. Warm up and cool down for eight to ten minutes before and after strength-training to reduce soreness and stress on the muscles. You can use the stretching exercises in Appendix B to get blood

flowing, loosen up the muscles, and increase flexibility. Stretch gradually and easily, with no bouncing.

2. Strength-train on alternate days, rather than every day, to give your muscles forty-eight hours to recover. If you don't let your muscles rest, they'll be constantly fatigued and subject to injury. (If you want to do some strength-training every day, alternate your training, concentrating on the upper body one day and the lower body the next.)

3. To determine your weight stack, or the maximum amount of weight you can lift properly, ask a staff member at your local health club or recreational facility to show you how to take a "one-repetition maximum" (1 RM) test on each piece of equipment you intend to use.

To do a 1 RM test, select a weight you think you can lift comfortably. Now add weight stacks and do one repetition with each stack until you can on longer lift properly. To get your starting weight, take the highest amount of weight you lifted properly and multiply that number by 70 percent. For example, if the maximum weight you lifted was one hundred pounds, your weight stack would be seventy pounds for that machine.

Do this for every piece of equipment you intend to use, resting at least thirty seconds between each lift, and two minutes between machines.

Repeat the 1 RM test for each piece of equipment every two weeks, or whenever you feel ready to move to a higher weight. The 1 RM will tell you if you're strong enough to handle more weight.

4. Consult the Generic/Home Strength Training section of the Thirty-Day Eating and Exercise Started Plan in Chapter 3, which will tell you the number of repetitions and sets to do for your color group.

5. Use the Generic/Home Strength and Training log in this section to keep track of your progress. Once you have completed all thirty days, go on to the Twenty-Week Generic/Home Strength Training Program chart in Chapter 4, starting with week five of that chart.

As you train, keep these safety tips in mind:

■ **Always warm up before you train, and cool down after your session.** It pays off in a safer, more comfortable workout.

■ **Pay attention to previous injuries.** If you have a knee problem, for example, get advice about how to compensate for that injury from the fitness director at your club, from a physician who specializes in sports medicine, or from a physical therapist.

■ **Stop training if you feel pain.** That's a signal you're overdoing it.

■ **Start with larger muscle groups and work down to the smaller ones.** When training the larger muscle groups, do so in the following order: abdominals to work the back and stomach muscles; the legs; then the chest and back.

To train the smaller muscle groups, start with the shoulders, work the biceps (front of upper arm), then finish with the triceps (back of upper arm). Strength-training circuits at most clubs are arranged in this order.

■ **Use proper posture.** When standing, make sure your feet are shoulder-width apart. Don't lock your elbows or knees; it puts undue strain on them. Keep weight well balanced, without leaning to one side or the other. Keep head and neck straight, making sure not to twist either. Keep your back flat and straight, making sure not to arch it or twist during any strength-training activity.

■ **Use only the proper muscles.** Avoid using muscles other than the one you're exercising. For example, if you're using the leg-curl machine, you should feel a pulling in the back of your thighs. If you feel it in your back as well, you're probably arching your back and using the wrong muscles.

■ **Lift with a smooth, dynamic motion.** You know your muscle is too tired when you can no longer lift smoothly.

■ **Breathe properly.** Exhale when lifting, inhale when returning. Whatever you do, don't hold your breath during any part of your training. Holding your breath tends to raise your blood pressure, which may result in dizziness or even a blackout.

■ **Take special care when using the back-extension machine (Roman chair).** Start with little or no weight, and add weight very gradually. While this machine can be very useful in building back muscles, using too much weight too soon can cause injury.

■ **Use common sense.** Pads and strapping are provided for your safety. Use them when provided. Follow diagrams on machines for proper use. If a strength-training machine is too big for you, find an alternative or get the proper instruction on how to use the appropriate free weights instead. If you use a machine that's too big, you'll be using all the wrong muscles, which can cause injury.

## The Home Program

Once you know your color group, go to Chapter 3 and follow the instructions for Generic/Home Strength Training in the exercise portion of the Thirty-Day Eating and Exercise Starter Plan. The exercise plan will tell you how often to do the following eleven exercises. Be sure to use the home strength training log in this section to keep track of your progress.

Once you have finished all thirty days, go on to the Twenty-Week Generic/Home Strength Training Program chart in Chapter 4. Start with week five, and continue until you've finished all twenty weeks.

Once you've completed this five-month program, you may want to continue at the same level, move to higher colors, add more exercises, get some instruction on proper use of free weights, or join a health club or recreational facility to use some strength-training equipment. Chapter 7 has tips for staying with your program.

Here are your strength-training exercises:

1. **Half curl-up.** Lie on your back, knees bent, feet close to buttocks. Cross your arms over your chest. Slowly curl your body forward, lifting your head, neck, shoulders, and upper back off the floor. Your lower back should remain flat, in contact with the floor. Then, in a smooth, slow motion, lower your body back down to the floor. One curl should take four seconds (two to curl up, two to lower). For the stomach and upper back.

2. **Alternating knee touch.** Lie on your back, hands behind head, fingers interlocked, elbows out. Now bend your knees and lift them so the lower portion of both legs are resting on a chair or bench. Keeping your lower back on the floor, slowly curl your upper body forward and rotate your trunk so your right elbow touches the left knee and vice versa. If you can't quite reach your knee with your elbow, move your knee in slightly so your elbow can reach it, allowing you to complete the exercise. For the waist and the stomach.

3. **Double flutter.** Lie on your stomach, hands resting comfortably under your chin, legs straight and together. Tighten your buttocks and slowly lift both feet two to six inches off the ground, then lower your feet slowly. For buttocks and thighs.

4. **Chest raise.** Lie on your stomach, hands behind head, fingers interlocked. Keeping your feet on the ground, slowly lift your head and upper body up from the floor. Hold for two seconds, and return to the ground slowly. If you can't do this alone, ask a partner to hold your feet down. For the lower back, buttocks, and hamstrings.

5. **Push-ups.** Do the same push-ups you did for the push-up test earlier in this section. For the arms, shoulders, and chest.

6. **Inverted push-ups.** Sit with your legs stretched out in front of you. Your palms are flat on the floor behind you, your arms are placed shoulder-width apart. Now raise yourself until your elbows are nearly straight but not locked, your legs are outstretched, and your toes are pointed. Lower yourself until your buttocks just touch the floor, and repeat. For the arms, shoulders, and upper back.

7. **Lunges.** Begin in a standing position, hands on hips. Step forward with the right foot, bending on one knee and dipping, with your left leg outstretched behind you. Step back to the starting position. Step forward with the right foot, repeating dipping and outstretching motions. For the thighs (quads and hamstrings).

8. **Three-way leg lift.** Stand near a wall or piece of furniture for support. While standing on your left leg with the knee straight but not

locked, slowly raise the right leg, with the toe pointed, straight up in front of you, six to twelve inches. Hold for two seconds.

In a smooth motion, return your leg to the side and slowly bring your extended leg out to the right, lifting six to twelve inches from the ground, toes pointed. Hold for two seconds.

Again in a smooth motion, return to the beginning position and slowly extend the leg out behind you, lifting six to twelve inches off the ground, toes pointed. Hold for two seconds. Return your leg to the beginning position.

Repeat with the left leg. You should gradually build to do this exercise without resting between position changes. For added resistance, use light ankle weights. For hips/buttocks and thighs (gluteals, quads, and hamstrings).

9. **Heel lifts.** Stand on one step, balancing on the balls of your feet, near a wall or railing. Slowly rise up onto your toes, hold for two seconds, then return to a balanced position. Now let your heels drop off the step, hold for one second, and return to a balanced position. This can also be done one foot at a time, or with ankle weights. For calves, ankles, and feet.

10. **Classic curl.** Stand with legs about shoulder width apart. Grasp a dumbbell with each hand, arms extended at the side, palms facing in. Bending at the elbows, curl the weight in toward your body, up to about shoulder height. Your palms should be facing you as you lift the weights. You can do both arms at the same time, or alternate. Remember to breathe smoothly as you lift. For front of the arms (biceps).

11. **Triceps teaser.** Standing with legs about shoulder-width apart, grasp the end of one dumbbell with both hands and place your arms above your head. Your elbows should be bent, your hands grasping the weight behind your head. Slowly extend both arms over your head, hold for two seconds, and return to the starting position. For back of the arms.

## LIFECIRCUIT STRENGTH TRAINING LOG

Name _____

Date (Day/Month) _____

| Machine | | | | | | | | | | | | | | | |
|---|---|---|---|---|---|---|---|---|---|---|---|---|---|---|---|
| **Seat** | | | | | | | | | | | | | | | |
| **Leg Extension** | Set up | | | | | | | | | | | | | | |
| | Tot. wt. | | | | | | | | | | | | | | |
| **Leg Curl** | Set up | | | | | | | | | | | | | | |
| | Tot. wt. | | | | | | | | | | | | | | |
| **Seated Row** | Set up | | | | | | | | | | | | | | |
| | Tot. wt. | | | | | | | | | | | | | | |
| **Chest Press** | Set up | | | | | | | | | | | | | | |
| | Tot. wt. | | | | | | | | | | | | | | |
| **Back Extension** | Set up | | | | | | | | | | | | | | |
| | Tot. wt. | | | | | | | | | | | | | | |
| **Abdominal** | Set up | | | | | | | | | | | | | | |
| | Tot. wt. | | | | | | | | | | | | | | |
| **Arm Curl** | Set up | | | | | | | | | | | | | | |
| | Tot. wt. | | | | | | | | | | | | | | |
| **Tricep Extension** | Set up | | | | | | | | | | | | | | |
| | Tot. wt. | | | | | | | | | | | | | | |

Comments:

## LIFECIRCUIT STRENGTH TRAINING LOG

Name _____

Date (Day/Month) _____

| Machine | | | | | | | | | | | | | | | |
|---|---|---|---|---|---|---|---|---|---|---|---|---|---|---|---|
| Seat | | | | | | | | | | | | | | | |
| Fly | Set up | | | | | | | | | | | | | | |
| | Tot. wt. | | | | | | | | | | | | | | |
| Shoulder Press | Set up | | | | | | | | | | | | | | |
| | Tot. wt. | | | | | | | | | | | | | | |
| Lat. Pulldown | Set up | | | | | | | | | | | | | | |
| | Tot. wt. | | | | | | | | | | | | | | |
| Leg Press | Set up | | | | | | | | | | | | | | |
| | Tot. wt. | | | | | | | | | | | | | | |
| | Set up | | | | | | | | | | | | | | |
| | Tot. wt. | | | | | | | | | | | | | | |
| | Set up | | | | | | | | | | | | | | |
| | Tot. wt. | | | | | | | | | | | | | | |
| | Set up | | | | | | | | | | | | | | |
| | Tot. wt. | | | | | | | | | | | | | | |
| | Set up | | | | | | | | | | | | | | |
| | Tot. wt. | | | | | | | | | | | | | | |

Comments:

# GENERIC STRENGTH TRAINING LOG

Name _____

Date (Day/Month)

| Machine | | | | | | | | | | | | | | | |
|---|---|---|---|---|---|---|---|---|---|---|---|---|---|---|---|
| Seat | | | | | | | | | | | | | | | |
| Leg Extension | Set up | | | | | | | | | | | | | | |
| | Tot. wt. | | | | | | | | | | | | | | |
| Leg Curl | Set up | | | | | | | | | | | | | | |
| | Tot. wt. | | | | | | | | | | | | | | |
| Seated Row | Set up | | | | | | | | | | | | | | |
| | Tot. wt. | | | | | | | | | | | | | | |
| Chest Press | Set up | | | | | | | | | | | | | | |
| | Tot. wt. | | | | | | | | | | | | | | |
| Lower Back | Set up | | | | | | | | | | | | | | |
| | Tot. wt. | | | | | | | | | | | | | | |
| Abdominal | Set up | | | | | | | | | | | | | | |
| | Tot. wt. | | | | | | | | | | | | | | |
| Bicep Curl | Set up | | | | | | | | | | | | | | |
| | Tot. wt. | | | | | | | | | | | | | | |
| Tricep Extension | Set up | | | | | | | | | | | | | | |
| | Tot. wt. | | | | | | | | | | | | | | |

Comments:

## HOME STRENGTH TRAINING LOG

Name _____

Date (Day/Month)

| | | | | | | | | | | | | | | | |
|---|---|---|---|---|---|---|---|---|---|---|---|---|---|---|---|
| Half curl-up | Sets | | | | | | | | | | | | | | |
| | Reps | | | | | | | | | | | | | | |
| Alternating knee-touch | Sets | | | | | | | | | | | | | | |
| | Reps | | | | | | | | | | | | | | |
| Double flutter | Sets | | | | | | | | | | | | | | |
| | Reps | | | | | | | | | | | | | | |
| Chest Raise | Sets | | | | | | | | | | | | | | |
| | Reps | | | | | | | | | | | | | | |
| Push-ups | Sets | | | | | | | | | | | | | | |
| | Reps | | | | | | | | | | | | | | |
| Inverted push-ups | Sets | | | | | | | | | | | | | | |
| | Reps | | | | | | | | | | | | | | |
| Lunges | Sets | | | | | | | | | | | | | | |
| | Reps | | | | | | | | | | | | | | |
| Three-way leg lift | Sets | | | | | | | | | | | | | | |
| | Reps | | | | | | | | | | | | | | |

Comments:

# Your Changing Vital Statistics

NAME _____ AGE _____ DATE _____

| | INITIAL TEST | 10 WKS. | 20 WKS. | CHANGE |
|---|---|---|---|---|
| **WEIGHT & CIRCUMFERENCES** | | | | |
| Weight | _____ | _____ | _____ | _____ |
| Waist (in.) | _____ | _____ | _____ | _____ |
| Abdomen (in.) | _____ | _____ | _____ | _____ |
| Buttocks (in.) | _____ | _____ | _____ | _____ |
| Mid Thigh (in.) | _____ | _____ | _____ | _____ |
| **AEROBIC CAPACITY** | | | | |
| Heart rate, rest (bpm) | _____ | _____ | _____ | _____ |
| Heart rate, total test time *Rockport Fitness Walking Test* (bpm) | _____ | _____ | _____ | |
| Heart rate, *Lifecycle FIT Test* (bpm) | _____ | _____ | _____ | |
| Heart rate, *Lifestep Electronic FIT Test* (bpm) | _____ | _____ | _____ | |
| **STRENGTH** | | | | |
| Push-up test (repeitions) | _____ | _____ | _____ | _____ |
| Sit-up test (repetitions) | _____ | _____ | _____ | _____ |

# For Further Reading

## General

*The American Heart Association Cookbook.* New York: David McKay Company, 1984.

Becker, Gail. *Heart-Smart: A Plan for Low-Cholesterol Living.* New York: Merrell Dow Publications, 1984.

Brody, Jane. *Jane Brody's Good Food Book: Living the High Carbohydrate Way.* New York: W. W. Norton & Company, 1985. Not specifically written for low-fat, low-cholesterol diets, but does contain many low-fat recipes.

Connor, Sonja, and William Connor. *The Best from the Family Hearts Kitchens.* Portland, OR: Oregon Health Sciences University, 1984.

————. *The New American Diet.* New York: Simon & Schuster, 1986.

Goor, Ron, and Nancy Goor. *Eater's Choice: A Food Lover's Guide to Lower Cholesterol.* Boston: Houghton Mifflin Company, 1987.

Kashiwa, Anne, and James Rippe. *Fitness Walking for Women.* New York: Perigee Books, 1987.

Piscatella, Joseph, and Bernie Piscatella. *Don't Eat Your Heart Out Cookbook.* New York: Workman Publishing Company, 1982.

Polak, Jeanne. *Fat and Calorie Controlled Meals.* Philadelphia: George F. Stickley Company, 1982.

Rippe, James M. *Dr. James M. Rippe's Fit for Success.* New York: Prentice Hall Press, 1989.

————, and Ann Ward. *Dr. James M. Rippe's Complete Book of Fitness Walking.* New York: Prentice Hall Press, 1989.

————, with Karla Dougherty. *The Rockport Walking Program.* New York: Prentice Hall Press, 1989.

## Metabolic Source Reference List
## Calculations for the exercise exchange lists in Chapter 5 were based on the following sources:

Alpert, J. S. *The Heart Attack Handbook.* Boston: Little, Brown, 1978.

American College of Sports Medicine. *Guidelines for Exercise Testing and Prescription,* 3rd and 4th eds. Philadelphia: Lea & Febinger, 1986, 1991.

Kashiwa, Anne, and James Rippe. *Fitness Walking for Women*. New York: Perigee Books, 1987.

McArdle, W. D., F. I. Katch, and V. L. Katch. *Exercise Physiology: Energy, Nutrition, and Human Performance*, 2nd ed. Philadelphia: Lea & Febinger, 1986.

Rippe, James, and Ann Ward. *A Professional's Guide to the Use of the Lifecycle Aerobic Trainer*. Unpublished manuscript, 1988.

Sharkey, B. J. *Physiological Fitness and Weight Control*. Missoula, MO: Mountain Press Publishing Company, 1974.

Ahlquist, L., Ward, A., Puleo, E., Rippe, J. *Energy Cost of Stepping on the Life Fitness Lifestep*. Unpublished manuscript, 1990.

## Strength Test/Home Program Reference List

Golding, L., C. Myers, and W. Sinning, *Y's Way to Physical Fitness*. Champaign, Ill.: Human Kinetics, 1989.

Myers, C. *The Official YMCA Physical Fitness Handbook*. New York: Popular Library, 1977.

Pearl, B. *Getting Stronger*. Revised. Bolinas, CA.: Shelter Publications, 1986.

Pollock, M., J. Wilmore, and S. Fox III. *Health and Fitness Through Physical Activity*. New York: John Wiley & Sons, 1978. Sit-up and push-up graph and test guide in Appendix F adapted from lists in this book.

# Index